EPILEPSY A TO Z

• • • • • •

A GLOSSARY OF EPILEPSY TERMINOLOGY

EPILEPSY A TO Z

· · · · · ·

A GLOSSARY OF EPILEPSY TERMINOLOGY

PETER W. KAPLAN, M.B., F.R.C.P.

PIERRE LOISEAU, M.D.

ROBERT S. FISHER, M.D., PH.D.

PIERRE JALLON, M.D.

demos vermande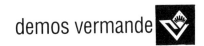

Demos Vermande, 386 Park Avenue South, New York, New York 10016

© 1995 by Demos Vermande. All rights reserved. This book is protected by copyright. No part of it may be reproduced, stored in a retrieval system, or transmitted in any form or by any means, electronic, mechanical, photocopying, recording, or otherwise, without the prior written permission of the publisher.

Library of Congress Cataloging-in-Publication Data

Epilepsy A to Z : a glossary of epilepsy terminology / Peter W. Kaplan
    ... [et al.].
         p.   cm.
      Includes index.
         ISBN 0-939957-75-2
      1. Epilepsy—Terminology.   2. Epilepsy—Dictionaries.
    3. Anticonvulsants—Dictionaries.   I. Kaplan, Peter W.
    RC372.E659   1995
    616.8'53'003—dc20   95-4234
                                                              CIP

Made in the United States of America

PREFACE

The purpose of this work is to provide health care personnel a convenient way to find brief answers to questions that arise regarding epilepsy. To this end, different terms used in epilepsy have been arranged alphabetically and annotated with comments. The intended level of detail is intermediate between a dictionary definition and a textbook discussion. The student should be able to gather a "nugget" of information pertaining to a phrase or topic, together with citations to further source material, which may include references from the authors' experience. Since this is a glossary, rare and common conditions are represented. No attempt is made, however, to be exhaustive.

The table of contents is arranged alphabetically. This number represents sequential headings in the glossary. Numbers in parentheses following or within the text represent useful references. References provided have been chosen because of their relative importance or because of their historic interest; almost all are in English excepting first descriptions and some by the authors. A number of important works have not been cited, as they may be found in more recent studies. The choice has been directed toward easily accessible journals as opposed to monographs.

Extensive cross-referencing has been used so the reader can easily find a subject. For example, a febrile seizure is cross-referenced under "Convulsions, (see also Febrile convulsions; Neonatal (S))," "Seizure, febrile (see Febrile seizure)," as well as "Febrile convulsions, seizure." The text phrase "see. . ." indicates that ". . ." is considered a relative synonym. The text phrase "see also. . . " suggests a related but not identical topic. For brevity, (S) denotes "seizure" and (E) "epilepsy." Naturally, these two terms are employed frequently.

Some abbreviations have been used throughout the text, typically:

Antiepileptic drug(s): AED(s)
Carbamazepine: CBZ
Phenobarbital: PB
Phenytoin: PHT
Valproic acid: VPA

The initial work was published in French. This English adaptation is primarily for physicians in the United States. Additional topics and English language literature citations were added, and others omitted. Antiepileptic drugs are listed by generic and common trade names, provided they are available or in clinical trials in the United States or the United Kingdom.

To paraphrase Albert Einstein, "simplify as much as possible, but no more." The authors assume responsibility for shortcomings in the direction of either oversimplification or insufficient brevity.

CONTENTS

ABDOMINAL EPILEPSY

The term "abdominal epilepsy" refers to paroxysmal episodes of colicky abdominal pain in conjunction with borborygmus, belching, nausea or vomiting, alterations in consciousness, and paroxysmal EEG abnormalities. These episodes have been associated with limbic or Sylvian foci or generalized epilepsies (1), and presumably represent vivid gastrointestinal auras of complex partial or simple partial seizures. Abdominal epilepsy occurs primarily in children (2). The differential diagnosis includes true abdominal disorders and epigastric pain associated with childhood migraine as well as functional illnesses. The occurrence of pain in these conditions led to the outdated, confusing, and misleading concept of "abdominal epilepsy" (3).

References

1. Gastaut H, Broughton R. *Epileptic seizures, clinical and electrographic features, diagnosis and treatment.* Springfield: Charles C. Thomas, 1972.
2. Sheeby B, Little S, Stone J. Abdominal epilepsy. *J Pediat* 1960;56:355–65.
3. Andermann F. Migraine-epilepsy relationships. *Epilepsy Res* 1987;1:213–16.

. . . . . .
ABSCESS, CEREBRAL

Cerebral abscesses are infrequent causes of seizures, although seizures are a common manifestation of cerebral abscesses, occurring in 36–72% (1,2). Common organisms include anaerobic or microaerophilic bacteria, streptococci, staphylococcus aureus, staphylococcus albans, gram negative enterobacteria, as well as parasites, fungi, and tubercle bacilli. The organism depends on the clinical setting, with staphylococci, for example, more common in surgical patients; pneumococcus more common with head trauma; pseudomonas aeruginosa, staphylococcus aureus, and Candida species in burn patients (3,4). With modern methods of diagnosis and therapy,

1

including head CT or MRI scanning (5), followed by stereotaxic drainage of the abscess (or full removal when judged necessary by neurosurgeons) and antibiotics (6), epileptic sequelae are much less frequent. AED prophylaxis is often employed when abscesses are diagnosed or after surgical treatment.

References

1. Legg NJ, Gupta PC, Scott DF. Epilepsy following cerebral abscess. *Brain* 1973;96:259–68.
2. Jefferson AA, Keogh AJ. Intracranial abscesses: a review of treated patients over 20 years. *Quart J Med* 1977;183:389–400.
3. Pendlebury WW, Perl DP, Munoz DG. Multiple microabscesses in the central nervous system: a clinicopathologic study. *J Neuropathol Exp Neurol* 1989;48:290–300.
4. Prasad JK, Feller I, Thompson PD. A ten-year review of Candida sepsis and mortality in burn patients. *Surgery* 1987;101:213– 16.
5. Haimes AB, Zimmerman RD, Morgello S, Weingarten K, Becker RD, Jennis R, Deck MD. MR imaging of brain abscesses. *Am J Roentgenol* 1989;152:1073–85.
6. Leys D, Christaens JL, Derambure PH, et al. Management of focal intracranial infections: is medical treatment better than surgery? *J Neurol Neurosurg Psychiatry* 1990;53:472–75.

· · · · · ·

ABSENCE SEIZURES, EPILEPSIES (SEE ALSO PETIT MAL)

Absences are characterized by an alteration in the level of consciousness without (simple absences) or with additional features (complex absences), associated with bursts of bilateral spike and slow waves on the EEG. Absences are a type of idiopathic generalized epilepsy, with onset almost invariably in childhood. Absence seizures may have additional features, such as prolonged duration or prominent automatisms.

Absence seizures produce a characteristic interruption in ongoing activities: a vacant stare, inability to answer, and inability to recall events. The usual duration is 3–10 seconds, ranging up to a few minutes. When absence seizures are very brief, an alteration in the level of consciousness is often difficult to document and ongoing activity may not be affected. The level of functioning during an absence depends on the duration of the seizure: seizures over about 10 seconds cause greater impairment in reaction time on tests requiring concentration (1,2). Recovery from absence occurs within a few seconds, whereas recovery from complex partial seizures is usually slower. Absence seizures may be precipitated by inactivity, emotional stimuli, intellectual effort, hypoglycemia, drowsiness, hyperventilation, visual stimulation, and interrupted ambient light.

Absences seizures may include (3–6):

Altered consciousness alone: With or without eye blinking and an EEG correlate of 3–4 per second spike and wave;

Clonic features: Sudden shock-like jerking movements involving the proximal extremities, neck, trunk, either in isolation or with forward jerking of the neck and upper limbs (myoclonic absence). These seizures may be difficult to distinguish from so-called impulsive petit mal (juvenile myoclonic epilepsy), the latter being somewhat more severe and occurring in an older age group;

Atonic features: Loss of body tone involving the head, trunk, and arms (atonic absence). Atonia may occur concurrently or shortly after spike and wave discharges;

Tonic features: Upward rolling of the eyes, conjugate eye and head deviation, or extension of the trunk (retropulsive or "hypertonic" absence). An asymmetric increase in tone may cause lateral truncal rotation;

Automatisms: A semi-purposeful continuation of ongoing activity, automatisms such as licking of the lips, lipsmacking and pursing of the lips, picking at the clothes, mumbling, swallowing, humming, etc. The incidence of automatisms varies with duration of the seizure (1).

Autonomic features: Alteration in respiration, blood pressure, heart rate, pupil size, bowel motility, and urinary incontinence.

Absence seizures may include several of the above features and one patient may evidence different types of absence seizures at different times (7).

During an absence seizure, the EEG shows bilateral, symmetric, synchronous, spike and slow wave bursts that vary between 150 and 1200 μv; at 3–4 Hertz. Bursts may be induced by hyperventilation and less often photic stimulation. Background EEG activity is normal. Clinical observation often underestimates the frequency of seizures, which are best quantified by routine EEG (7) or ambulatory EEG monitoring (8).

Differential diagnosis and associated conditions: Differential diagnosis of typical absence includes complex partial seizures, atypical absence, inattention or attention deficit disorder in school children, transient global amnesia in the middle-aged and elderly, simple memory lapses, or "blackout spells" from alcohol abuse. Some patients with various psychiatric disorders or the mentally retarded may appear to be staring or "absent" while being, as it were, in their own world. Absence seizures may be a clinical feature seen in a number of syndromes, e.g., absence seizures of infancy, juvenile onset absence seizures, juvenile myoclonic epilepsy (9), and other idiopathic generalized seizure disorders in which absence spells are one of several manifestations. Categorizing absence seizures under a single clinical entity has no heuristic value (10).

ABSENCE, ATYPICAL (3)

Clinical features: Compared to typical absence, atypical absence produces a more gradual alteration in the level of consciousness with a variable duration, usually 1–2 minutes. As with typical absence, common features include staring, eyelid fluttering, interruption of activity or conversation with immediate resumption following cessation of the spell. Complex automatisms, sudden loss of postural tone, head drop, and falls are more common in atypical absence. Absence seizures associated with falls may be classified as atonic, myoclonic, or myoclonic-atonic.

EEG features: Atypical absence seizures are associated with a high-frequency discharge at approximately 20 Hz; a high-voltage discharge at 10 Hz; or a slow (less than 3 per second) spike and wave pattern. The background EEG activity is abnormal, showing slowing, disorganization, and frequent runs of generalized spikes, polyspikes, or 1.5–3/second spike-wave complexes.

Differential diagnosis and associated conditions: Atypical absence can be difficult to distinguish from complex partial seizures, or even nonepileptic events by observation alone. Absence tends to have onset in a younger age group (but there is overlap), evidence quicker recovery of cognition, show more generalized spike-wave EEG patterns, and respond better to ethosuximide or valproic acid. Mental retardation and marked behavioral disturbances often make clinical diagnosis difficult, and video-EEG monitoring is sometimes required (11). Atypical absence seizures may be associated with generalized epilepsies, e.g., the Lennox-Gastaut syndrome and other static or progressive encephalopathies of childhood; perinatal injury; progressive, metabolic, or storage diseases of the central nervous system; or they may be cryptogenic.

References

1. Porter RJ, Penry JK, Dreifuss FE. Responsiveness at the onset of spike wave bursts. *Electroenceph clin Neurophysiol* 1973;34:239–45.
2. Mirsky AF, Duncan CC, Myslobodsky MS. Petit mal epilepsy: a review and integration of recent information. *J Clin Neurophysiol* 1986;3:179–208.
3. Gastaut H, Broughton R. *Epileptic seizures, clinical and electrographic features, diagnosis and treatment.* Springfield: Charles C. Thomas, 1972.
4. Janz D. *Die Epilepsien.* Stuttgart: G. Thieme Verlag, 1969.
5. Penry JK, Porter RJ, Dreifuss FE. Simultaneous recording of absence seizures with video tape and electroencephalography: a study of 374 seizures in 48 patients. *Brain* 1975;98:427–40.
6. Holmes GH, McKeeve RM, Adamson M. Absence seizures in children: clinical and electroencephalographic features. *Ann Neurol* 1987; 26:268–73.
7. Browne TR, Dreifuss FE, Penry JK. Clinical and EEG estimates of absence seizure frequency. *Arch Neurol* 1983;40:468–72.

8. Keilson MJ, Hauser WA, Magrill JP, Tepperberg J. Ambulatory cassette EEG in absence epilepsy. *Ped Neurol* 1987;3:273–76.
9. Panayiotopoulos CP, Obeid T, Waheed G. Absence in juvenile myoclonic epilepsy: a clinical and video-electroencephalographic study. *Ann Neurol* 1989;25:391–97.
10. Olsson I. Epidemiology of absence epilepsy. I: concept and incidence. *Acta Paediat Scand* 1988;77:860–66.
11. Metrick ME, Ritter FJ, Gates JR, Jacobs MP, Skare SS, Loewenson RB. Nonepileptic events in childhood. *Epilepsia* 1991;32(3):322–28.

• • • • • •
ACETAZOLAMIDE (DIAMOX®)

Tablets 250 mg; capsules 500 mg (sustained release).

A carbonic anhydrase inhibitor used with variable results in atypical absences, generalized tonic-clonic seizures, perimenstrual (catamenial), and myoclonic seizures (1). The drug half-life is 6–12 hours, and it is 90% protein-bound. Effective plasma concentrations range from 1 to 22 mg/L (2), but they are not usually measured. Tolerance to the antiepileptic effect is common. Significant side effects are rare, but may include increased urination, paresthesias, anorexia, drowsiness, headache, rash, confusion, renal calculi, and rare instances of agranulocytosis, leukopenia, and thrombocytopenia.

References

1. Resor SR Jr, Resor LD. Chronic acetazolamide monotherapy in the treatment of juvenile myoclonic epilepsy. *Neurology* 1990;40:1677–81.
2. Oles KS, Penry JK, Cole DL, Howard G. Use of acetazolamide as an adjunct to carbamazepine in refractory partial seizures. *Epilepsia* 1989;30:74–78

• • • • • •
ADRENOCORTICOTROPIC HORMONE (ACTH)

Symptomatic generalized and severe cryptogenic epilepsies (e.g., West syndrome, Lennox-Gastaut syndrome, ESES) have been treated with corticosteroids since 1958. A wide variety of steroids and dosages may be used (1):

ACTH: natural or synthetic; the latter is thought to have more side effects.

Hydrocortisone; Prednisone; Prednisolone (Medrol®); *Dexamethasone* (Decadron®).

There is great variability in the duration and modality of treatment; from 3–8 weeks to 6–8 months. Corticosteroids may be preferable to ACTH as they may be given orally. ACTH is purported to have a rapid effect, but with relapses (1). No significant incremental benefit of ACTH levels above 30 units per day has been found (2).

Marked side effects occur: lowered immune resistance with increased infections, Cushingoid facies, obesity, gastrointestinal disturbances, electrolyte abnormalities, hyperglycemia, hypertension, agitation, insomnia, adrenal suppression and insufficiency.

References

1. Sneyd DC, Benton JW, Myers GJ. ACTH and prednisone in childhood seizure disorders. *Neurology* 1983;33:566–970.
2. Kellaway P, Frost JD Jr, Hrachovy RA. Infantile spasms. In: Morselli PL, Pippenger CE, Penry JK (eds.). *Antiepileptic drug therapy in pediatrics.* New York: Raven Press, 1983:115–36.

• • • • • • •
ADRENOLEUKODYSTROPHY (ALD)

ALD is an hereditary disorder of very long-chain fatty acid (24–30 carbon-chain length) metabolism associated with lignoceroyl CoA synthetase deficiency, resulting in deposition of fatty acids in the central nervous system (1,2). Transmission is primarily by X-linked inheritance, with a different clinical expression in males and females. Children are most frequently affected. Older age groups have a progressive neuropathy and spastic paraplegia, occasionally with dementia or psychosis (3). In women, the myelopathic clinical form predominates. The neonatal syndrome shows an autosomal recessive inheritance and may resemble West syndrome.

Leukodystrophy, Addison's disease, blindness, dysarthria, emotional lability, and encephalopathy are frequent; a myeloneuropathic form may be seen (4). Diagnosis may be made using clinical characteristics (1), measurement of very long-chain fatty acid serum and tissue concentrations (2), and MRI (5). The phenotypic presentation is variable, but in the juvenile form in males, seizures are usually a secondary manifestation with relatively later onset. Dietary therapeutic lowering of VLCFA levels over 1–2 years using Lorenzo oil does not measurably improve CNS dysfunction (6,7).

References

1. Moser HW, Moser AE, Singh I, O'Neill BP. Adrenoleukodystrophy: survey of 303 cases: biochemistry, diagnosis, and therapy. *Ann Neurol* 1984;16:628–41.
2. Naidu S, Moser HW. Peroxisomal disorder. *Neurol Clin* 1990;8:507–19.

3. James ACD , Kaplan PW, Lees AJ, Bradley JJ. Schizophreniform psychosis and adrenomyeloneuropathy. *J Roy Soc Med* 1984;77:882–84.
4. Griffin JW, Goren E, Schaumburg H, Engel WK, Loriaux L. Adreno-myeloneuropathy: probable variant of adrenoleukodystrophy. *Neurology* 1977; 27:1107–13.
5. Young IR, Randell CP, Kaplan PW, James A, Bydder GM, Steiner RE. Nuclear magnetic resonance (NMR) imaging in white matter disease of the brain using spin-echo sequences. *J Comput Assist Tomogr* 1983; 7:290–94.
6. Kaplan PW, Tusa RJ, Shankroff J, Heller J, Moser HW. Visual evoked potentials in adrenoleukodystrophy: a trial with glycerol trioleate and Lorenzo oil. *Ann Neurol* 1993;34:169–74.
7. Kaplan PW, Tusa RJ, Moser HW, Shankroff J, Fittro K. Somatosensory evoked potentials in adrenolenkodystrophy. *J Neurology* 1992;239:586.

• • • • • •

AFFECTIVE (SEIZURES)

Affective seizures are characterized by a change in affect, typically an unpleasant one (fear, anxiety, panic), but more rarely with pleasurable symptomatology, e.g., euphoria, ecstasy, contentment. EEG manifestations at the scalp may be absent, but limbic or cingulate gyrus discharges have been recorded. Clinical manifestations include hallucinations or poorly described subjective sensations of unreality.

Affective symtoms are seen in simple or complex partial seizures and in cryptogenic and symptomatic localization-related epilepsies.

Reference

Gastaut H, Broughton R. *Epileptic seizures, clinical and electrographic features, diagnosis and treatment.* Springfield: Charles C. Thomas, 1972.

• • • • • •

AGE OF ONSET (OF SEIZURES)

The age of onset is significant in establishing both a diagnosis and classification of certain epileptic syndromes, determining the etiology of a particular epilepsy, initiating treatment, and providing a prognosis (1).

Epidemiological studies show a bimodal distribution of the incidence of epilepsy (recurrent, unprovoked seizures): 69.9/100,000 in children less than 10 years of age; 36.6/100,000 in adolescents and young adults; 82/100,000 in the elderly. For all seizures, these values are: 122/100,000 in children of less than 10 years of age, 50/100,000 in adolescents, and 144/100,000 in older patients, respectively (2). A similar distribution was noted for first seizures (3). In developing countries, a higher incidence was noted in adolescents and young adults (4). Certain epileptic syndromes have a predilection toward a specific age of onset, for example, West syndrome, Lennox-Gastaut syndrome, absence epilepsies, febrile convulsions.

The age of onset of the first seizure also directs attention toward an underlying cause: neonatal anoxia in children, cerebral tumors, or metabolic disturbances (e.g., toxins or substances of abuse) in midlife, and strokes in the aged.

The age of seizure onset or of an epileptic syndrome has prognostic value. In children, there is a favorable progression with later onset (5). This may be partially due to the poor prognosis of neonatal seizures and of epilepsies with an onset before age 1 year and the spontaneous remission of some of the idiopathic childhood epilepsies. Absence epilepsy of adolescence remits more frequently.

References

1. Hauser WA, Hesdorffer DC. *Epilepsy: frequency, causes and consequences.* New York: Demos, 1990:1–378.
2. Hauser WA, Kurland LT. The epidemiology of epilepsy in Rochester, Minnesota, 1935 through 1967. *Epilepsia* 1975;16:1–66.
3. Loiseau J, Loiseau P, Guyot M, Duché B, Dartigues J-F, Aublet B. Survey of seizure disorder in the French southwest. I. Incidence of epileptic syndromes. *Epilepsia* 1990;31:391–96.
4. Jallon P, Dartigues JF. Epidémiologie descriptive des épilepsies. *Rev Neurol* (Paris) 1987;143:341–50.
5. Brorson LO, Wranne L. Long term prognosis in childhood epilepsy: survival and seizure prognosis. *Epilepsia* 1987;28: 324–30.

• • • • • •

AGRANULOCYTOSIS
(SEE ALSO ANEMIA)

Agranulocytosis, also referred to as granulocytopenia, is a severe deficiency of granulocytes (white blood cells). Granulocyte counts may fall lower than 500 per cubic mm and predispose to infected mucosal ulcers or other opportunistic infections. Agranulocytosis is an uncommon complication of AED therapy.

Reference

Schmidt D. *Adverse effects of antiepileptic drugs.* New York: Raven Press, 1982:1–226.

. . . . . .
AICARDI'S SYNDROME

This epileptic syndrome is only seen in girls. It usually appears in the first year of life, but occasionally in the neonatal period. Typically, the syndrome presents with flexor spasms that may be asymmetric, isolated, or associated with other seizure types; partial or total agenesis of the corpus callosum and multiple chorio-retinal lacunes (2). Other associated cerebral malformations have been reported: ventricular heterotopia, microgyria, and pachygyria. Vertebral malformations have been seen in 50% of cases.

The EEG shows a burst-suppression pattern independently in both hemispheres (3). The prognosis is almost invariably poor.

The syndrome must be distinguished from certain familial forms of agenesis of the corpus callosum associated with infantile spasms (4).

References

1. Aicardi J, Chevrie JJ, Rousseli F. Le syndrome spasmes en flexion, agénésie calleuse, anomalies chorio-retiniennes. *Arch Fr Pediatr* 1969;26:1103–20.
2. Lacey DJ. Agenesis of the corpus callosum: clinical features in 40 children. *AJDC* 1985; 139:953–55.
3. Fariello RG, Chun RW, Doro JM, Buncic R, Prichard JS. Recognition of Aicardi's syndrome. *Arch Neurol* 1977;34:563–66.
4. Cao A, Cianchetti C, Signorini E, Loi M, Sanna G, de Vergilis S. Agenesis of corpus callosum, infantile spasms, spastic quadriplegia, microcephaly and severe mental retardation in three siblings. *Clin Genet* 1977;12:290–96.

. . . . . .
ALCOHOL, EFFECTS OF

The pathophysiological mechanisms relating alcohol and seizures are under extensive study, but remain incompletely understood. In clinical practice, alcohol remains one of the most important causes of seizures and epilepsy. Several issues are of clinical relevance.

THE ROLE OF ALCOHOL IN THE APPEARANCE OF SEIZURES

Seizures can occur during the acute phase of alcohol intake (8). Blood alcohol levels are always raised.

Alcohol withdrawal seizures are seen after partial or complete alcohol withdrawal in a setting of chronic alcohol abuse (1). Single or multiple generalized tonic-clonic seizures occur. Less frequently, partial seizures are seen (2,3).

Seizure onset usually occurs between the 12th and 24th hour of withdrawal, more frequently between the 7th and 72nd hour. It is frequently seen at the end of the weekend. The EEG is usually normal or shows nonspecific abnormalities that may also be found in alcohol abusers who have never had seizures. These alcohol withdrawal seizures may herald the appearance of delirium tremens in 3–4% of cases (4). Seizures appearing during delirium tremens (approximately 18% of cases) usually have a more complex pathogenesis (metabolic disturbances) (5).

RISK OF EPILEPSY IN THE ALCOHOL ABUSER

There is a clear risk of epilepsy associated with alcohol consumption (6,7), which is related to the amount of alcohol being consumed (8). Seizures tend to be infrequent (1–2/year) and are unrelated to any other epileptogenic disorder (9). It should be recognized that alcohol abusers are at higher risk for head trauma and intracranial infections, which may themselves predispose to epilepsy (2).

Status epilepticus may be the first presentation of alcohol-related seizure in 44% of patients (10).

ALCOHOL INTAKE IN PATIENTS WITH EPILEPSY

Excessive intake of alcohol can increase the frequency of seizures by a number of mechanisms: metabolic changes (hypoglycemia, hyponatremia), variation in the levels of some AEDs (increased phenytoin clearance), sleep deprivation during bouts of drinking, and poor compliance with antiepileptic medication. Some studies have shown that acute alcohol intake (11) or "social" drinking (12) do not affect seizure frequency or produce EEG abnormalities in patients with epilepsy.

THE RISK OF ALCOHOLISM IN PATIENTS WITH EPILEPSY

Alcoholism is more frequent in patients with epilepsy than in those without (possibly as a reaction to their chronic condition). The frequency of alcoholism in adults may result in diagnostic errors such as attributing seizures to alcoholism and not to the possible presence of intracranial lesions (13).

PREVENTING ALCOHOL-WITHDRAWAL SEIZURES

The use of AEDs to prevent alcohol withdrawal seizures is controversial. While some investigators have advocated their use in individuals who have had recent seizures or previous bouts of seizures in conjunction with alcohol withdrawal (14), others have argued against prophylaxis. The argument against therapy derives from two lines of evidence: 1. Alcohol-withdrawal seizures tend to occur in brief clusters (1); 2. Treatment is likely to be ineffective (15). Chronic AED therapy is usually futile, since compliance is poor in this setting. Barbiturates, in particular, should be avoided because of their synergism with alcohol to depress respiration.

References

1. Victor M, Brausch V. The role of abstinence in the genesis of alcoholic epilepsy. *Epilepsia* 1967;8:1–20.
2. Earnest MP, Yarnell PR. Seizure admissions to a city hospital: the role of alcohol. *Epilepsia* 1976;17:387–93.
3. Bartolomei F, Nicoli F, Gastaut J-L. Partial complex epileptic seizures provoked by ingestion of alcohol. *J Neurol* 1993;240:232–34.
4. Hillbom ME. Occurrence of cerebral seizures provoked by alcohol abuse. *Epilepsia* 1980;21:459–66.
5. Isbel H, Fraser HF, Wilker A, Belleville RE, Eisebman AJ. An experimental study of the etiology of "rum fits" and delirium tremens. *J Stud Alcohol* 1985;16:1–33.
6. Devetag F, Mandich G, Zaiotti G, Toffolo GG. Alcoholic epilepsy: review of a series and proposed classification and etiopathogenesis. *Ital J Neurol Sci* 1983;3:275–84.
7. Chan WK. Alcoholism and epilepsy. *Epilepsia* 1985;26:323–33.
8. Hauser WA, Ng SKC, Brust JCM. Alcohol, seizures and epilepsy. *Epilepsia* 1988;29 (Suppl 2): S66–S78.
9. Ng SKC, Hauser WA, Brust JCM, Susser M. Alcohol consumption and withdrawal in new-onset seizures. *N Engl J Med* 1988;319: 666–73.
10. Alldredge BK, Lowenstein DH. Status epilepticus related to alcohol abuse. *Epilepsia* 1993;34:1033–37.
11. Mattson RH, Sturman JK, Gronowski ML, Goici H. Effects of alcohol intake in non-alcoholic epileptics. *Neurology* 1975;25:361–62.
12. Hoppener RJ, Kuyer A, Van der Lugt PJM. Epilepsy and alcohol: influence of social alcohol intake on seizures and treatment in epilepsy. *Epilepsia* 1983;24:459–71.
13. Earnest MP, Feldman M, Marx JA, Harris JA, Biletch M, Sullivan LP. Intracranial lesions shown by CT scans in 259 cases of first alcohol-related seizures. *Neurology* 1988;38:1561–65.
14. Sampliner R, Iber FL. Diphenylhydantoin control of alcohol withdrawal seizures: results of a controlled study. *JAMA* 1974;230:1430–32.
15. Alldredge BK, Lowenstein DH, Simon RP. Placebo-controlled trial of intravenous diphenylhydantoin for short-term treatment of alcohol withdrawal seizures. *Am J Med* 1989;87:645–48.

• • • • • •
ALOPECIA

Alopecia is the loss or thinning of hair. A small percentage of patients on valproic acid, and even fewer patients taking carbamazepine, ethosuximide, or other AEDs, may experience alopecia. Hair usually regrows with reduction or discontinuation of medication.

• • • • • •
ALPERS' (DISEASE) (DIFFUSE PROGRESSIVE DEGENERATION OF THE CEREBRAL GRAY MATTER)

Alpers' disease is a degenerative disease of uncertain etiology (speculatively a mitochondrial encephalopathy) seen in children, with onset usually before the age of one year. The syndrome is characterized by progressive hypotonia, psychomotor retardation, respiratory problems, and hepatic insufficiency. Seizures, of a myoclonic, partial, and generalized tonic-clonic type, may ensue and come to dominate the clinical picture. The patient may develop focal status epilepticus. EEG interictally and ictally may demonstrate high-voltage spikes and slow waves (2). Most often, the disease is rapidly progressive and fatal, but prolonged survival has occurred (3).

References

1. Alpers BJ. Diffuse progressive degeneration of the cerebral gray matter. *Arch Neurol Psychiatry* 1931;25:466–72.
2. Brick JF, Westmoreland BF, Gomez MR. The electroencephalogram in Alpers' disease. *Electroenceph clin Neurophysiol* 1984;58:31P (abstract).
3. Harding BN. Progressive neuronal degeneration of childhood with liver disease (Alpers-Huttenlocher syndrome): a personal review. *J Child Neurol* 1990;5:273–87.

• • • • • •
ALPHA RHYTHM (SEE ALSO EEG)

The alpha rhythm is a pattern seen in the normal EEG of children and adults. The frequency of alpha ranges from 8–13 Hertz, and amplitude is maximal in the relaxed, eyes-closed awake state and is blocked by eye opening. It is best detected over the posterior portions of the head and is part of the background activity. Slowing or disruption of the alpha rhythm may suggest an underlying diffuse or posterior cerebral disturbance. Idiopathic epilepsies are characterized by a normal alpha rhythm; symptomatic epilepsies by abnormally slow background frequencies. Slowing of the alpha activity may be seen with some AED toxicity. Preservation of alpha rhythm during a generalized seizure is supportive evidence for pseudo-seizures (psychogenic seizures).

Reference

Kellaway P. An orderly approach to visual analysis: characteristics of the normal EEG of adults and children. In: Daly DD, Pedley TA (eds.). *Current practice of clinical electroencephalography,* 2nd edition. New York: Raven Press, 1990.

• • • • • • •
AMBULATORY EEG

Ambulatory EEGs permit recording of EEG patterns for prolonged periods (e.g., 24 hours) at home, work, or school (1,2). Up to 16 channels of EEG, ECG, or event marker signals may be recorded on analog tape and correlated by digital clock to events of interest. The tape is scanned on a computerized reader in accelerated time, and segments of interest analyzed on an oscilloscope screen or paper output. In some settings, the diagnostic yield for detection of seizures approaches that of inpatient video-EEG intensive monitoring (3); however, artifact identification and ability to localize seizure discharges are better with intensive inpatient monitoring. The ambulatory EEG technique is limited by lack of video-correlate to assist with interpretation of the many movement artifacts, high cost relative to routine EEG, and the need to capture a clinical episode. Nevertheless, ambulatory EEG can be of value in the diagnosis of frequently recurrent "spells."

References

1. Bridges SL, Ebersole JS. The clinical utility of ambulatory cassette EEG. *Neurology* 1985;35:166–73.
2. Aminoff MJ, Goodin DS, Berg BO, Compton MN. Ambulatory EEG recordings in epileptic and nonepileptic children. *Neurology* 1988;38:558–62.
3. Ebersole JS, Bridges SL. Direct comparison of 3- and 8-channel ambulatory cassette EEG with intensive inpatient monitoring. *Neurology* 1985;35:846–54.

• • • • • • •
AMMONIA

Ammonia is generated by the metabolism of urea and amino acids. Individuals with inherited hyperammonemias are more prone to seizures (1). The antiepileptic drug valproic acid (VPA) may increase serum ammonia by inhibition of ammonia transport across mitochondrial and cell membranes, possibly contributing to an encephalopathy (2). This may occur without increases in serum hepatic transaminase levels. Asymptomatic rises of serum ammonia levels from VPA are of uncertain clinical significance. Carnitine, a substance with few side effects, can facilitate transport across mitochondrial membranes and reduce symptoms from hyperammonemia (3).

References

1. Batshaw ML. *Hyperammonemia: current problems in pediatrics.* Chicago: Chicago Year Book Publishers, 1984.
2. Batshaw ML, Brusilow SW. Valproate-induced hyperammonemia. *Ann Neurol* 1982;11:319–21.
3. Matsuda I, Ohtani Y, Ninomiya N. Renal handling of carnitine in children with carnitine deficiency and hyperammonemia associated with valproate therapy. *J Pediatr* 1986;109:131–34.

• • • • • •
AMYGDALA

The amygdala comprises a complex of grey matter nuclei in the anterior-medial temporal lobe, classified as part of the limbic system, and of the olfactory system. The amygdala is situated immediately anteriorly to the hippocampal formation. Considerable study has been devoted to the phenomenon of kindling (see Kindling), which is best elicited by repeated electrical stimulation of the amygdala. Seizures arising from the amygdala are characterized by a sensation of rising epigastric discomfort, nausea, oral automatisms, chewing, fear, panic, and marked autonomic features: facial flushing, pupillary dilatation, belching, and borborygmus (see also Abdominal (E)). Depth wire EEG recording has revealed seizure spread from the amygdala to the hypothalamus, fronto-orbital region, and the hippocampal formation. The etiologies of amygdalar seizures are the same as those for seizures arising from the temporal lobe.

Reference

Maldonado HM, Delgado-Escueta AV, Walsh GO, Swartz BE, Rand RW. Complex partial seizures of hippocampal and amygdalar origin. *Epilepsia* 1988;29:420–35.

●●●●●●
ANEMIA (SEE ALSO AGRANULOCYTOSIS)

Mild, transient leukopenia—approximately 10%—(1) or more severe, irreversible (2) aplastic anemias may be seen with carbamazepine (1–3), ethosuximide (4), or very rarely with phenytoin (5). When aplastic anemia supervenes, the mortality rate may reach 33–50% (2,3), with a case incidence of 0.5/100,000 treatment-years (2). Recently, several cases of aplastic anemia have occurred with felbamate (see Felbamate), leading to restriction in its use. Megaloblastic anemias may be seen with carbamazepine, phenytoin, primidone, and phenobarbital (5).

References

1. Livingston S, Pauli LL, German W. Carbamazepine in epilepsy. Nine years' follow-up with special reference on unwanted reactions. *Dis Nerv Syst* 1974;35:103–107.
2. Hart RG, Easton JD. Carbamazepine and hematological monitoring. *Ann Neurol* 1982;11:309–12.
3. Pisciotta AV. Hematological toxicity of carbamazepine. *Adv Neurol* 1975;11: 355–68.
4. Dreifuss F. Ethosuximide toxicity. In: Levy RH, Dreifuss FE, Mattson RH, Meldrum BS, Penry JK (eds.). *Antiepileptic drugs,* 3rd edition. New York: Raven Press, 1989:701–702.
5. Reynolds EH. Phenytoin toxicity. In: Levy RH, Dreifuss FE, Mattson RH, Meldrum BS, Penry JK (eds.). *Antiepileptic drugs,* 3rd edition. New York: Raven Press,1989.

●●●●●●
ANESTHESIA

No changes in AED dosage are required before or after general anesthesia. Oral intake of AEDs suspended during the procedure may be resumed when the patient awakens and bowel motility is restored. The dose immediately preceding anesthesia can be doubled to ensure higher AED blood levels.

Some anesthetics are contraindicated in patients with epilepsy: enflurane, ketamine, methohexitone, althesin, and propanidid (1).

There is no risk with local anesthesia (2). Local anesthetics have been used parenterally for the treatment of status epilepticus (see Lidocaine).

Seizures have rarely been reported with epidural anesthesia (bupivacaine) when the agent has entered the intravascular or intrathecal compartments.

References

1. Evans DM. Anesthesia and the epileptic patient. *Anaesthesia* 1975;30:34–45.
2. Davis JAH, Gill SS, Weber JCP. Intravenous regional analgesia using bupiva-caine. *Anaesthesia* 1981;36:331.

• • • • • •

ANEURYSMS, ARTERIAL

Unlike with angiomas, seizures do not occur with aneurysms excepting with giant aneurysms or aneurysmal rupture and hemmorhage.

Seizures occur in 10–25% of patients who have undergone surgical intervention for aneurysm repair. A higher incidence of seizures is seen with larger aneurysms, particular localizations (medium-sized cerebral arteries), the presence of a hematoma, postoperative vasospasm, and hydro-cephalus (1,2), often providing a relative indication for the use of pro-phylactic AED therapy (six months to three years).

References

1. Keranen T, Tapaninaho A, Hernesniemi J, Vapalahti M. Late epilepsy after aneurysm operations. *Neurosurgery* 1985;17:897–900.
2. Richardson AE, Uttley D. Prevention of postoperative epilepsy. *Lancet* 1980;i: 650.

• • • • • •

ANIMAL MODELS OF THE EPILEPSIES

There are ethical and practical limits on study of epilepsy in patients. Much of what is known about mechanisms of epilepsy and of potential antiepilep-tic drugs has been learned via animal models of the epilepsies (1,2). No one animal model suffices for study, since none perfectly replicates the clinical epilepsies and different types of epilepsy require different models. An experimenter chooses a model based on the experimental question, familiarity, cost, and the availability of information about the model.

Acute partial seizures have been modeled in rodents, cats, and mon-keys by deposition of a variety of convulsant compounds on the surface of the brain. Penicillin, which antagonizes GABA receptors, is common-ly employed in acute focal models (3). Metals, including aluminum, cobalt, tungsten, and iron, can produce chronically recurring partial seizures (4).

Complex partial epilepsies, involving temporal-limbic discharges, have been modeled by several methods. The excitotoxic glutamate analogue, kainic acid, can be injected systemically, intraventricularly, or intrahippocampally to produce seizure discharges originating primarily in hippocampus (5). Kindling is a process by which repeated, brief electrical stimulations of brain (often amygdala) result in progressively more complex afterdischarges, and eventually seizures originating from the limbic system (6). Kindling can serve as a model not only of epilepsy, but of plastic changes in brain leading to genesis of epilepsy. Considerable advances in our understanding of epilepsy mechanisms have derived from study of the *in vitro* hippocampal slice model system (7,8). Brainslice model systems sacrifice realism for control over numerous experimentally important variables, but have been pivotal in the development of several important hypotheses.

Generalized seizures have been modeled sucessfully by maximal electroshock in rats and mice, which predicts a putative anticonvulsant's efficacy against tonic-clonic epilepsy (9,10). Generalized seizures can also be produced by systemic administration of chemoconvulsant drugs, such as pentylenetetrazol (11), picrotoxin (12), strychnine (13), bemegride (14), bicuculline (15), allylglycine (16), methionine sulfoximine (17), certain general anesthetics, and a variety of other agents. Since certain epilepsies have a genetic component (see Genetics), study of genetically prone strains of mice (18) and rats (19) has been of particular interest as models of absence and tonic-clonic seizures. These studies have demonstrated that a gene mutation at a single locus is able to produce a complex syndrome of epilepsy and neurological deficits (20). Parenteral administration of penicillin in cats produces spike-wave EEG discharges and behavioral manifestations similar to absence seizures (21,22). Gamma-hydroxybutyrate (GHB) is a GABA metabolite used to model absence seizures (23).

Despite the existence of many models for the epilepsies, only listed here in abbreviated form, there is still a great need for more accurate and convenient models.

References

1. Fisher RS. Animal models of the epilepsies. *Brain Res Rev* 1989;14:245–78.
2. Löscher WL, Schmidt D. Which animal models should be used in the search for new antiepileptic drug? A proposal based on experimental and clinical considerations. *Epilepsy Res* 1988;2:145–81.
3. Matsumoto H, Ajmone-Marsan C. Cortical cellular phenomena in experimental epilepsy: interictal manifestations. *Exp Neurol* 1964;9:286–304.
4. Ward AA. Topical convulsant metals. In: Purpura DP, Penry JK, Woodbury DM, Tower DB, Walter RD (eds.). *Experimental models of epilepsy—a manual for the laboratory worker.* New York: Raven Press, 1972:13–35.

5. Nadler V. Kainic acid as a tool for the study of temporal lobe epilepsy. *Life Sci* 1981;29:2031–42.

6. Goddard GV. Development of epileptic seizures through brain stimulation at low intensity. *Nature* 1967;214:1020–21.

7. Dingledine R (ed.). *Brain slices.* New York: Plenum Press, 1984.

8. Schwartzkroin PA, Wheal HV (eds.). *Electrophysiology of epilepsy.* New York: Academic Press, 1984.

9. Merritt HH, Putnam TJ. A new series of anticonvulsant drugs tested by experiments on animals. *Arch Neurol Psychiatry* 1938;39:1003–15.

10. Swinyard EA. Electrically-induced convulsions. In: Purpura DP, Penry JK, Woodbury DM, Tower DB, Walter RD (eds.). *Experimental models of epilepsy—a manual for the laboratory worker.* New York: Raven Press, 1972: 435–58.

11. Starzl TE, Niemer WT, Dell M, Forgave PR. Cortical and subcortical electrical activity in experimental seizures induced by metrazol. *J Neuropathol Exp Neurol* 1953;12:262–76.

12. Hahn F. Analeptics. *Pharmacol Rev* 1960;12:447–530.

13. Bigler ED. Comparison of effects of bicuculline, strychnine, and picrotoxin and those of pentylenetetrazol on photically evoked after discharges. *Epilepsia* 1977;18:465–70.

14. Rodin EA, Rutledge LT, Calhoun HD. Megimide and metrazol: a comparison of their convulsant properties in man and cat. *Electroenceph clin Neurophysiol* 1958;10:719–23.

15. Meldrum BS, Horton RW. Convulsive effects of 4–deoxypyridoxine and of bicuculline in photosensitive baboons (Papio papio) and in rhesus monkeys (Macaca mulatta). *Brain Res* 1971;35: 419–36.

16. Meldrum BS, Horton RW, Brierly JB. Epileptic brain damage in adolescent baboons following seizures induced by allylglycine. *Brain* 1974;97:407–18.

17. Harris B. Cortical alterations due to methionine sulfoximine *Arch Neurol* 1964;11:388–407.

18. Seyfried TN, Glaser GH. A review of mouse mutants as genetic models of epilepsy. *Epilepsia* 1985;26:143–50.

19. Reigel CE, Dailey JW, Jobe PC. The genetically epilepsy-prone rat: an overview of seizure-prone characteristics and responsiveness to anticonvulsant drugs. *Life Sci* 1986;39:763–74.

20. Noebels JL. A single gene error of noradrenergic axon growth synchronizes central neurones. *Nature* 1984;310:409–11.

21. Fisher RS, Prince DA. Spike-wave rhythms in cat cortex induced by parenteral penicillin. I. Electroencephalographic features. *Electroenceph clin Neurophysiol* 1977;42:608–24.

22. Gloor P. Generalized epilepsy with spike-and-wave discharge: a reinterpretation of its electrographic and clinical manifestations. *Epilepsia* 1979;20:571–88.

23. Snead OC III. Gamma-hydroxybutyrate model of generalized absence seizures: further characterization and comparison with other absence models. *Epilepsia* 1988;29:361–68.

• • • • • •
ANOXIA/HYPOXIA

Severe, diffuse anoxia in adults produces a variety of neurological disorders and seizures (see also Hypoxia). These include focal, generalized tonic-clonic, and myoclonic seizures for which EEG may provide diagnostic and prognostic information (1,2).

In neonates, hypoxic-ischemic insult is the commonest cause of seizures in the first 48 hours of life (3), accounting for 50–75% of cases. Isolated seizures are usually followed by clusters or volleys of seizures, contributing to 75–85% of the incidence of status epilepticus in the newborn.

The interictal EEG is abnormal with bursts of epileptiform activity or with bilateral suppression. The prognosis is poor, with only 16–50% of children developing normally. There is a five-fold increase in the incidence of epilepsy (4).

References

1. Krumholtz A, Stern BJ, Weiss HD. Outcome from coma after cardiopulmonary resuscitation: relation to seizures and myoclonus. *Neurology* 1988;38:401–405.
2. Wijdicks EFM, Parisi JE, Sharbrough FW. Prognostic value of myoclonus status in comatose survivors of cardiac arrest. *Ann Neurol* 1994;35:239–43.
3. Volpe JJ. Neonatal seizures. *Lancet* 1989;ii:135–37.
4. Bergamasco B, Benna P, Ferrero P, Gavinelli R. Neonatal hypoxia and epileptogenic risk: a clinical prospective study. *Epilepsia* 1984;25:131–36.

• • • • • •
ANTICONVULSANT/ANTIEPILEPTIC DRUG (AED) LEVELS (1,2)

AED levels may be obtained from whole blood, plasma, serum, blood cells, saliva, tears, urine, cerebrospinal fluid, or tissues. Blood levels are usually used to monitor therapeutic AED intake.

For every drug, there is an optimal concentration for maximal effectiveness and minimal toxicity, the so-called "therapeutic" zone. Levels above this zone are likely to produce side effects (so-called "toxic" levels).

Brain and blood concentrations are supposed to be similar. In fact, they may differ among different (pathological) brain regions. The dosage in mg/kg needed to provide optimal blood levels may vary, however, from patient to patient. When multiple AEDs are used, drug interactions may be predicted in general, but the degree of interaction cannot. Certain pathological states, including hypoalbuminemia, hepatic or renal insufficiency, may change the equilibrium or disappearance rate of AEDs.

AED noncompliance is rarely admitted to, and AED monitoring is essential in verifying compliance.

METHODS OF AED MONITORING

- Chromatography, radioimmunoassay, immuno-enzymatic monitoring.
- Usually, the total plasma AED levels are measured, which do not distinguish between the free and protein-bound fractions.
- If there are reasons to believe an increase in the free fraction of a particular AED, free or unbound drug levels may be measured. Such tests may be needed in patients on renal dialysis in whom saliva and tear AED levels may be measured. When blood samples are difficult to obtain (e.g., in children), salivary levels can be helpful (3).
- Measurement of drug metabolites—usually in blood or urine—is difficult and is usually done for research purposes.

AED TEST RESULTS

Laboratory values must always be interpreted in the light of the patient's clinical state:

- Noncompliance may produce lower than expected blood levels, as may poor gastrointestinal absorption, increased clearance (genetic factors, enzyme induction, measurement taken before steady state is achieved), or the normal expected fluctuation occurring during the course of the day.
- Higher than expected levels may be seen due to faulty compliance, decreased clearance (genetic factors, drug interactions, hepatic insufficiency, renal insufficiency).
  Epilepsy control can be much improved by the repeated use of AED monitoring.
- At present, levels of the newer AEDs (felbamate, gabapentin, and lamotrigine) are not generally measured.

DRAWBACKS

- Therapeutic or toxic drug levels are statistical concepts derived from the evaluation of large groups of patients. Certain patients may be controlled with levels considered as subtherapeutic, whereas others may require so-called toxic levels. Some patients have side effects at low or mid-therapeutic levels; others may tolerate high therapeutic or toxic levels. The goal of treatment is to eliminate seizures, not to produce a therapeutic AED drug value (4).

- As drug level determinations may be costly, patients who are well-controlled and without side effects may not require testing (5).
- Laboratory testing is subject to error; a possible mismatch of AED level obtained to clinical status should be kept in mind (5,6).

ASSAYS

Assays are now routinely available for most AEDs excepting felbamate, gabapentin, and lamotrigine, although these can be determined. AED levels are helpful in several clinical situations (7):

1. monitoring patient compliance;
2. correlating objective or subjective problems attributable to drug toxicity to a measurable blood level (see Antiepileptic drug toxicity);
3. determining which drug is responsible for drug toxicity in the presence of polypharmacy;
4. helping to determine therapeutic ineffectiveness before considering switching to other AEDs;
5. evaluating the possiblility of subtherapeutic AED levels when "breakthrough" seizures occur.

"Therapeutic ranges" are provided by the laboratory performing AED assays. These may be used as guidelines in management, but treatment must be adapted to the patient's needs. Not infrequently, higher or lower than "therapeutic level" ranges are needed in controlling an individual's seizures or avoiding toxicity. Often, supratherapeutic levels may be reached without clinical toxicity, but which provide the requisite seizure control.

In certain metabolic states such as renal insufficiency, AED levels may not correlate with seizure control or toxicity. In uremia, for example, the free (unbound) and therefore active fraction of phenytoin may be significantly raised, resulting in toxicity, even though total phenytoin levels are within the therapeutic range. Similarly, half the "therapeutic level" of total phenytoin may be sufficient to control seizures. Assays for the free fraction of an AED are often available.

References

1. Levy RH, Dreifuss FE, Mattson RH, Meldrum BS, Penry JK (eds.). *Antiepileptic drugs*, 3rd edition. New York, Raven Press, 1989.
2. Commission on Antiepileptic Drugs, International League Against Epilepsy. Guidelines for therapeutic monitoring on antiepileptic drugs. *Epilepsia* 1993; 34:585–87.

3. Henkes GK, Eadie MJ. Possible roles for frequent salivary antiepileptic drug monitoring in the management of epilepsy. *Epilepsy Res* 1990;6:146–54.
4. Woo E, Chan YM, Yu YL, Chan YW, Huang CY. If a well-stabilized epileptic patient has a subtherapeutic antiepileptic drug level, should the dose be increased? A randomized prospective study. *Epilepsia* 1988;29:129–39.
5. Choonara IA, Rane A. Therapeutic drug monitoring of anticonvulsants. State of the art. *Clin Pharmacokin* 1990;28:318–28.
6. Pippenger CE, Penry JK, White BG, Daly DD, Buddington R. Interlaboratory variability in determination of plasma antiepileptic drug concentrations. *Arch Neurol* 1976;33:351–55.
7. Engel J Jr. *Seizures and epilepsy. General principles of treatment.* Philadelphia: F.A. Davis, 1989:380–409.

• • • • • • •
ANTICONVULSANT/ANTIEPILEPTIC DRUG MECHANISMS

Historically, there have been three general approaches to the development of antiepileptic drugs: serendipity, mass screening of barbiturate analogues, and designer drugs based on research into mechanisms of the epilepsies. The earliest antiepileptic drug, bromide, was discovered on the basis of an erroneous theory relating epilepsy to sexual dysfunction (1). The second antiepileptic drug, phenobarbital, was discovered by "informed serendipity," from observations on a medication designed to serve another function. Merritt and Putnam introduced the electroshock screening method for anticonvulsants in 1938, along with their discovery of the anticonvulsant properties of phenytoin (2). Over 20,000 chemical compounds have been screened for activity against electroshock or chemoconvulsant models of epilepsy (3). Recently, an understanding of basic mechanisms of the epilepsies (see Basic mechanisms of the epilepsies) has allowed antiepileptic drug development to be based on rational theory. The calcium channel antagonists, such as flunarizine (4), the GABA degradation inhibitors, such as vigabatrin (5), and other GABAergic agents, such as progabide, have been developed with this mechanistic approach.

Since most antiepileptic drug development has been empirical, understanding of drug mechanisms remains rudimentary (6). Several possible mechanisms exist, and many drugs may involve more than one mechanism. Enhancement of GABAergic synaptic inhibition appears to be an important mechanism of action of benzodiazepines (7,8) and barbiturates (9,10). Phenytoin, carbamazepine, valproic acid, and phenobarbital can inhibit sustained repetitive firing of neurons in a seizure focus (11). Several of these drugs can also inhibit calcium currents in certain model systems, perhaps relating to their antiepileptic actions (12). Block of sodium channels also appears important in inhibiting epileptiform cellular bursting (13). Lamotrigine appears to work on voltage-sensitive sodium channels to inhibit presynaptic release of glutamate. The anti-absence agent, ethosuximide, appears to inhibit a particular calcium current in thalamic neurons involved in rhythmic thalamic activity (14).

Valproic acid can antagonize metabolic degradation of GABA, but it probably requires supratherapeutic concentrations to do so (15). Gabapentin has no effect on the GABA or other known neurotransmitter systems, but may act on a gabapentin-specific binding site similar to the L-amino acid transport system to modulate seizure activity. Better evidence is available for vigabatrin as an irreversible inhibitor of GABA breakdown, thus increasing brain GABA levles (5).

A recent class of drugs able to antagonize excitatory amino acid transmission has come under intense study (16). A prototype of this class is MK-801 (17). Whether excitatory amino acid antagonists will be effective for clinical epilepsy remains to be seen. Certain anticonvulsants, such as phenytoin, may in some circumstances diminish seizure propagation without eliminating synchronous epileptiform discharge at the focus.

AED research is a rapidly growing field. The hope is that further advances in this area will facilitate effective therapies for the millions of people whose epilepsy is not controlled by current medication.

References

1. Friedlander WJ. Who was 'the father of bromide treatment of epilepsy'? *Arch Neurol* 1986;43:505–507.
2. Merritt HH, Putnam TJ. A new series of anticonvulsant drugs tested by experiments on animals. *Arch Neurol Psychiatry* 1938;39:1003–15.
3. Porter RJ, Cereghino JJ, Gladding GD, Hessie BJ, Kupferberg HJ, Scoville B, White BG. Antiepileptic drug development program. *Cleve Clin Q* 1984; 51:293–305.
4. Froscher W, Bulau P, Burr W. Double-blind placebo-controlled trial with flunarizine in therapy-resistant epileptic patients. *Clin Neuropharmacol* 1988;11:232–40.
5. Schechter PJ, Hanke NFJ, Grove J, Huebert N, Sjoerdsma A. Biochemical and clinical effects of gamma-vinyl GABA in patients with epilepsy. *Neurology* 1984;34:182–86.
6. DeLorenzo RJ. Mechanisms of action of anticonvulsant drugs. *Epilepsia* 1988;2(Suppl 29):S35–S47.
7. Macdonald RL, Barker JL. Benzodiazepines specifically modulate GABA-mediated postsynaptic inhibition in cultured mammalian neurones. *Nature* 1978;271:563–64.
8. Tallman J, Gallager D. The GABA-ergic system: a locus of benzodiazepine action. *Annual Rev Neurosci* 1985;8:21–44.
9. Evans RH. Potentiation of the effects of GABA by phenobarbitone. *Brain Res* 1979;171:113–20.

10. Study RE, Barker JL. Diazepam and (±) pentobarbital: fluctuation analysis reveals different mechanisms for potentiation of gamma-aminobutyric acid responses in cultured central neurons. *Proc Natl Acad Sci USA* 1981;78:180–84.
11. Macdonald RL. Antiepileptic drug actions on neurotransmitter receptors and ion channels. In: Fisher RS, Coyle JT. *Neurotransmitters and epilepsy.* New York: Wiley-Liss, Inc., 1991:231–45.
12. Ferrendelli JA, Daniels-McQueen S. Comparative actions of phenytoin and other anticonvulsant drugs on potassium- and veratridine-stimulated calcium uptake in synaptosomes. *J Pharmacol Ther* 1982;220:29–34.
13. Courtney KR, Etter EF. Modulated anticonvulsant block of sodium channels in nerve and muscle. *Eur J Pharmacol* 1983;88:1–9.
14. Coulter DA, Huguenard JR, Prince DA. Characterization of ethosuximide reduction of low-threshold calcium current in thalamic neurons. *Ann Neurol* 1989;25:582–93.
15. Macdonald RL, Bergey GK. Valproic acid augments GABA-mediated post-synaptic inhibition in cultured mammalian neurons. *Brain Res* 1979;167:323–36.
16. Croucher MJ, Collins JF, Meldrum BS. Anticonvulsant action of excitatory amino acid antagonists. *Science* 1982;216:899–901.
17. Troupin AS, Mendius JR, Cheng F, Risinger MW. MK-801. In: Meldrum BS, Porter RJ (eds.). *New anticonvulsant drugs.* London: John Libbey Eurotext, 1986:191–201.

• • • • • •

ANTIEPILEPTIC DRUGS (AEDS) (1)

There are several AEDs available for long-term use in outpatient control of epilepsy and, in the hospital setting, for control of status epilepticus (1). Drugs of choice vary with experience, personal preference, desire to avoid particular side effects, cost convenience issues, and seizure type. The following list of suggested drugs of choice is therefore not unique. Simple partial and complex partial seizures, with or without secondary generalization, are best treated with carbamazepine (Tegretol®), phenytoin (Dilantin®, Epanutin®), or valproic acid (Depakene®); Divalproex sodium (Depakote®). Drugs of choice for primary generalized tonic-clonic epilepsies include valproic acid, carbamazepine, or phenytoin. Absence seizures may be treated with ethosuximide or valproic acid. Myoclonic seizures are usually treated with valproic acid or benzodiazepines. Second-line drugs for a variety of seizure types include the barbiturates, phenobarbital (Luminal®, Gardenal®), mephobarbital (Mebaral®), and primidone (Mysoline®). Primidone degradation products include phenylethylmalonic acid (PEMA) and phenobarbital, each with antiepileptic properties. Antiepileptic benzodiazepines include diazepam (Valium®), clonazepam (Klonopin®), clorazepate (Tranxene®), lorazepam (Ativan®), and midazolam (Versed®).

Recently developed AEDs are now available in the United States as add-on therapy for partial seizures with secondary generalization. Felbamate (Felbatol®) (also effective in Lennox-Gastaut syndrome) may still have a role as a second-line drug in the AED armamentarium, but has been associated with aplastic anemia and liver failure and probably should be used advisedly in patients in whom epilepsy outweighs the medical risks of drug side effects. Gabapentin (Neurontin®) and Lamotrigine (Lamictal®) are useful second-line drugs for partial and secondarily generalized seizures. Other AEDs that are not yet available in the United States include progabide (Gabrene®), clobazam (Urbanyl®), vigabatrin (Sabril®), and flunarizine (Sibelium®).

ANTIEPILEPTIC DRUGS (AEDS) AVAILABLE FOR CLINICAL USE IN THE UNITED STATES

(* = of major clinical importance)

Hydantoins
Phenytoin* (Dilantin®)
Ethotoin (Peganone®)
Mephentoin (Mesantoin®)

Barbiturates
Phenobarbital* (Luminal®)
Primidone* (Mysoline®)
Mephobarbital (Mebaral®)
Methabarbital (Gemonil®)

Carboxamides
Carbamazepine* (Tegretol®)

Succinimides
Ethosuximide* (Zarontin®)
Methsuximide (Celontin®)
Phensuximide (Milontin®)

Carbamates
Felbamate* (Felbatol®)

Triazine derivative
Lamotrigine (Lamictal®)

Oxazolidinediones
Paramethadione (Paradione®)
Trimethadione (Tridione®)

Phenylureas
Phenacemide (Phenurone®)

Carboxylic acids
Valproic acid* (Depakene®)

Carbonic anhydrase inhibitor
Acetazolamide (Diamox®)

Benzodiazepines
Diazepam* (Valium®)
Clonazepam* (Klonopin®)
Lorazepam (Ativan®)
Chlorazepate (Tranxene®)
Midazolam (Versed®)

GABA analog
Gabapentin (Neurontin®)

MECHANISM OF ACTION

Despite considerable research, the mechanism of action of most of the AEDs remains poorly understood (see Anticonvulsant/Antiepileptic drug mechanisms).

ANTICONVULSANT/ANTIEPILEPTIC DRUG PHARMOCOKINETICS

Pharmacokinetics is the study and mathematical expression of the fate of drugs in the body, including absorption, distribution, metabolism, and excretion (2).

Absorption: After the ingestion of a single dose, the half-life of an AED can be extrapolated from absorption and decay curves obtained from repeated blood levels. The highest point of the curve represents peak concentration and the speed of absorption, whereas the area under the curve reflects bioavailability. Intravenous AED administration produces total and immediate absorption. Oral ingestion requires penetration of the gastrointestinal mucous membrane and passage through entero-hepatic circulation before reaching the systemic circulation. This process usually involves passive diffusion of the nonionized portion of the anticonvulsant. Many factors affect distribution: molecular size, lipid solubility, membrane concentration of anticonvulsant, gastrointestinal contents, gastric emptying. Solubility may vary from one formulation of a drug to another. Bioavailability of an AED may be determined by measuring the area under the curve produced by intravenous or oral administration. Rectal administration of some drugs in solution results in excellent absorption. Conversely, certain AEDs (e.g., phenytoin when given intramuscularly) may bind to muscle proteins, thus creating irregular absorption.

Distribution: In blood, distribution is a balance of absorption, excretion, and entry into the extravascular tissue compartment. Immediately after intravenous injection, blood drug concentrations fall exponentially, since it is the total plasma volume that is cleared in a given time. After oral administration, the serum concentration increases and subsequently decreases by the same mechanism. For most AEDs, the rate of clearance is proportional to the serum concentration (first order kinetics). For other AEDs (e.g., phenytoin at high serum concentrations), clearance is limited by the rate of biotransformation, with a clearance rate independent of serum concentration (zero order kinetics). In circumstances of zero order kinetics, high serum levels may take a much greater time to clear than lower levels.

When a medication is taken frequently in repeated doses, some portion remains in the intravascular compartment, thus leading to an accumulation or increase in blood concentration. With first order kinetics, clearance is proportional to the concentration, and equilibrium is achieved between input and output. With zero order kinetics, and with an intake that exceeds the maximum rate of clearance, serum concentrations continue to rise. Whatever the means of administration or the number of doses, concentration falls when intake stops. The apparent clearance half-life is the time needed for the serum concentration to fall by one half. As a general rule, achievement of steady-state on the rising phase of drug administration requires about five half-lives.

For any given medication, an equilibrium is produced between a free and a protein- or tissue-bound fraction. The free fraction is the ratio of the free concentration to the total concentration. Molecules bound to proteins provide a "drug reservoir" and may disassociate so as to maintain a constant free drug level. Only the free fraction can cross the vascular endothelium to reach brain.

The apparent volume of distribution (Vd) is the hypothetical volume required to produce the same concentration as in the blood compartment. Vd represents the proportion of the blood concentration to the amount administered. For a given drug, this varies according to physiological states (e.g., pregnancy) or pathological ones (e.g., obesity, hypoalbuminemia).

In the extravascular compartment, the free fraction distributes itself into the various organs. AEDs are distributed evenly between the blood and intracerebral compartments.

Clearance: Elimination of a drug from the body proceeds in the form of biotransformation (metabolism) and clearance (excretion). Biotransformation of AEDs begins in the liver with oxidation, reduction, and hydrolysis. Drugs are transformed into numerous metabolites, some active, some inactive, and some potentially toxic. The cytochrome P450 system of the hepatic endoplasmic reticulum plays a major role in metabolism. Age, humoral and genetic factors may all modify the activity of the P450 system. After hepatic metabolism, the water-soluble (usually conjugated) metabolites are renally excreted by glomerular filtration and tubular secretion.

Drug Interactions: Many drug interactions occur between the various AEDs, as well as between AEDs and other drugs (3). Absorption of some AEDs can be diminished by certain antacids. Competition may exist between drugs for a protein binding site: e.g., with bilirubin, aspirin, nonsteroidal anti-inflammatory drugs, heparin, and several others. One drug may increase the free fraction of another without significantly altering the total level. During biotransformation, drug interactions may occur via induction of the hepatic cytochrome P450 system and increased metabolism of other drugs. Phenobarbital, phenytoin, and carbamazepine are

potent P450 inducers. Conversely, certain drugs can inhibit the biotransformation of others, either by competition for the same enzyme system or
by inhibition of a metabolic enzyme. Valproic acid increases serum barbiturate levels by about 30% via inhibition of barbiturate metabolism. Felbamate increases phenytoin, valproate, and carbamazepine-epoxide levels while lowering carbamazepine levels. During excretion, modifications
in urinary pH may alter clearance.

ANTIEPILEPTIC DRUG TOXICITY

AEDs are generally less toxic than many other drug groups. Side effects
may be grouped according to the drug responsible, the target organ, or the
parent mechanism.

Dose-dependent side effects: Acute or subacute overdosage: When too
high a dose is prescribed, too large a dose is taken, or unexpected decreases
in clearance occur, for example by interaction with another drug (e.g., CBZ
and erythromycin (4)), toxicity may occur. Intercurrent infection such as
hepatitis may also result in drug accumulation and toxicity. Typical clinical signs include drowsiness, dizziness, ataxia, nystagmus, and occasionally a paradoxical increase in seizure frequency.

Chronic overdosage: An individual patient's tolerance of AEDs may be
more important than the amount of drug taken. In most cases, signs of
toxicity are seen with high doses and high serum levels. In some susceptible patients, these signs and symptoms may appear even when doses and
AED levels lie within the the so-called therapeutic range. Therapeutic
ranges are based on monotherapy, and polypharmacy may lead to the
accumulation of metabolites with consequent side effects. Patients may
appear sedated, lethargic, and somnolent with decreased verbal output and
psychomotor retardation. All the above features may adversely affect professional or scholastic performance.

These effects are more commonly seen with phenobarbital and primidone than with valproic acid or carbamazepine (5,6).

Side effects may appear insidiously and be attributed to other factors,
e.g., epilepsy, environmental or psychological factors.

Side effects may be noted only when the drug is stopped and symptoms
resolve. Other side effects reported include weight gain or loss, gastrointestinal problems, endocrine abnormalities, acne, a fall in serum folate,
leukopenia, macrocytosis, osteoporosis, and an increase in hepatic enzymes
(gamma GT). (See individual AEDs for profile of side effects.)

Idiosyncratic side effects (7). These are rare, unpredictable, and frequently
serious side effects occasionally leading to death: leukopenia and aplastic anemia (see also Anemia, Agranulocytosis), severe exfoliative dermatitis (occa-

sionally leading to Stevens-Johnson syndrome), hepatitis, pancreatitis; serum sickness may appear 1 to 8 weeks after starting treatment and occasionally resolves if the drug is stopped immediately. Recently, felbamate, an AED approved by the FDA, was found to be associated with aplastic anemia and liver failure when much larger populations were exposed to the drug (see Felbamate (Felbatol®)). Steroids may be helpful.

References

1. Levy RH, Mattson RH, Meldrum BS, Penry JK, Dreifuss FE (eds.). *Antiepileptic drugs,* 3rd edition. New York: Raven Press, 1989.
2. Gomeni R, Latini R. Basic concepts of pharmacokinetics. In: Morselli PL (ed.). *Drug disposition during development.* New York: Spectrum Publications, 1977:1–49.
3. Pisani F, Perruca E, DiPerri R. Clinically relevant antiepileptic drug interactions. *J Int Med Res* 1990;18:1–15.
4. Turner PV, Renton KW. The interaction between carbamazepine and erythromycin. *Can J Physiol Pharmacol* 1989;67:582–86.
5. Smith DB, Mattson RH, Cramer JA, Collins JF, Novelly RA, Craft B, and the V.A. Epilepsy Cooperative Study Group. Results of a nationwide Veterans Administration Cooperative Study comparing the efficacy and toxicity of carbamazepine, phenobarbital, phenytoin and primidone. *Epilepsia* 1987;28 (Suppl 3):S50–S58.
6. Meador KJ, Loring DW, Allen ME, Zamrini EY, Moore EE, Abney OL, King DW. Comparative cognitive effects of carbamazepine and phenytoin in healthy adults. *Neurology* 1991;41:1537–40.
7. Booker HE. Idiosyncratic reactions to the antiepileptic drugs. *Epilepsia* 1975; 16:171–81.

• • • • • •

APHASIA/EPILEPSY; LANDAU-KLEFFNER SYNDROME

This rare syndrome (1) beginning in early childhood results in progressive deterioration in language function over several years. The EEG may show bilateral synchronous epileptiform discharges or more focal temporal ictal activity. Over several years, epileptiform activity becomes more continuous, and focal or generalized seizures appear in about 70% of patients. Although seizures remit in adolescence, AEDs may be useful in the younger age group.

This syndrome may share clinical features with "epilepsy with continuous spikes and waves during slow sleep" or "epilepsy with electrical status epilepticus during slow sleep" (ESES) (see also this heading) (2).

References

1. Landau, WM, Kleffner FR. Syndrome of acquired aphasia with convulsive disorder in children. *Neurology* 1957;7:523–30.

2. Roulet E, Deonna T, Gaillard F, Peter-Favre C, Despland PA. Acquired apha-
    sia, dementia and behavior disorder with epilepsy and continuous spikes and
    waves during sleep in a child. *Epilepsia* 1991;32:495–503.

• • • • • • •
APNEA (SEE ALSO RESPIRATION)

Apnea may be seen in complex partial seizures and is frequently associated with autonomic symptoms. It is a constant feature of the tonic-clonic
phase of generalized convulsions.

Apnea may be the only clinical correlate of seizures in infants and the
newborn (see Neonatal seizures).

• • • • • • •
ARACHNOID CYSTS

Arachnoid cysts are intra-arachnoidal collections of CSF with little or no communication with normal arachnoid spaces. They are seen in the temporo-
Sylvian, suprasellar, and posterior fossa regions. Cysts may remain asymptomatic, an incidental finding on scanning (especially in adults), or may
present with intracranial hypertension or seizures (especially in childhood).
Seizures may be the presenting feature in 20% (1) to 25% (2) of cases.

Indications for surgical excision depend on the size or rate of growth
of the cysts as well as the presence of progressive neurological signs. Shunting procedures from the cyst to the peritoneal cavity are also performed.
Cyst evacuation may not necessarily cure seizures (3).

References

1. Galassi E, Piazza G, Gaist G, et al. Arachnoid cyst of the middle cranial fossa:
    a clinical and radiological study of 25 cases treated surgically. *Surg Neurol*
    1980;14:211–19.
2. Choux M, Raybaud C, Pinsard N, et al. Intracranial supratentorial cysts in
    children excluding tumors and parasitic cysts. *Child's Brain* 1978;4:15–32.
3. Gandy SE, Heier LA. Clinical and magnetic resonance features of primary
    intracranial arachnoid cysts. *Ann Neurol* 1987;21:342–48.

• • • • • • •
ARRHYTHMIA

Cardiac dysrhythmias may be the result of excessive autonomic nervous
system discharge with consequences ranging from benign to lethal (1,2) (see

also Mortality). Additionally, cardiac dysrhythmias resulting in loss of consciousness (Stokes-Adams attacks) may rarely simulate epileptic seizures (see also Syncope). (See also Autonomic seizures.)

References

1. Howell SJL, Blumhardt LD. Cardiac asystole associated with epileptic seizures: a case report with simultaneous EEG and ECG. *J Neurol Neurosurg Psychiatry* 1989;52:795–98.
2. Frysinger AC, Engel J, Harper RM. Interictal heart rate patterns in partial seizure disorders. *Neurology* 1993;43:2136–39.

• • • • • •
ARTERIOVENOUS MALFORMATION (AVM)

Arteriovenous malformations usually come to light when they bleed, although seizures may be a presenting feature. Seizures may occur at the time of hemorrhage or after surgical intervention. Seizures have been reported to lead to the discovery of AVMs in 18% (1) to 31% (2) of cases; older reports cite 17–40%. Sixty percent of AVMs may give rise to seizures (2), the risk increasing with the size and superficial localization of the AVM and the youth of the patient. Surgical resection may (1) or may not (2) increase the incidence of seizures, which may rise from 18% to 57% after 20 years (3). Poorly controlled seizures may be seen in about 50% of patients (2); others have obtained good control in a similar proportion of patients (4). AVMs have been implicated in secondary epileptogenesis in the mesiotemporal regions, anatomically distant from the malformation (5).

References

1. Crawford PM, West CR, Shaw MDM, Chadwick DW. Cerebral arteriovenous malformations and epilepsy: factors in the development of epilepsy. *Epilepsia* 1986;27:270–75.
2. Murphy MJ. Long-term follow-up of seizures associated with cerebral arteriovenous malformations. Results of therapy. *Arch Neurol* 1985;42:477–79.
3. Crawford PM, West CR, Chadwick DW, Shaw MDM. Arteriovenous malformations of the brain: natural history of unoperated patients. *J Neurol Neurosurg Psychiatry* 1986;49:1–10.
4. Heros RC, Korosue K, Diebold PM. Surgical excision of cerebral arteriovenous malformations: late results. *Neurosurgery* 1990;26:570–78.
5. Yeh H-S, Privitera MD. Secondary epileptogenesis in cerebral arteriovenous malformations. *Arch Neurol* 1991;48:1122–24.

• • • • • •
ARTERITIS, CEREBRAL

Cerebral arteritis may predispose to seizures. Seizures may be seen in systemic lupus erythematosus with cerebral involvement (44% of cases) (1) and may be a presenting feature of disease onset. An AED-induced lupus syndrome may occur in patients known to have epilepsy (2), but drug-induced lupus syndromes infrequently cause CNS problems.

References

1. Kogeorgos J, Scott DF. Neuropsychiatric and EEG features in 74 cases of systemic lupus erythematosus with cerebral involvement. *Electroenceph clin Neurophysiol* 1982;53:1P(abstract).
2. Benton JW, Tynes B, Register HB, Alford C, Holley HL. Systemic lupus erythematosus occurring during anti-convulsant drug therapy. *JAMA* 1962; 180:115–18.

• • • • • •
ASPARTAME

Aspartame (Nutrasweet®), which is produced from L-phenylalanine and aspartame, is an extremely popular low-calorie peptide used as a sweetener in the United States. It is estimated that many millions of Americans consume aspartame every year. Because aspartame is chemically related to excitatory amino acids (glutamate and aspartate—see these headings) that can cause seizures and neurotoxic changes (1), concern has been raised about the use of aspartame by individuals with epilepsy (2). Aspartame may increase EEG spike-waves in absence epilepsy (3), and in massive amounts might precipitate seizures (4). Review of the animal and clinical literature to date provides no evidence for convulsive or neurotoxic effects of aspartame when used in reasonable quantities (5).

References

1. Olney JW, Collins RC, Sloviter RS. Excitotoxic mechanisms of epileptic brain damage. *Adv Neurol* 1986;44:857–77.
2. Wurtman RJ. Aspartame: possible effect on seizure susceptibility. *Lancet* 1985;2:1060.
3. Camfield PR, Camfield CS, Dooley JM, Gordon K, Jollymore S, Weaver DF. Aspartame exacerbates EEG spike-wave discharge in children with generalized absence epilepsy. A double-blind controlled study. *Neurology* 1992;42: 1000–1003.
4. Eshel Y, Saro-Pinhas I. Aspartame and seizures. *Neurology* 1993;43:2154–55.
5. Fisher RS. Aspartame, neurotoxicity, and seizures: a review. *J Epilepsy* 1989; 2:55–64.

• • • • • •
ASPARTATE

Aspartate is a four-carbon dicarboxylic amino acid found in high concentrations in the brain, spinal cord, and other tissues. Aspartate and glutamate are believed to be important excitatory neurotransmitters (see also Glutamate-aspartate).

Reference

Cotman CW, Nadler JV. Glutamate and aspartate as hippocampal transmitters: biochemical and pharmacological evidence. In: Roberts PJ, Storm-Mathisen J, Johnston JAR (eds.). *Glutamate: transmitter in the central nervous system.* New York: John Wiley and Sons, 1981:117–54.

• • • • • •
ASTATIC (SEIZURES)

This is a vague term now in disuse (see Atonic (S)).

Reference

Gastaut H. *Dictionary of epilepsy. Part 1: Definitions.* Geneva: World Health Organization, 1973.

• • • • • •
ASTROCYTOMA

Patients with slow-growing, locally invasive tumors (see also Tumors) may present with persistent focal or generalized seizures (1). Seizures may precede other clinical features, such as headache or focal weakness, by several years. Malignant change to glioblastoma may occur over time. The optimal management, resective surgery with or without radiotherapy versus conservative treatment in patients presenting with long histories of epilepsy, has not been resolved (2).

References

1. Boon PA, Williamson PD, Fried I, Spencer DD, Novelly RA, Spencer SS, Mattson RH. Intracranial, intraaxial, space-occupying lesion in patients with intractable partial seizures: an anatomical, neuropsychological, and surgical correlation. *Epilepsia* 1991;32:467–76.

2. Smith DF, Hutton JL, Sandemann D, Foy PM, Shaw MDM, Williams IR, Chad-
    wick DW. The prognosis of primary intracerebral tumours presenting with
    epilepsy: the outcome of medical and surgical management. *J Neurol Neuro-
    surg Psychiatry* 1991;54:915–20.

• • • • • •
ATAXIA

Ataxia is a frequent presenting complaint in patients with AED toxicity.
Phenytoin, carbamazepine, and primidone are the more frequent causative
agents, although a newer agent, gabapentin, may also do so. Ataxia may
not strictly correlate with AED levels in or outside the therapeutic range.
Patients with therapeutic levels may be ataxic; conversely, supratherapeutic levels may not give rise to ataxia.

Ataxia may be seen as part of certain syndromes that also include
seizures (see also Alpers' disease, Baltic myoclonus, Cerebellum, Ceroid-
lipofuscinoses, Dyssynergia cerebellaris myoclonica, or Ramsay Hunt syndrome).

• • • • • •
ATIVAN® (LORAZEPAM)

IV solutions are used in status epilepticus. Oral preparations are rarely used
for chronic seizure prophylaxis.

Tablets 0.5 mg, 1 mg, 2 mg
Vials (injectable after dilution) 1 ml @ 2 mg per mL, or 4 mg per mL.
(See also Lorazepam.)

• • • • • •
ATONIC (SEIZURES)

There are two kinds (1):

- Brief drop attacks or atonic seizures which may involve the sudden
  forward drop of the head. Postural skeletal muscles may be
  involved, resulting in an abrupt fall. EEG recordings show the loss
  of tone to occur with the onset of polyspike and wave discharges.
  Myoclonic-atonic seizures (2,3) with bilateral myoclonus and polyspike activity on the EEG occur in the Lennox-Gastaut syndrome as
  well as in myoclonic-astatic seizures of childhood;

- Prolonged atonic seizures with loss of consciousness and generalized hypotonia lasting several minutes. The child may fall to the ground and remain immobile. The EEG shows irregular spike waves, or slow spike and waves. These seizures are seen in the Lennox-Gastaut syndrome (cataplectic seizure, apoplectic seizure, inhibitory seizures, and akinetic seizures are terms no longer used). (See also Absence seizures/epilepsy-atonic features.)

Drop attacks also occur in simple partial seizures of frontal lobe origin.

The differential diagnosis includes cataplexy, narcolepsy, and syncope.

References

1. Gastaut H. *Dictionary of epilepsy. Part 1: Definitions.* Geneva: World Health Organization, 1973.
2. Gastaut H, Broughton R. *Epileptic seizures, clinical and electrographic features, diagnosis and treatment.* Springfield: Charles C. Thomas, 1972.
3. Gastaut H, Regis H. On the subject of Lennox's "akinetic" Petit Mal. *Epilepsia* 1961;2:298–305.

● ● ● ● ● ● ●
AUDITORY (SEIZURES)

Seizures may cause a subjective perception of sounds (1,2).

These include:

Simple sounds: The dulling of sounds, whistles, rhythmic or rumbling sounds likened to the sound of a motor or a cicada. Abnormalities may involve Heschl's gyrus in the first temporal convolution.

Illusional: Sound perception is altered with respect to intensity, distance, rhythm, tonality, and timbre. This may be due to lesions in the superior temporal cortex near the auditory association areas.

Hallucinatory: There is the perception of words, sentences, conversations, songs, and melodies. Cortical localization is in the auditory association areas adjoining Heschl's gyrus.

References

1. Gloor P, Olivier, A, Quesney LP, Andermann T, Horowitz S. The role of the limbic system in experiential phenomena of temporal lobe epilepsy. *Ann Neurol* 1982;12:129–44.
2. Bancaud J. Sémiologie clinique des crises épileptiques d'origine temporale. *Rev Neurol* (Paris) 1987;143:392–400.

• • • • • •
AURA

Although commonly used, this term has been "officially" discarded since 1973. It referred to symptoms preceding the loss of consciousness in complex partial seizures or in secondarily generalized seizures. At present, these clinical features are thought to represent a simple partial seizure.

Reference

Porter RJ. Recognizing and classifying epileptic seizures and epileptic syndromes. *Neurolog Clin* 1986;4:495–508.

• • • • • •
AUTOMATISMS

Automatisms are involuntary movements occurring during a seizure (ictal automatisms) or following the seizure (postictal automatisms). Video-EEG recording may be required to distinguish nonictal, ictal, or postictal automatisms. In the work-up for seizure surgery, implanted electrodes may show localization when scalp EEG is nonlocalizing (1).

Automatisms may be categorized as follows:

1. According to their appearance, e.g., carrying out a sequence of patterned movements: normally, poorly, clumsily, or too vigorously (dyspractic or apractic automatisms).
2. Representing a continuation of an ongoing activity or the appearance of a new pattern of activity (*de novo* automatisms).
3. Stereotypical patterned movement or movements in response to exterior stimuli.
4. According to characteristic patterns (2,3):
   a. Eating automatisms are the most frequent. Activities such as lip-smacking, licking of the lips, or chewing represent seizures involving the amygdala; swallowing movements are seen with seizures involving the supra-insular region.
   b. Automatisms that reflect the emotional state of the patient.
   c. Automatisms with simple gestures such as scratching, fidgeting, or fumbling with an object are seen in seizures involving the limbic circuits.
   d. Complex gestures, e.g., buttoning and unbuttoning, smoothing clothing, moving objects, arranging objects, or organized movements of the hands and feet, may be seen in frontal lobe seizures or in the more advanced phases of limbic seizures.

e. Simple or complex verbal automatisms localizing to the temporal lobe. Verbal automatisms with repetitive violent movements and little or no impairment of consciousness localizing to the fronto-orbital regions (1).

f. Walking automatisms: When of short duration, may represent ictal phenomena; when prolonged, are frequently postictal (see Fugue).

Differential diagnosis: Sleepwalking, hypersomnias with automatic walking (4); transient global amnesia; anger; night terrors; emotional crises; extreme agitation or confusional states, or delirium with psychiatric manifestations possibly due to metabolic or toxic encephalopathies.

The term "automatisms" is not a synonym for partial seizures (e.g., absence seizures may present with automatisms) or of temporal lobe seizures (frontal lobe seizures may include automatisms) (1–3). Generally, chewing or lip-smacking automatisms are seen in temporal lobe seizures, whereas complex gestural automatisms occur with frontal lobe seizures; simple gestures may be seen in both. Automatisms occurring during complex partial seizures cannot be recalled. They may, however, involve no alteration in the level of consciousness (1,2). In frontal lobe seizures, patients may complain of movements or gestures not under their control (forced automatisms) (3).

References

1. Chang C-N, Ojemann LM, Ojemann GA, Lettich E. Seizures of fronto-orbital origin: a proven case. *Epilepsia* 1991;32:487–91.
2. Munari C, Stoffels C, Bossi L, Bonis A, Talairach J, Bancaud J. Automatic activities during frontal and temporal lobe seizures: are they the same? In: Dam M, Gram G, Penry JK (eds.). *Advances in Epileptology, XIIth Epilepsy International Symposium.* New York: Raven Press, 1981:287–91.
3. Geier S, Bancaud J, Talairach J, Bonis A, Enjelvin M, Hossard-Bouchaud H. Automatisms during frontal epileptic seizures. *Brain* 1976;99:447–58.

• • • • • •

AUTONOMIC (SEIZURES)

Autonomic disturbances are frequently a component of simple partial seizures. Autonomic phenomena include oropharyngeal and epigastric discomfort, sweating, flushing, pallor, pupillary dilatation, piloerection, salivation, bradycardia and tachycardia, and changes in respiratory rate and blood pressure. Previously, when some of these features occurred before progression to complex partial seizures, they were referred to as auras (see also Abdominal (E); Aura).

Autonomic dysfunction may also be seen with absence, complex partial, and tonic-clonic seizures; pallid and cyanotic syncope; and psychiatric disorders. Seizure-induced cardiac dysrhythmias have been implicated in sudden death (see also Arrhythmia; Mortality; Syncope).

● ● ● ● ● ●
AXON

The axon is a specialized, elongated neuronal process involved in the signaling of information over relatively long distances. The axonal membrane consists of a lipid bi-layer, with embedded protein molecules that serve as ionic channels and enzymes. Axons may be coated with further lipid material known as myelin, serving to insulate the axon and provide greater efficiency of electrical conduction. The internal milieu of the axon is composed of high concentrations of potassium, chloride, and inorganic anions. The extra-axonal fluid consists of high concentrations of sodium, calcium, and chloride. Axonal membrane permeability to cations markedly increases during the process known as the action potential. Hodgkin and Huxley described the equations governing axonal membrane permeability in the generation of the action potential. Despite its importance in neuronal signaling, action potentials are little reflected in the EEG because of their brief duration (less than 2 msec) and limited synchrony.

References

1.   Katz B. *Nerve, muscle, and synapse.* New York: McGraw-Hill, 1966:193.
2.   Koaster J. Voltage-gated ion channels and the generation of the action potential. In: Kandel ER, Schwartz JH, Jessell TM (eds.). *Principles of neuroscience.* New York: Elsevier, 1991:104–18.

BALTIC MYOCLONUS

Baltic myoclonus is a form of progressive myoclonic epilepsy identified in Finland (1,2) with a prevalence of 1 in 20,000. The clinical presentation is similar to that of the Unverricht-Lundborg syndrome.

Inheritance is by an autosomal recessive pattern. Onset occurs between age 6 and 15 years (mean 10.8). The myoclonic movements are characteristic: segmental, widespread, and induced by effort, movement, stress, or sensory stimuli. Generalized tonic-clonic seizures are also frequently seen.

Intention and rest cerebellar ataxias usually appear late in the course. Mental decline is slowly progressive. The EEG is abnormal with slow and disorganized background rhythms, spikes, polyspikes, and slow waves (3). Degenerative lesions are found, but no Lafora bodies are seen. Its existence as a separate syndrome is arguable, as similar clinical pictures have been described in other regions in the world (4).

References

1. Koskiniemi M, Donner M, Majuri H, Haltia AM, Norio R. Progressive myoclonus epilepsy: a clinical and histopathological study. *Acta Neurol Scand* 1974; 50:307–52.
2. Norio R, Koskiniemi M. Progressive myoclonus epilepsy: genetic and nosological aspects with special reference to 107 Finnish patients. *Clin Genet* 1979;15:382–98.
3. Koskiniemi M, Toivakka E, Donner M. Progressive myoclonus epilepsy: electroencephalographic studies. *Acta Neurol Scand* 1974;50:333–59.
4. Marseille Consensus Group. Classification of progressive myoclonus epilepsies and related disorders. *Ann Neurol* 1990;28:113–16.

BARBITURATES

Two groups of barbiturates with variable duration of action are used in the treatment of seizures: (a) Intermediate-onset barbiturates used in *status epilepticus* (see Status epilepticus); (b) Long-acting barbiturates used in chronic epilepsies. Of the latter, phenobarbital is the oldest (1,2) and the most prescribed AED. Other long-acting barbiturates are used in other countries (e.g., mephobarbital). Ultra short-acting barbiturates such as methohexital or thiopental may have a convulsant effect.

References

1. Hauptmann A. Luminal bei Epilepsie. *Munch Med Wochenschr* 1912;59: 1907–1909.
2. Feely M, O'Callagan M, Duggan B, Callaghan N. Phenobarbitone in previously untreated epilepsy. *J Neurol Neurosurg Psychiatry* 1980;43:365–68.

• • • • • • •
BASIC MECHANISMS OF THE EPILEPSIES

Thousands of studies have been published regarding basic mechanisms of the epilepsies, and many volumes written (1); nevertheless, the basic mechanisms of clinical epilepsy remain largely unknown. Limitations in our understanding arise from several sources. First, animal models of the epilepsies are imperfect representations of the clinical disorder, especially in the case of primary generalized epilepsies (2). Second, the clinical epilepsies are heterogeneous disorders, not one disease. Findings in one type of epilepsy do not necessarily apply to another variety of epilepsy. Third, epilepsy is an extremely complex disorder. A full understanding of epilepsy will require major advances in the neurosciences (3). Despite these limitations, certain general principles have been established.

Epilepsy reflects an imbalance between excitation and inhibition, such that certain populations of neurons fire synchronously. The most important excitatory influence is the excitatory postsynaptic potential, mediated primarily in the forebrain by glutamate or aspartate. Excitatory neurotransmitters open membrane channels (ionophores) and allow influx of sodium ions and depolarization of the neuronal membrane. Inhibitory neurotransmitters such as gamma aminobutyric acid (GABA) open chloride channels and hyperpolarize neurons.

In certain focal seizures, GABA-mediated inhibition can be shown to be decreased (4). Manipulations that decrease inhibition can induce epileptiform activity (5,6). Nevertheless, disinhibition does not appear to be the mechanism in all types of epilepsy. In absence and certain nonconvulsive seizures, inhibitory function may be increased (7,8), possibly because inhibition plays a crucial role in synchronizing neuronal populations. Synchronization of neuronal populations may be more important than an absolute level of inhibition or excitation.

Cellular mechanisms underlying seizures are complex. Intracellular recordings from cortical neurons in experimental seizure foci show giant depolarizations called "paroxysmal depolarization shifts" or PDSs (9). These PDSs represent a combination of synchronous EPSPs from neurons in the focus (10) and of intrinsic membrane calcium currents activated by neuronal depolarization (11). A few neurons with bursting behavior and recurrent excitatory collaterals to neighboring neurons can recruit a large population of cells into participation in a seizure discharge (12). Interictal-ictal transitions may occur when a critical mass is achieved, when inhibitory mechanisms become insufficient to limit spread of the discharge, or via a variety of other synaptic and extra-synaptic mechanisms (13). A seizure produces major ionic changes in the extracellular milieu, with a rise of potassium and a fall of sodium and calcium concentrations (14). These ionic changes may depolarize neighboring neurons and contribute to seizure elaboration and spread.

The brain possesses a variety of inhibitory processes, including GABA-mediated and non-GABA mediated synaptic inhibition, post-burst after-hyperpolarizations dependent upon calcium-activated potassium currents (15,16), and metabolically-mediated inhibitory ionic pumps (17). Which of these inhibitory processes are most involved in termination of seizures remains uncertain.

References

1. Delgado-Escueta AV, Ward AA Jr, Woodbury DM, Porter RJ. New wave of research in the epilepsies. *Adv Neurol* 1986;44:3–55.
2. Fisher RS. Animal models of the epilepsies. *Brain Res Rev* 1989;14:245–78.
3. Dichter MA. Cellular mechanisms of epilepsy and potential new treatment strategies. *Epilepsia* 1989;30(Suppl 1):S3–S12.
4. Ribak CE, Harris AB, Vaughn JE, Roberts E. Inhibitory GABAergic nerve terminals decrease at sites of focal epilepsy. *Science* 1979;205:211–14.
5. Dingledine R, Gjerstad L. Reduced inhibition during epileptiform activity in the in vitro hippocampal slice. *J Physiol* 1980;305:297–313.
6. Wong RKS, Prince DA. Dendritic mechanisms underlying penicillin-induced epileptiform activity. *Science* 1979;204:1228–31.
7. Babb TL, Brown WJ. Neuronal, dendritic and vascular profiles of human temporal lobe epilepsy correlated with cellular physiology "in vivo." *Adv Neurol* 1986;44:949–66.
8. Roberts RC, Ribak CE. Anatomical changes of the GABAergic system in the inferior colliculus of the genetically epilepsy-prone rat. *Life Sci* 1986;39:789–98.
9. Prince DA. Neurophysiology of epilepsy. *Annual Rev Neurosci* 1978;1:395–415.
10. Johnston D, Brown TH. Giant synaptic potential hypothesis for epileptiform activity. *Science* 1981;11:294–97.
11. Schwartzkroin PA, Prince DA. Changes in excitatory and inhibitory synaptic potentials leading to epileptogenic activity. *Brain Res* 1980;183:61–76
12. Traub RD, Wong RKS. Cellular mechanisms of neuronal synchronization in epilepsy. *Science* 1982;216:745–47.

13. Jensen MS, Yaari Y. The relationship between interictal and ictal paroxysms in an in vitro model of focal hippocampal epilepsy. *Ann Neurol* 1988;24:591–98

14. Heinemann U, Lux HD, Gutnick M. Extracellular free calcium and potassium during paroxysmal activity in the cerebral cortex of the cat. *Exp Brain Res* 1977;27:237–43

15. Alger BE, Nicoll RA. Epileptiform burst after hyperpolarization: calcium-dependent potassium potential in hippocampal CA1 pyramidal cells. *Science* 1980; 210:1122–24.

16. Hotson JR, Prince DA. A calcium-activated hyperpolarization follows repetitive firing in hippocampal neurons *J Neurophysiol* 1980;43: 409–19

17. Haglund MM, Schwartzkroin PA. Role of Na-K pump potassium regulation and IPSPs in seizures and spreading depression in immature rabbit hippocampal slices. *J Neurophysiol* 1990;63:225–39

● ● ● ● ● ●
BATTEN-VOGT-SPIELMEYER SYNDROME

Batten-Vogt-Spielmeyer syndrome was the first of the ceroid-lipofuscinoses (see this heading) to be described (1903) (1), and is the juvenile form of this disorder (2).

Transmitted as an autosomal recessive trait, the onset is approximately at age 5, marked by a decrease in visual acuity due to retinitis pigmentosa, and behavioral problems. Myoclonic and generalized tonic-clonic seizures occur later.

Progression is slow, with death usually occurring 6–8 years after the onset of symptoms (3).

The histological diagnosis is based on finding intracellular and curvilinear inclusions with fingerprint inclusions, believed to represent an accumulation of lipo-pigments.

References

1. Batten FE. Cerebral degeneration with symmetrical changes in the maculae in two members of a family. *Trans Ophtalmol Soc UK* 1903;23:386–90.

2. Batten FE. Family cerebral degeneration with macular changes (so-called juvenile form of family amaurotic idiocy). *Q J Med* 1914;7:444–54.

3. Dyken PR. The neuronal ceroid lipofuscinosis. *J Child Neurol* 1989;4:165–74.

● ● ● ● ● ●
BEHAVIOR (ABNORMALITIES OF)

Most patients with epilepsy exhibit normal behavior.

Some typical behavioral problems may be classified as follows:

- Directly correlated with seizures: automatisms, inappropriate behavior, either ictally (complex partial seizures or complex partial status epilepticus, petit mal status) or postictally as part of a confusional state.
- Interictal: Multifactorial behavior problems may be due to the underlying cortical lesion, involvement of neighboring cerebral areas from repeated seizure spread, particularly to limbic or frontal structures (1–4), AED side effects (5,6), poor self-image in patients with epilepsy (7), rejection or overprotectiveness by family or friends (8), and repeated stressful experiences. The stress involved includes: seizures with a strong affective component of fear, seizures that occur in public, the constant need for antiepileptic medication, and the effect of consequent professional or scholastic frustrations and failures (9,10).
- Behavioral abnormalities: In the past, physicians identified "the epileptic personality," characterized by several of the following features: verbosity, hypergraphia, obsequiousness, viscosity, adhesiveness, humorlessness, dependence, obsessional tendencies, exaggerated interest in particular ideas or concepts, hyperreligiosity, interest in philosophic or cosmic themes, hyposexuality, moodiness, irritability, explosiveness and violence (see also Violence). Although this picture may occur, it is a rare phenomenon in its complete form (11). Isolated characteristics as described above may be found in people with chronic epilepsy. Personality disorders have been attributed, particularly to epilepsies involving the temporal lobe, since the limbic system and temporal lobes are involved in affect (12,13), but data suggest that personality problems are as frequent in idiopathic generalized epilepsies and in non-epileptic patients with psychiatric problems as in patients with temporal foci (14). There is no "epileptic personality" per se.

Behavioral abnormalities may be due to low IQ. Widespread cortical lesions may account for both seizures and mental retardation; the epilepsy itself need not be the cause. Patients with seizures have variable IQs, ranging in different reports from 35 to 165.

Other patients may present with mood disorders: sadness, anxiety, hypochondriasis, disappointment, neuroses, and multifactorial depressive states (15), which may warrant psychiatric intervention. Emotional problems are three times as frequent in patients with epilepsy than in people without epilepsy (7), although the Minnesota Multiphasic Personality Inventory (MMPI) has failed to show an increased incidence of psychopathology in patients with epilepsy (16).

References

1. Geschwind N. Behavioral changes in temporal lobe epilepsy. *Psychol Med* 1979;9:217–19.
2. Rausch R, Lieb JP, Crandall PH. Neuropsychologic correlates of depth spike activity in epileptic patients. *Arch Neurol* 1978;35:699–705.
3. Wieser HG, Landis T. Is the "interictal behavior syndrome of temporal lobe epilepsy" really an interictal phenomenon? *Neurologia and Psychiatria* 1983;6:70–78.
4. Boone KB, Miller BL, Rosenberg L, Durazo A, McIntyre H, Weil M. Neuropsychological and behavioral abnormalities in an adolescent with frontal lobe seizures. *Neurology* 1988;38:583–86.
5. Trimble MR, Thompson PJ. Anticonvulsant drugs, cognitive function, and behavior. *Epilepsia* 1983;24 (Suppl 1):S55–S63.
6. Trimble MR. Anticonvulsant drugs and cognitive function: a review of the literature. *Epilepsia* 1987;28 (Suppl 3):S37–S45.
7. Britten N, Wadsworth MEJ, Fenwick PBC. Stigma in patients with early epilepsy: a national longitudinal survey. *J Epidemiol and Community Health* 1984;38:291–95.
8. Grunberg P, Pond DA. Conduct disorders in epileptic children. *J Neurol Neurosurg Psychiatry* 1955;20:65–68
9. Ryan R, Kempner K, Emlen AC. The stigma of epilepsy as a self-concept. *Epilepsia* 1980;21:433–44.
10. Schneider JW, Conrad P. In the closet with illness: epilepsy, stigma potential and information control. *Social Problems* 1980;28:32–44.
11. Hoeppner JB, Garron DC, Wilson RS, Koch-Weser MP. Epilepsy and verbosity. *Epilepsia* 1987;28:35–40.
12. Bear DM. Temporal lobe epilepsy. A syndrome of sensory-limbic hyperconnection. *Cortex* 1979;15:357–84.
13. Waxmann SG, Geschwind N. The interictal behavior syndrome of temporal lobe epilepsy. *Arch Gen Psychiat* 1975;32:1580–86.
14. Master DR, Toone BK, Scott DF. Interictal behavior in temporal lobe epilepsy. In: Porter RJ et al. (eds.). *Advances in Epileptology: XVth Epilepsy International Symposium.* New York: Raven Press, 1984:557–65.
15. Robertson MM, Trimble MR. Depressive illness in patients with epilepsy. A review. *Epilepsia* 1983;24 (Suppl 2): S109–S116.
16. Whitman S, Hermann BP, Gordon AC. Psychopathology in epilepsy: how great is the risk? *Biological Psychiatry* 1984;29:213–36.

● ● ● ● ● ●

BEMEGRIDE® (MEGIMIDE)

A seizure-inducing substance or convulsant used to activate clinical or EEG seizures so as to diagnose and evaluate seizure disorders (1). This drug, as with pentylenetetrazol, has been used to induce both clinical and electrographic seizures. Because of false-positive effects produced in the normal population, these drugs have fallen into disuse in the evaluations of the nature, diagnosis, and localization of seizures (1–4).

References

1. Feuerstein J, Kurtz D, Rohmer F. Activation by means of Megimide. *Epilepsia* 1966;7:220–27.
2. Bancaud J. EEG activation by Metrazol and Megimide in the diagnosis of epilepsy. In: Remond A (ed.). *Handbook of electroencephalography and clinical neurophysiology,* Vol. 3C. Amsterdam: Elsevier, 1976:105–20.
3. Wieser HG, Bancaud J, Talairach J, Bonis A, Szikla G. Comparative value of spontaneous and chemically and electrically induced seizures in establishing the lateralization of temporal lobe seizures. *Epilepsia* 1979;20:47–59.
4. Kaplan PW, Lesser RP. Long-term monitoring. In: Daly DD, Pedley TA (eds.). *Current practice of clinical electroencephalography,* 2nd edition. New York: Raven Press, 1990:513–34.

● ● ● ● ● ●
BENIGN EPILEPSIES

The benign nature of an epileptic disorder is ultimately determined by its outcome. This would include 1) the permanent remission of seizures, either spontaneously or noted after an extended period without treatment; 2) complete seizure control enabling normal social integration even on treatment. Certain partial epilepsies of childhood possess clinical and EEG characteristics indicating a more benign course.

1. Certain idiopathic localization-related epilepsies of childhood possess clinical and EEG characteristics that indicate an excellent prognosis (see also Rolandic (E); Occipital (E)). They share in common seizure onset between the ages of 2 and 10; a normal neurological examination and intelligence prior to presentation; seizures brought on by drowsiness or sleep; normal EEG background with focal epileptiform abnormalities brought out by slow-wave sleep, and few seizures that respond well to treatment. However, even with frequent and drug-resistant seizures, the long-term outcome is excellent, and patients may be considered as cured over age 16.
2. Many cases of idiopathic generalized epilepsies such as absence epilepsies, juvenile myoclonic epilepsy, and grand mal epilepsies with childhood or adolescent onset have seizures that remit on

AED therapy. Patients may have a normal life-style, at least when on treatment.

3. Cryptogenic epilepsies with rapid seizure control after onset. Benign epilepsies account for less than a third of all epilepsies; an idiopathic or cryptogenic epilepsy is not synonymous with a benign epilepsy. Some of the latter may be very difficult to treat.

● ● ● ● ● ●

BENZODIAZEPINES

Benzodiazepines are drugs of choice in the treatment of status epilepticus, flurries of seizures, and prolonged seizures. They are adjunctive therapies in the chronic epilepsies, especially myoclonic epilepsies. They have the following characteristics (1):

PHARMACOKINETICS

Oral bioavailability ranges from 75 to 100%. Peak plasma levels are reached 1–4 hours after oral intake, depending on the formulation, more rapidly with solutions than with tablets or syrups. Protein binding is 80–98%; half-life ranges from 20 to 95 hours. Steady state levels are achieved in 4–7 days. Hepatic enzyme induction is usually minimal. Metabolism is increased by liver enzyme-inducing drugs and decreased by cimetidine.

DOSAGE

The dose depends on the type of benzodiazepine. Typical regimens vary from once to four times per day, depending on the half-life. A gradual increase in dose over 2–4 weeks is often required to minimize sedative side effects.

SIDE EFFECTS

1. Sedation (10–50% of patients): problems with attention and memory are often seen;
2. Attention deficits, excitation in children, and a hyperkinetic state;
3. Acute psychotic episodes;
4. Increased bronchial secretions;
5. Weight gain;

6. Very rarely may cause seizures (2–5);
7. Dependence, tolerance, and tachyphylaxis.

INDICATIONS

Diazepam, clonazepam, clobazam, clorazepate, nitrazepam (see these headings) are used in chronic epilepsy. Diazepam is less useful when used chronically because of its sedative effect; clobazam appears to be less sedating.

Although benzodiazepines have a striking, immediate effect on seizures, they typically lead to tolerance and breakthrough seizures within six months of therapy. Breakthrough seizures may be seen as early as the second week in half the patients. Increasing the dose usually does not decrease seizures, but merely increases the possibility of toxicity (6,7). Furthermore, the occurrence of seizures after abrupt withdrawal of benzodiazepines often necessitates discontinuing this form of therapy. One indication for their use is to diminish the seizure frequency in resistant epilepsy (6). Lorazepam IV and midazolam IM are effective in status epilepticus and are generally available in the United States. In Europe, clonazepam and diazepam are the drugs of first choice for the treatment of status epilepticus, frequent seizures with brief intervals between them, and prolonged seizures in childhood (8).

References

1. Levy RH, Dreifuss FE, Mattson RH, Meldrum BS, Penry JK (eds.). *Antiepileptic drugs,* 3rd edition. New York: Raven Press, 1989.
2. DiMario FJ Jr, Clancy RR. Paradoxical precipitation of tonic seizures by clonazepam in a child with atypical absence seizures. *Pediatr Neurol* 1988;4:249–51.
3. Prior PM, MacLaine M, Scott DF, Laurence M. Tonic status epilepticus precipitated by intravenous diazepam in a child with Petit Mal status. *Epilepsia* 1972;13:467–72.
4. Somerville ER, Bruni J. Tonic status epilepticus presenting as confusional state. *Ann Neurol* 1983;13:549–51.
5. Tassinari CA, Dravet C, Cano JP, Gastaut H. Tonic status epilepticus precipitated by intravenous benzodiazepine in five patients with Lennox-Gastaut syndrome. *Epilepsia* 1972;13:421–35.
6. Scott DF, Moffett A. The long-term effect of clobazam as adjunctive therapy in epilepsy. *Acta Neurol Scand* 1988;77:498–502.
7. Haigh JRM, Gent JP, Garratt JC, Pullar T, Feely M. Disappointing results of increasing benzodiazepine dose after the development of anticonvulsant tolerance. *J Neurol Neurosurg Psychiatry* 1988;51:1008–1009.
8. Treiman DM. Pharmacokinetics and clinical use of benzodiazepines in the management of status epilepticus. *Epilepsia* 1989;30 (Suppl 2):S4–S10.

• • • • • •
BETA ACTIVITY (SEE ALSO EEG)

Beta activity refers to EEG activity in the frequency range above 13 Hertz. It is a normal component of the waking and sleeping EEG, often increased by sedative medications. Diffuse decrease in beta activity may suggest a diffuse encephalopathy, and focal decrease, a local cortical disturbance. High-voltage beta activity occurs with some cortical dysplasias.

• • • • • •
BILATERAL SYNCHRONY, PRIMARY

Primary bilateral synchrony refers to an EEG pattern seen with generalized tonic-clonic or absence seizures. Spikes and slow waves appear nearly simultaneously (within about 50 msec) over both sides of the head. The presumption is of a deep pacemaker for these rhythms, the precise nature of which remains unknown (see Bilateral synchrony, secondary; Centrencephalic (S)).

• • • • • •
BILATERAL SYNCHRONY, SECONDARY

Secondary bilateral synchrony (SBS) is an electroencephalographic concept generated by Jasper, Gastaut, and Niedermeyer, denoting the situation in which a focal discharge rapidly spreads to both hemispheres. The disappearance of generalized seizures and bilateral spike and slow wave discharges after ablation of a focal lesion is the best argument in favor of SBS.

The most clearly delineated examples of SBS are seen with frontal and especially parasagittal lesions, followed by temporal lesions, but may also be seen with more posterior lesions (1).

Longitudinal EEG studies may reveal the appearance of a contralateral focus in patients originally having a unilateral focus. After 6–15 years, 51% of parasagittal foci and 35% of temporal foci become bilateral (2). Although these findings raise the issue of secondary epileptogenesis (see this heading), delayed maturation of a parallel focus must also be considered.

References

1.   Chevrie JJ, Specolo N, Aicardi J. Secondary bilateral synchrony in unilateral pial angiomatosis: successful surgical treatment. *J Neurol Neurosurg Psychiatry* 1988;51:663–70.

2. Hughes JR. Long-term clinical and EEG changes in patients with epilepsy. *Arch Neurol* 1985;42:213–23.

· · · · · · ·
BIOFEEDBACK

This involves training patients by means of feedback from EEG recording to achieve a level of cerebral activity believed to raise the seizure threshold (1). Although initial investigations were promising, this technique has not been widely accepted or practiced (2).

References

1. Sterman MB, Friar L. Suppression of seizures in an epileptic following sensorimotor EEG feedback training. *Electroenceph clin Neurophysiol* 1972;33:89–95.
2. Engel J Jr. *Seizures and epilepsy.* Philadelphia: F.A. Davis, 1989:465.

· · · · · · ·
BRAIN

The brain is the physical substrate for behavior and for disorders of behavior and physiology, such as epilepsy. Regional variations in brain function correlate with different manifestations of partial (focal) seizures, for example, motor seizures with abnormal electrical discharges in the pre-central gyrus; visual distortions with occipital seizures; inappropriate memories and emotions with deep temporal foci. John Hughlings Jackson, the father of modern epileptology, called epilepsy a "spotlight on the brain," since clinical observation of seizures could provide insight into brain function.

· · · · · · ·
BREAST-FEEDING

Most AEDs taken by the mother are found in breast milk to a variable degree, depending on protein binding: valproate (5–10% of maternal serum levels), phenytoin (19%), carbamazepine (41%), phenobarbital (36%), primidone (70%), and benzodiazepines (small) (1). Some obstetricians discourage breast-feeding by mothers on AEDs, but others believe the benefits of breast-feeding outweigh potential problems from the small amount of medication reaching the breast milk. Sedative AEDs, such as phenobarbital, may lead to sedation in the baby with consequent difficulties in feeding. Discontinuation of barbiturates and benzodiazepines can lead to withdrawal problems (1,2). If the baby appears sedated, serum levels can be performed and the desirability of breast-feeding reassessed.

References

1. Kaneko S, Suzuki K, Sato T, Ogaway Y, Nomura Y. The problems of antiepileptic medication in the neonatal period: is breast feeding advisable?. In: Janz D, Dam M, Richens A, Bossi L, Helge H, Schmidt S (eds.). *Epilepsy, pregnancy and the child*. New York: Raven Press, 1982:343–48.
2. Nau H, Kuhnz W, Egger HJ, Rating D, Helge H. Anticonvulsants during pregnancy and lactation. *Clin Pharmacokinet* 1982; 7:508–43.

● ● ● ● ● ●
BREATHHOLDING SPELLS

Breathholding spells are non-epileptic paroxysmal events seen in approximately 4% of children less than five years of age (1). Episodes present as cyanotic syncope brought on by fear, pain, surprise, anger, or frustration. After several wails, respiration halts in the expiratory phase with loss of consciousness, flacidity, cyanosis of the lips, and a few brief clonic movements before consciousness is regained. The EEG may show diffuse slow waves typical of any transient cerebral anoxic event. The syndrome may also include pallid syncope (reflex anoxic seizure) brought on by benign trauma, resulting in loss of consiousness with or without crying, marked pallor, tonic spasm, and asystole (2,3). (see also Atonic seizures).

References

1. Lombroso CT, Lerman P. Breathholding spells (cyanotic and pallid infantile syncope). *Pediatrics* 1967;39:563–81.
2. Stephenson JBP. Reflex anoxic seizures and ocular compression. *Dev Med Child Neurol* 1980;22:381–86.
3. Stephenson JBP. *Fits and faints*. Philadelphia: J.B. Lippincott Co., 1990.

● ● ● ● ● ●
BROMIDES

Bromides are the first known AEDs, originally instituted to decrease sexual drive in individuals with epilepsy and mental disorders (Locock, 1857). Although occasionally effective, bromides can have marked side effects, such as sedation, behavior disturbance, acne, and unstable serum sodium levels. Bromides fell out of favor in 1912, after the discovery of phenobarbital. Recently, interest has been renewed for use of bromides in early generalized seizures of childhood resistant to other AEDs (1,2) and in porphyria, where other AEDs have known porphyrogenic potential (3).

References

1. Ernst JP, Doose H, Baier WK. Bromides were effective in intractable epilepsy with generalized tonic/clonic seizures and onset in early childhood. *Brain Dev* 1988;10:385–88.
2. Scheunemann W. Bromides—a therapeutic possibility for early infancy grand mal-epilepsy. *Epilepsia* 1984;15:369 (abstract)
3. Kaplan PW, Lewis DV. Juvenile acute intermittent porphyria with hypercholesterolemia and epilepsy: a case report and review of the literature. *J Child Neurol* 1986;1:38–45.

C

• • • • • • •

CALCIUM CHANNEL BLOCKERS

Calcium's role in epileptogenesis is linked to its capacity as a second messenger (1,2):

- Calcium exerts effects on membrane plasticity: activation of phospholipases A2 and C, which in turn trigger enzymatic lipid degradation involved in phosphatidyl inositol metabolism, thus activating proteolytic enzymes;
- Calcium directly affects synaptic transmission, since presence of calcium in the presynaptic terminal is required for release of synaptic vesicles. Calcium is also involved in synaptic re-uptake of glutamate and GABA. Certain inhibitory potentials, such as the post-burst afterhyperpolarization, are dependent upon calcium influx into the postsynaptic neuron. Calcium thus exerts complex excitatory and inhibitory actions on neural systems. Certain calcium channel blockers (3), including verapamil, nifedipine, cinnarizine, and flunarizine, have a demonstrable anticonvulsant property in animal models of epilepsy. Nifedipine (4,5), nimodipine (6), and flunarizine (7) have variable antiepileptic effects in man.

References

1. Greenberg DA. Calcium channels and calcium channel antagonists. *Ann Neurol* 1987;21:317–30.
2. Rasmussen H. The calcium messenger system. *N Engl J Med* 1986;314: 1094–1101,1164–70.
3. Wong WS, Rahwan RG. Examination of the potential antiepileptic activity of calcium antagonists with different sites of action. *Gen Pharmacol* 1989;20:309–12.
4. Sander JWAS, Trevisol-Bittencourt PC. Nifedipine as an add-on drug in the management of refractory epilepsy. *Epilepsy Res* 1990;6:82–84.
5. Larkin JG, Besag FMC, Williams J, Brodie MJ. Nifedipine for epilepsy? A double-blind, placebo-controlled trial. *Epilepsia* 1992;33:346–52.
6. de Falco FA, Bartiromo U, Majello L, Di Geronimo G, Mundo P. Calcium antagonist nimodipine in intractable epilepsy. *Epilepsia* 1992;33:343–45.
7. Starreveld E, de Beukelaar F, Wilson AF, McLean DR, Findlay HP. Double-blind, cross-over, placebo controlled study of flunarizine in patients with therapy resistant epilepsy. *Can J Neurol Sci* 1989;16:187–90.

● ● ● ● ● ● ●
CALLOSOTOMY

Section of the corpus callosum is a palliative operation performed to decrease uncontrolled atonic and tonic-clonic seizures in patients with secondary generalized epilepsies or severe multifocal seizures. Partial (anterior) and total section of the corpus callosum have each been advocated. Section of the anterior two-thirds section of the corpus callosum appears to induce little neuropsychological impairment; conversely, total section may result in more severe deficit. Variability in surgical technique, and pre- and post-operative evaluation according to different reports, hamper accurate evaluation of the results. According to some authors, secondary generalization of seizures may be prevented in up to 75% of cases. Best results are seen in patients with focal or unilateral lesions; the worst results in patients with diffuse lesions or severe mental retardation (1–3). Atonic seizures with injuries are the most likely to respond to this approach. The neurological and neuropsychological operative side effects have been evaluated (4).

References

1. Makari GS, Holmes GL, Murro AM, et al. Corpus callosotomy for the treatment of intractable epilepsy in children. *J Epilepsy* 1989;2:1–7.
2. Purves SJ, Wada JA, Woodhurst WB, Moyes PD, Strauss E, Kosaka B, Li D. Results of anterior corpus callosum section in 24 patients with medically intractable seizures. *Neurology* 1988;38:1194–1201.
3. Spencer SS. Corpus callosum section and other disconnection procedures for medically intractable epilepsy. *Epilepsia* 1988;29 (Suppl 2):S85–S99.
4. Sass KJ, Spencer DD, Spencer SS, Novelly RA, Williamson PD, Mattson RH. Corpus callosotomy for epilepsy. 2. Neurologic and neuropsychological outcome. *Neurology* 1988;38:24–28.

● ● ● ● ● ● ●
CARBAMAZEPINE (CBZ, TEGRETOL®) (1)

Carbamazepine is an AED related to tricyclic antidepressants and is useful in the treatment of partial and secondarily generalized seizures. There are three formulations: Tegretol®, Tegretol-OROS (osmotic release oral system, a long-acting preparation in clinical trial in the United States), and Tegretol® suspension.

PHARMACOKINETICS

Linear kinetics: There is uneven absorption following oral administration (70–75%), resulting in peak plasma levels 2–8 hours after ingestion, but as long as 24 hours later. Marked variability in blood levels may occur between two doses. About 70–75% of the ingested dose is bound to protein. Carbamazepine half-life is 5–16 hours for adults, 8–19 hours for children. Steady state serum levels are reached in three days. The volume of distribution (Vd) is 0.8–2 L/kg. As an enzyme inducer, Tegretol increases the biotransformation of other drugs, both endogenous and exogenous, and also induces its own metabolism during the first month of therapy (a dose increase may be required). Clearance may be diminished by isoniazid, macrolide antibiotics: triacetyloleandomycine (2) and erythromycin (3), and propoxyphene with a risk for toxic serum levels. The major metabolite is a carbamazepine 11–epoxide which has AED properties, but potentially is more toxic than CBZ (4–6).

Carbamazepine is taken twice a day, although 3–4 times a day may be required with breakthrough seizures. Suggested therapeutic blood levels are 4–12 mg/L.

SIDE EFFECTS

- Acute or subacute overdose: dizziness, diplopia, nausea, nystagmus, ataxia, "drunkenness," obtundation, and confusion (7);
- General fatigue, lightheadedness, and malaise;
- Skin rashes may appear 8–10 days after onset of treatment in 5–10% of cases. Because of the risk of bullous epidermolysis, hypersensitivity syndromes (8), and Stevens-Johnson syndrome, the treatment should be stopped, or the patient followed extremely closely;
- Hepatotoxic reaction (9);
- Alteration in immune system;
- A lupus-like syndrome occasionally occurs (10), which rarely involves the CNS;
- Dyskinesias (11,12);
- A worsening of seizures in secondary generalized epilepsies (13,14);
- Inappropriate ADH secretion with hyponatremia, occasionally with headaches and vomiting;
- Mild leukopenias frequently seen, rare agranulocytoses (about 40/million in incidence) (15).

INDICATIONS

Carbamazepine has the same effectiveness as other first-line AEDs for different seizure types (with the exception of typical absence seizures) (16). It is an AED of first choice in partial seizures because of the paucity of side effects (17).

References

1. Levy RH, Dreifuss FE, Mattson RH, Meldrum BS, Penry JK (eds.). *Antiepileptic drugs,* 3rd edition. New York: Raven Press, 1989.
2. Dravet C, Mesdjian E, Cenraud B, Roger J. Interaction between carbamazepine and triacetyloleandomycin. *Lancet* 1977;1:810–11.
3. Hedrick R, Williams N, Morin R, Lamb WA, Cate JC. Carbamazepine-erythromycin interaction leading to carbamazepine toxicity in four epileptic children. *Ther Drug Monitor* 1983;5:405–407.
4. Theodore WH, Narang PK, Holmes MD, Reeves P, Nice FJ. Carbamazepine and its epoxide: relation of plasma levels to toxicity and seizure control. *Ann Neurol* 1989;15:194–96.
5. Gillham RA, Williams N, Wiedmann K, Butler E, Larkin JG, Brodie MJ. Concentration-effect relationships with carbamazepine and its epoxide on psychomotor and cognitive function in epileptic patients. *J Neurol Neurosurg Psychiatry* 1988;51:929–33.
6. Tomson T, Almkvist O, Nilsson B, Svensson J-O, Bertilsson L. Carbamazepine-10,11-epoxide in epilepsy. A pilot study. *Arch Neurol* 1990;47:888–92.
7. Fisher RS, Cysyk B. A fatal overdose of carbamazepine: case report and review of literature. *J Toxicol Clin Pharmacol* 1988;26:477–86.
8. Ray-Chaudhuri K, Pye IF, Boggil DM. Hypersensitivity to carbamazepine presenting with a leukemoid reaction, eosinophilia, erythroderma, and renal failure. *Neurology* 1989;39:436–38.
9. Horowitz S, Patwardhan R, Marcus E. Hepatotoxic reactions associated with carbamazepine therapy. *Epilepsia* 1988;29:149–54.
10. Oner A, Topalollu R, Beibas N, Topalollu H. Carbamazepine-induced systemic lupus erythematosus: another warning. *Clin Neurol Neurosurg* 1990;92:261–62.
11. Aguglia U, Zappia M, Quatrone A. Carbamazepine-induced non-epileptic myoclonus in a child with benign epilepsy. *Epilepsia* 1987;28:515–18.
12. Ambrosetto G, Riva R, Baruzzi A. Hyperammonemia in asterixis induced by carbamazepine: two case reports. *Acta Neurol Scand* 1984;69:186–89.
13. Shields WD, Saslow E. Myoclonic atonic and absence seizures following institution of carbamazepine therapy in children. *Neurology* 1983;33:1487–89.
14. Snead OC, Hosey LC. Exacerbation of seizures in children by carbamazepine. *N Engl J Med* 1985;313:916–21.
15. Sobotka JL, Alexander B, Cook BJ. A review of carbamazepine's hematologic reactions and monitoring recommendations. *DICP Ann Pharmacother* 1990;24:1214–19.
16. Mattson RH, Cramer JA, Collins JF, et al. Comparison of carbamazepine, phenobarbital, phenytoin and primidone in partial and secondarily generalized tonic-clonic seizures. *N Engl J Med* 1985;313:145–51.
17. Smith DB, Mattson RH, Cramer JA, Collins JF, Novelly RA, Craft B, and the V.A. Epilepsy Cooperative Study Group. Results of a nationwide Veterans Administration Cooperative Study comparing the efficacy and toxicity of carbamazepine, phenobarbital, phenytoin and primidone. *Epilepsia* 1987;28 (Suppl 3):S50–S58.

• • • • • •
CATAMENIAL (SEIZURES) (1,2)

Catamenial seizures refer to seizures clustered around the time of menstruation, presumably related to the changes in hormonal and fluid status and the possible variation in AED levels during the menstrual cycle. Estrogens and progestogens possess convulsant and anticonvulsant properties, and it has been believed that correction of the underlying endocrine flux might lead to effective treatment. In practice, some patients have exacerbations in seizure control with breakthrough seizures before, during, or after the onset of ovulation or menstruation, suggesting that no constant relationship to particular hormone levels is responsible (3). Hormone therapy—the use of various contraceptive pills—has been unsatisfactory. Benzodiazepines such as clobazam (4) and adjunctive therapy with acetazolamide started 10 days before and continued during and after menstruation may be effective. A premenstrual increase in standard AED therapy has also been advocated.

References

1. Newmark ME, Penry JK. Catamenial epilepsy: a review. *Epilepsia* 1980;21: 281–300.
2. Schachter SC. Hormonal considerations in women with seizures. *Arch Neurol* 1988;45:1267–70.
3. Newmark ME. Catamenial epilepsy: a neurologic myth persisting for more than 100 years. *Epilepsia* 1989;30:704.
4. Feely M, Gibson J. Intermittent clobazam for catamenial epilepsy: tolerance avoided. *J Neurol Neurosurg Psychiatry* 1984;47:1279–82.

• • • • • •
CATAPLEXY

Cataplexy is the sudden fall to the ground from a brief loss of body tone. Attacks may be brought on by strong emotional stimuli such as surprise, anger, or pleasure. Seen as part of the tetrad of symptoms of patients with narcolepsy (see also this heading), it occurs in about half. Cataplexy may be distinguished from atonic seizures by its characteristic precipitants and preservation of consciousness.

• • • • • •
CAVERNOMAS, CAVERNOUS HEMANGIOMAS, CAVERNOUS ANGIOMAS

These vascular malformations are hamartomas consisting of an abnormal mixture of normal tissue elements (1) which may then develop subsequent calcification, thrombosis, microhemorrhages, or frank bleeds. CNS cavernomas are multiple in 25% of patients. Most are supratentorial (1), predominantly in the temporal or Rolandic regions. Cavernomas produce seizures as a presenting or even sole feature (2); the clinical picture depends on seizure localization and spread. Seizures are usually focal or secondarily generalized and tend to occur in flurries, occasionally associated with micro-bleeds. Response to AEDs is poor. For a long time, cavernomas were thought to be rare. Between 1976 and 1978, there was a marked increase in cases reported in the literature with the advent of head CT scans (3,4). Other imaging techniques such as angiography may be negative and skull x-rays show calcifications in only a minority of cases. CT head scan frequently reveals focal hyperdensity surrounded by an area of decreased density. MRI of the head (5) is more sensitive than CT for diagnosis and shows increased signal intensity around the zone of calcification on the T1–weighted image, whereas on the T2–weighted image, centrally increased signal intensity is surrounded by low signal intensity. These quasi-pathognomonic MRI findings are produced by the hemosiderin deposits (6). Treatment is frequently surgical. How much tissue requires removal is in dispute, but several surgeons have argued for a conservative removal of only the cavernoma and visibly abnormal surrounding rim of tissue.

References

1. Voigt K, Yasargil MG. Cerebral cavernous hemangiomas or cavernomas. Incidence, pathology, localization, diagnosis, clinical features and treatment. *Neurochirurgia* 1976;2:59–68.
2. Farmer JP, Cosgrove GR, Villemure JG, Meagher-Villemure K, Tampieri D, Melanson D. Intra-cerebral cavernous angiomas. *Neurology* 1988;38:1699–1704.
3. Requena I, Arias M, Lopez-Ibor L, Pereiro I, Barba A, Alonso A, Monton E. Cavernomas of the central nervous sysem: clinical and neuroimaging manifestations in 47 patients. *J Neurol Neurosurg Psychiatry* 1991;54:590–94.
4. Simard JM, Garcia-Bengachea F, Ballinger WE, Mickle JP, Quisling RC. Cavernous angioma: a review of 126 collected and 12 new clinical cases. *Neurosurgery* 1986;18:162–72.
5. Dunn GD, Finn JP, Moseley IF. Cerebral cavernous malformations. Letter to the Editor. *N Engl J Med* 1988;319:1414.

6. Lemme-Plaghos G, Kutcharczyk W, Branot-Zawadzki M, Uske A, Edwards M, Norman D, Newton TH. MRI of angiographically occult vascular malformations. *Amer J Roentgenol* 1986;146:1223–28.

• • • • • • •
CENTRENCEPHALIC (SEIZURES)

Centrencephalic is a term referring to anatomical localizations introduced by Penfield and Jasper (1) involving the nonspecific thalamus, the diencephalon, the mesencephalon, and the rhombencephalon. Certain seizure types were ascribed to discharges in the deeper structures, although this has never been proven. Idiopathic and cryptogenic generalized epilepsies (see Classification of seizures and epilepsies) are examples of centrencephalic seizures. The term "centrencephalic" is falling from use, replaced by the term "cortico-reticular" epilepsies, emphasizing the systems nature of generalized epilepsies (2).

References

1. Penfield W, Jasper H. *Epilepsy and the functional anatomy of human brain.* London: J and A Churchill Ltd., 1954.
2. Gloor P. Generalized epilepsy with spike and wave discharge reinterpretation of its electrographic and clinical manifestations. *Epilepsia*1979;20:571–88.

• • • • • • •
CEREBELLUM

The cerebellum is one of the very few regions of the brain lacking the capacity to sustain seizure activity, since most synaptic interactions in cerebellar circuits are inhibitory. Nevertheless, the cerebellum is important in epilepsy because several syndromes combine seizures and cerebellar deficits (see also Alpers' disease, Baltic myoclonus). Furthermore, the cerebellum can be injured by seizures and possibly by AEDs (see also Ataxia).

CEREBELLAR SYNDROMES IN PATIENTS WITH EPILEPSY

1. Progressive encephalopathies with epilepsy, myoclonus, and cerebellar signs are seen in progressive myoclonic epilepsies (see also Myoclonic epilepsies progressive), Alpers' disease, and childhood and adult ceroid-lipofuscinoses.

2. Nonprogressive cerebellar abnormalities may be seen in chronic epilepsy: some infantile encephalopathies, e.g., Lennox-Gastaut syndrome (1), where cerebellar signs appear intermittently or permanently.

3. Progressive cerebellar disorders with kinetic or static ataxias may be seen in chronic epilepsies in which seizures are frequent, prolonged, and ongoing for many years. Pyramidal, extrapyramidal, and neuropathic features are often associated.

4. Transient "cerebellar" signs may be seen in chronic epilepsies as a result of chronic or acute phenytoin intake.

5. Irreversible cerebellar signs may be seen after acute overdose of phenytoin (2) or chronic phenytoin intake (3–5).

CEREBELLAR PATHOLOGY IN EPILEPSY

Anatomical abnormalities of the cerebellum in patients with epilepsy may be manifest or subclinical. The cerebellum may be atrophied. The most characteristic abnormality involves Purkinje cell degeneration, atrophy of cerebellar cortex, and occasionally vermian atrophy.

Causes include (6):

- Anoxia as a result of seizures;
- Perinatal anoxic insult with diffuse cerebral edema and recurrent insult during seizures;
- Diffuse lesions of the cortex and vermis from phenytoin treatment—this is probably rare (7);
- Unilateral lesions, often contralateral to the seizure focus, attributed to transneuronal degeneration (6,8);
- Lesions from anoxia due to terminal events that have affected neuropathologic interpretation.

References

1. Mencke HJ. Pathology of childhood epilepsies. *Cleve Clin J Med* 1989;56: S111–S120.

2. Masur H, Fahrendorf G, Oberwittler C, Reuther G. Cerebellar atrophy following acute intoxication with phenytoin. *Neurology* 1990;40:1800–1801.

3. Iivanainen M, Viukari M, Helle E-P. Cerebellar atrophy in phenytoin-treated mentally retarded epileptics. *Epilepsia* 1977;18:375–86.

4. McLain LW Jr, Martin JT, Allen JH. Cerebellar degeneration due to chronic phenytoin therapy. *Ann Neurol* 1980;7:18–23.

5. Ghatak NR, Santoso RA, McKinney WM. Cerebellar degeneration following long-term phenytoin therapy. *Neurology* 1976;26:818–20.

6. Gessaga EC, Urich H. The cerebellum of epileptics. *Clin Neuropathol* 1985; 4:238–45.

7. Dam M. The density and ultrastructure of the Purkinje cells following diphenyl-hydantoin treatment in animals and man. *Acta Neurol Scand* 1972;49 (Suppl): 3–65.

8. Dunan R, Patterson J, Hadley DM, Bone I. Unilateral cerebellar damage in focal epilepsy. *J Neurol Neurosurg Psychiatry* 1990;53:436–37.

● ● ● ● ● ● ●
CEREBROVASCULAR ACCIDENTS AND SEIZURES

Isolated or recurrent seizures may be seen following cerebrovascular accidents (CVAs), including infarcts, hemorrhagic infarcts, or cerebral hemorrhages.

1. Seizure Association With Cerebrovascular Accidents

Prodromal seizures. Seizures may precede the obvious manifestations of cerebral infarction. The incidence of prodromal seizures is 4–7% (1). Sensory, motor, or mixed partial seizures are typical in this setting, sometimes with secondary generalization; rarely with a postictal deficit. Seizures may appear singly or in clusters. Since CT scans and MRI often show old infarcts (1–3), prodromal seizures may well be related to earlier silent embolic infarcts (2).

Seizures occurring with cerebral infarction. Approximately 5% of cerebral infarcts present simultaneously with a seizure, accounting for 33% of the seizures seen following cerebral infarction (4). Most commonly, they are simple partial seizures or generalized seizures. A jacksonian march suggests localization to the Sylvian region; a presentation that may be triggered by metabolic abnormalities such as hyperglycemia. The incidence of early seizures (within two weeks of the stroke) is about 6% (5). The seizures do not necessarily herald an epileptic sequela (6,7), but status epilepticus has a poor prognosis.

Late seizures after cerebral infarction. Late seizures appear from the second week to 18 years after a cerebral infarction (7), occurring in about 3–10% (5,8). A high risk for seizures exists after cortical infarcts, especially those in the territory of the middle cerebral artery (9), and are a frequent cause of epilepsy in the aged (10). The pathogenesis is poorly understood, but may be due to glial scarring, iron deposition, or hemodynamic factors. In the absence of clinical abnormality, neuroimaging may reveal infarction (2,3).

2. Seizures and Intracerebral Hemorrhage

Early seizures may herald the onset of hemorrhage or may follow it by several hours. They correlate to the lobar localization of hemorrhage or cortical extension, or the presence of blood in the meningeal or intraventricular regions (11,12). Seizures are usually generalized, and status epilepticus is frequent.

Late seizures occurring after cerebral hemorrhage are relatively infrequent (2.5–6.5%) (12,13), but usually require AED treatment.

3. Seizures and Subdural Hematomas

Although subdural hematomas are caused by head injury in most cases, the incidence of seizures is low: 2 of 56 patients not on AEDs; 0 of 73 patients on AEDs (14).

4. Neonatal Cerebral Infarction or Hemorrhage

With the advent of head CT scans, there has been an increase in the early identification of neonatal infarction. Partial or generalized seizures, occurring singly or in clusters, usually have a good response to treatment (15). Neurological examination may confirm the presence of cerebral infarction, typically in the territory of the middle cerebral artery. There may be an eventual progression to a chronic epilepsy.

Seizures are more frequent after intracerebral hemorrhage than with infarction, occurring in up to one quarter of cases (15).

References

1. Shinton RA, Gill JS, Zezulka AV, Beevers DG. The frequency of epilepsy preceding stroke. Case-control study in 230 patients. *Lancet* 1987;1:11–13
2. Roberts RC, Shorvon S, Cox TCS, Gilliatt RW. Clinically unsuspected cerebral infarction revealed by computed tomography scanning in late onset epilepsy. *Epilepsia*1988;29:190–94.
3. Chodosh EH, Foulkes MA, Kase CS, Hier DB, Price TR, Furtado JG. Silent stroke in the NINCDS Stroke Data Bank. *Neurology* 1988;38:1674–79.
4. Gupta SR, Naheedy MH, Elias D, Rubino FA, Post-infarction seizures. A clinical study. *Stroke* 1988;19:1477–81.
5. Sung CY, Chu NS. Epileptic seizures in thrombotic stroke. *J Neurology* 1990; 237:166–70.
6. Lesser RP, Luders H, Dinner DS, Morris HH. Epileptic seizures due to thrombotic and embolic cerebrovascular disease in older patients. *Epilepsia* 1985; 26:622–30.
7. Danielle O, Mattaliano A, Tassinari CA, Natale E. Epileptic seizures and cerebrovascular disease. *Acta Neurol Scand* 1989;80:17–22.
8. Olsen TS, Hogenhaven H, Thage O. Epilepsy after stroke. *Neurology* 1987; 37:1209–11.
9. De Carolis P, D'Alessandro Ferrara R, Andreoli A, Sacquegna T, Lugaresi E. Late seizures in patients with internal carotid and middle cerebral artery occlusive disease following ischemic events. *J Neurol Neurosurg Psychiatry* 1984;47: 1345–47.
10. Loiseau J, Loiseau P, Duche B, Guyot M, Dartigues JF, Aublet B. A survey of epileptic disorders in Southwest France: seizures in elderly patients. *Ann Neurol* 1990;27:232–37.
11. Berger AR, Lipton RB, Lesfer ML, Lantos G, Portenoy RK. Early seizures following cerebral hemorrhage: implications for therapy. *Neurology* 1988;38: 1363–65.

12. Faught E, Peters D, Bartoluccia A, Moore L, Miller PC. Seizures after primary intracerebral hemorrhage. *Neurology* 1989;39:1089–93.
13. Sung CY, Chu NS. Epileptic seizures in intracerebral haemorrhage. *J Neurol Neurosurg Psychiatry* 1989;52:1273–76.
14. Ohno K, Maehara T, Ichimura K, Suzuki R, Hirakawa K, Monma S. Low incidence of seizures in patients with chronic subdural haematoma. *J Neurol Neurosurg Psychiatry* 1993;56:1231–33.
15. Levy SR, Abroms IF, Marshall PC, Rosquette EE. Seizures and cerebral infarction in the full-term newborn. *Ann Neurol* 1985;17:366–70.

• • • • • •
CEROID-LIPOFUSCINOSES

Ceroid-lipofuscinosis is a term introduced in 1969 for a group of neurological disorders (1). These genetic diseases present at different ages, and are all characterized by the accumulation of lipo-pigments in lysosomes (2). The etiology is unknown, and no universal enzyme defect has been identified. The clinical and EEG features are those of a progressive myoclonic epilepsy. Depending on the age of onset, there are four classic syndromes: early infantile (Santavuori-Haltia), late infantile (Janski-Bielchowsky), juvenile (Batten-Vogt-Spielmeyer), and an adult form (Kufs disease) (see under these headings). Other variations have also been described. The diagnosis is made by finding inclusion bodies in different organs, e.g., sweat glands, muscle, rectal mucosa, and neurons. These inclusions contain excessive amounts of ceroid or lipofuscin lipo-pigments (3).

References

1. Zeman W, Dyken PR. Neuronal ceroid-lipofuscinosis (Batten's disease). Relationship to amaurotic familial idiocy? *Pediatrics* 1969;44:570–83.
2. Dyken PR. The neuronal ceroid-lipofuscinoses. *Child Neurology* 1989;4:165–74.
3. Carpenter S, Karpati G, Andermann F, Jacob JC, Andermann E. The ultrastructural characteristics of the abnormal cytosomes in Batten's and Kufs disease. *Brain* 1977;60;137–56.

• • • • • •
CHOREA (SEE DYSKINESIAS)

AEDs may cause choreiform movements. Although phenytoin is most commonly mentioned, phenobarbital and carbamazepine have been implicated.

• • • • • • •
CHOREOATHETOSIS, PAROXYSMAL

In the syndrome of paroxysmal choreoathetosis, abnormal movements begin in childhood or adolescence. Attacks are brief, lasting 1–2 minutes, occur daily, and are brought on by sudden movement of the legs, e.g., upon standing, beginning to walk, or accelerating pace. Often abnormal movements present distally in one foot with tonic intorsion, followed by spread up the leg with flexion or extension of the knee; elbow flexion, hemifacial spasm, and impairment of speech. In more prolonged episodes, there may be torsion, chorea, and athetosis. Consciousness is usually preserved and ictal and interictal EEG recordings are normal. The neurological examination is normal. Half of the published cases have a family history. Attacks usually cease by 20–40 years of age.

Paroxysmal choreoathetosis was previously thought to be a variety of movement-induced reflex epilepsy because of its resemblance to partial motor seizures and response to AEDs; however, current thinking supports its classification as an extrapyramidal syndrome rather than as an epilepsy.

Reference

Lance JW. Familial paroxysmal dystonic choreoathetosis and its differentiation from related syndromes. *Ann Neurol* 1977;2:285–93.

• • • • • • •
CLASSIFICATION OF SEIZURES AND EPILEPSIES

The International League Against Epilepsy has proposed several classifications of seizures (1) and epileptic syndromes (2). These schemes replace those suggested by Gastaut in 1970 (3).

CLASSIFICATION OF SEIZURES (1981)

Principle: To distinguish convulsive or nonconvulsive generalized primary generalized seizures from partial seizures using clinical and EEG criteria.

- Simple partial seizures do not affect the level of consciousness;
- Complex partial seizures, either initially or during the seizure, affect the level of consciousness or attention;
- Because of the absence of sufficient information, a number of seizures cannot be classified.

Advantages: To provide a common language for all epileptologists, thus simplifying research and epidemiology.

Disadvantages: The difficulty in obtaining sufficient information from the history and the paucity of ictal EEG evaluation (with the exception of video-EEG capture) of an event. There are difficulties in determining change in the level of consciousness, whether generalized seizures are primary or secondary, and problems in interpretation of interictal epileptiform events. Difficulties arise when using particular signs or symptoms to determine whether seizures spread through several areas simultaneously or successively. Apparent alteration in responsiveness, vigilance, attention, or consciousness may result from various anatomical involvements and similar clinical presentations may arise from variable physiopathological processes. Clinical anatomical correlations do not clearly correlate with the seizure type.

I.   PARTIAL (FOCAL, LOCAL) SEIZURES
    A. Simple partial seizures (consciousness not impaired)
        (1) With motor signs:
            (a) Focal motor without march
            (b) Focal motor with march (jacksonian)
            (c) Versive
            (d) Postural
            (e) Phonatory (vocalization or arrest of speech)
        (2) With somatosensory or special-sensory symptoms (simple hallucinations, e.g., tingling, light flashes, buzzing):
            (a) Somatosensory
            (b) Visual
            (c) Auditory
            (d) Olfactory
            (e) Gustatory
            (f) Vertiginous
        (3) With autonomic symptoms or signs (including epigastric sensation, pallor, sweating, flushing, piloerection, and pupillary dilatation).
        (4) With psychic symptoms (disturbance of higher cerebral function). These symptoms rarely occur without impairment of consciousness and more commonly occur as complex partial seizures.
            (a) Dysphasic
            (b) Dysmnesic (e.g., déjà-vu)
            (c) Cognitive (e.g., dreamy states, distortions of time sense)
            (d) Affective (fear, anger, etc.)
            (e) Illusions (e.g., macropsia)
            (f) Structured hallucinations (e.g., music, scenes)

    B. Complex partial seizures (with impairment of consciousness)
        (1) Simple partial onset followed by impairment of consciousness:
            (a) With simple partial features (A1–A4) followed by impaired consciousness
            (b) With automatisms
        (2) When they start with impairment of consciousness:
            (a) With impaired consciousness only
            (b) With automatisms
    C. Partial seizures with secondary generalization
        (1) Simple partial seizures (A) evolving to generalized seizures
        (2) Complex partial seizures (B) evolving to generalized seizures
        (3) Simple partial seizures evolving to complex partial seizures, evolving to generalized seizures.
II. GENERALIZED SEIZURES
    A. Absence type seizures
        (1) Typical absence seizures:
            (a) Impairment of consciousness only
            (b) With mild clonic components
            (c) With atonic components
            (d) With tonic components
            (e) With automatisms
            (f) With autonomic components
        (2) Atypical absence: May have:
            (a) Changes in tone more pronounced than in A1
            (b) More gradual onset and/or cessation
    B. Myoclonic seizures
    C. Clonic seizures
    E. Tonic-clonic seizures
    F. Atonic seizures (astatic)
III. UNCLASSIFIED EPILEPTIC SEIZURES

CLASSIFICATION OF EPILEPTIC SYNDROMES (1989) (1–5)

Principles: To organize epileptic seizures based on EEG and clinical criteria of the seizures and their localization. "An epileptic syndrome is an epileptic disorder characterized by a cluster of signs and symptoms customarily occurring together; these include such items as type of seizure, etiology, anatomy, precipitating factors, age of onset, severity, chronicity, diurnal and circadian cycling, and sometimes prognosis" (2). Epileptic syndromes are empirically defined and may not share common etiologies.
    These are:

- EEG and clinical characteristics of the seizures indicating a focal or generalized disturbance;

- Etiological considerations;
- Idiopathic epilepsies (previously called primary epilepsies). These generalized epilepsies have specific clinical and EEG characteristics, are age-dependent and without known cause. They appear to be genetically linked;
- Cryptogenic epilepsies have no underlying cause that can be determined using present diagnostic techniques;
- Symptomatic epilepsies are caused by known or suspected, static or progressive lesions or are secondary to inborn errors of metabolism.

Advantages: The classification of epileptic syndromes codifies on an empiric basis the most common epileptic syndromes, thus providing a common scientific basis for research. This allows comparison between studies and a standardized approach to prognosis and treatment.

Disdvantages:

- The classification does not necessarily take into account the underlying mechanisms for the seizures, multifactorial causes, or any "gray areas" of overlap between epileptic "syndromes";
- In attempting to be complete and exhaustive, it includes, on the one hand, rare syndromes; on the other, syndromes that are being discarded. Furthermore, the different syndromes overlap;
- Its complexity makes epidemiological studies, student teaching, and the education of the public more difficult;
- It does not take into account more recent advances in molecular biology and the understanding of inherited forms of epilepsy.

The classification includes (2):

1. LOCALIZATION-RELATED (FOCAL, LOCAL, PARTIAL) EPILEPSIES AND SYNDROMES
   1.1. Idiopathic (with age-related onset)
   - Benign childhood epilepsy with centrotemporal spikes;
   - Childhood epilepsy with occipital paroxysms;
   - Primary reading epilepsy.
   1.2. Symptomatic
   - Chronic progressive epilepsia partialis continua of childhood (Kojewnikow's syndrome);
   - Syndromes characterized by seizures with specific modes of precipitation;
   - Temporal lobe epilepsies;
   - Frontal lobe epilepsies;
   - Parietal lobe epilepsies;
   - Occipital lobe epilepsies.

1.3. Cryptogenic

Cryptogenic epilepsies are presumed to be symptomatic, but with unknown etiology. This category thus differs from the previous one by a lack of demonstrable etiology.

2. GENERALIZED EPILEPSIES AND SYNDROMES

2.1. Idiopathic (with age-related onset—listed in order of age)
- Benign neonatal familial convulsions;
- Benign neonatal convulsions;
- Benign myoclonic epilepsy of childhood;
- Childhood absence epilepsy (pyknolepsy);
- Juvenile absence epilepsy;
- Juvenile myoclonic epilepsy (Impulsive Petit Mal);
- Epilepsy with grand mal (GTCS) seizures on awakening;
- Other generalized idiopathic epilepsies not defined above;
- Epilepsies with seizures precipitated by specific modes of activation.

2.2. Cryptogenic or symptomatic
- West syndrome (infantile spasms, Blitz-Nick-Salaam Krampfe);
- Lennox-Gastaut syndrome;
- Epilepsy with myoclonic-astatic seizures;
- Epilepsy with myoclonic absences;

2.3. Symptomatic

2.3.1) nonspecific etiology
- Early myoclonic encephalopathy;
- Early infantile epileptic encephalopathy with burst suppressions;
- Other symptomatic generalized epilepsies not defined above.

2.3.2) Specific syndromes
- Epileptic seizures may complicate many disease states. These include diseases in which seizures are a presenting or dominant feature.

3. EPILEPSIES AND SYNDROMES UNDETERMINED WHETHER FOCAL OR GENERALIZED

3.1. With both generalized and partial seizures
- Neonatal seizures;
- Severe myoclonic epilepsy of childhood;
- Epilepsy with continuous spike waves during slow wave sleep;
- Acquired epileptic aphasia (Landau-Kleffner syndrome);
- Other undetermined epilepsies not defined above.

3.2. Without unequivocal generalized or focal features.

This includes generalized tonic-clonic seizures in which clinical and EEG findings do not permit their classification as being either clearly generalized or localization-related.

4. SPECIAL SYNDROMES
    4.1. Situation-related seizures
        • Febrile convulsions
        • Seizures occurring only with acute metabolic or toxic dis-
          turbances due to factors such as alcohol, drugs, eclampsia,
          or nonketotic hyperglycemia.
    4.2. Isolated seizures or status epilepticus
Definitions of these epileptic syndromes can be found in reference (2).

References

1. Commission on Classification and Terminology of the International League Against Epilepsy. Proposal for revised clinical and electroencephalographic classification of epileptic seizures. *Epilepsia* 1981;22:489–501.
2. Commission on Classification and Terminology of the International League Against Epilepsy. Proposal for revised classification of epilepsies and epileptic syndromes. *Epilepsia* 1989;30:389–99.
3. Gastaut H. Clinical and electroencephalographic classification of epileptic seizures. *Epilepsia*1970;11:102–13.
4. Inherited forms of epilepsy. *Epilepsia* 1993;34 (Suppl 3):S1–S78.
5. Molecular genetics and epilepsy: foundation for therapeutic advances. *Epilepsia* 1994;35 (Suppl 1):S1–S62.

• • • • • •
CLINICAL TRIALS

These trials are essential in the development of new AEDs. Until the 1970s, many clinical trials lacked precision (1), but there have been significant methodological improvements in the interval (2,3). The International League Against Epilepsy has established several guidelines (4). For new drugs, an initial trial of their effectiveness as an AED and the absence of toxic side effects must be established in animal studies. The drug is then administered to man in a sequence of stages:

• Phase I, early. The purpose is to determine the pharmacokinetics of the drug in man and the maximal tolerated dose. Healthy adult volunteers take various amounts of the drug either as a single dose or in repeated doses for four weeks;
• Phase I, late. The purpose is to evaluate the antiepileptic effectiveness, toxicity, pharmacokinetics, and interactions with other drugs. In adults with uncontrolled seizures, the new drug is used as an add-on treatment in either open or closed study conditions for one to two months;

- Phase II, early. The objective is to confirm the effectiveness of the new drug. Controlled trials using double-blind, placebo-controlled design are made with the new drug as add-on therapy in poorly controlled adult patients with epilepsy. These last three to four months and are performed in parallel groups or as a crossover study;
- Phase II, late. The objective is to determine the effectiveness and toxicity of the new drug, and the absence of tolerance when used as monotherapy. These are randomized trials in a) previously untreated adults and children, or b) patients on other AEDs providing insufficient seizure control, in which there is introduction of the new drug and diminution in the previous ineffective medication;
- Phase III. The objective is to determine clinical indications for the new AED within the therapeutic armamentarium, its long-term effectiveness and side effects, and its specific role in treatment of epilepsy syndromes. These open-label trials usually involve large numbers of patients (100–150) tested for at least a year against placebo or a reference AED.

In all these trials, patients are examined according to specific standards that determine drug toxicity and effectiveness, thus ensuring patient safety. The inclusion and exclusion criteria are strictly defined, usually with the exclusion of a large number of patients with epilepsy from particular studies.

After the drug reaches the market, phase IV investigations may be used to evaluate the advantages and disadvantages of the AED under community conditions.

References

1. Coatsworth JJ. Studies on the clinical efficacy of marketed antiepileptic drugs. NINDS monograph n 12. Washington, D.C.: U.S. Government Printing Office, 1971.
2. Delgado-Escueta AV, Mattson RH, Smith DB, Cramer JK, Collins JF. Principles in designing clinical trials for antiepileptic drugs. *Neurology* 1983;33 (Suppl 1): 8–13.
3. Mattson RH, Cramer JA, Delgado-Escueta AV, Smith DB, Collins JF. A design for the prospective evaluation of the efficacy and toxicity of antiepileptic drugs in adults. *Neurology* 1983;33 (Suppl 1):14–25.
4. Commission on Antiepileptic Drugs of the International League Against Epilepsy. Guidelines for clinical evaluation of antiepileptic drugs. *Epilepsia*1989; 30:400–408.

•••••••
CLOBAZAM (URBANYL®)

Clobazam is a 1,5–benzodiazepine, less sedative than other benzodiazepines (see Benzodiazepines). In Europe, it is used as a drug of second choice or as adjunctive therapy in typical absence seizures and in partial epilepsies. It is usually divided into two doses per day. Excellent short-term results have been achieved with clobazam (1,2), but relapses occur due to tolerance (2–4). An intermittent course of therapy may be helpful (5). If there has been little response after 1–3 months, further use is probably unhelpful (6).

References

1. Koeppen D, Baruzzi A, Capozza M, et al. Clobazam in therapy-resistant patients with partial epilepsy: a double-blind placebo-controlled crossover study. *Epilepsia* 1987;28:495–506.
2. Gastaut H, Low MD. Antiepileptic properties of clobazam, a 1–5 benzodiazepine in man. *Epilepsia* 1979;20:437–46.
3. Robertson M. Current status of the 1,4—and 1,5—benzodiazepines in the treatment of epilepsy: the place of clobazam. *Epilepsia* 1986;27 (Suppl)1:27–41.
4. Shorvon SD. Benzodiazepines. Clobazam. In: Levy RH, Mattson RJ, Meldrum BS, Penry JK, Dreifuss FE (eds.). *Antiepileptic drugs,* 3rd edition. New York: Raven Press, 1989;821–40.
5. Feely M, Gibson J. Intermittent clobazam for catamenial epilepsy: tolerance avoided. *J Neurol Neurosurg Psychiatry* 1984;87:1279–82.
6. Buchanan N. Clobazam in the treatment of epilepsy: prospective followup of 8 years, *J Roy Soc Med* 1993;86:378–80.

•••••••
CLONAZEPAM (KLONOPIN®, RIVOTRIL®)

Clonazepam is a benzodiazepine frequently used in chronic epilepsies (see Benzodiazepines). It is usually given as one evening dose. Particularly useful in myoclonic epilepsies (benign and progressive) and in photosensitive seizures, its effectiveness in other seizure types is variable. Studies in children with severe epilepsies treated with multiple AEDs have shown it to be ineffective in 75% of cases, effective in 7.5% of cases, and associated with worsening of seizures in 15%. Withdrawal seizures occur upon discontinuation of clonazepam in 47% (1). In Europe, clonazepam is a drug of first choice in the treatment of status epilepticus, impending status epilepticus, frequent seizures, prolonged seizures, and febrile convulsions. Administration of clonazepam in the emergency setting is by slow intravenous injection over 2–5 minutes because of the possibility of precipitation in bags or plastic tubing. The drug may also be given per rectum. Bronchial obstruction has been noted in children and the elderly.

References

1. Specht U, Boenigk HE, Wolf P. Discontinuation of clonazepam after long-term treatment. *Epilepsia* 1989;30:458–63.
2. Levy RH, Dreifuss FE, Mattson RH, Meldrum BS, Penry JK (eds.). *Antiepileptic drugs,* 3rd edition. New York: Raven Press, 1989.

• • • • • •
CLONIC (SEIZURES)

Clonic seizures are characterized by rhythmic jerks, usually generalized, although with variations in amplitude, frequency, and distribution during a single seizure. Over the age of three, the clonic movements are predominantly regular and symmetric. In the younger age groups, unilateral or asymmetric jerks may be seen (hemibody jerks, unilateral, hemiclonic). Jerks may shift from one side to the other. The EEG correlate of clonic seizures is often one of irregular spikes and slow waves. Clonic seizures may last seconds to hours. Bilateral seizures cause an immediate loss of consciousness followed by marked autonomic problems. In hemiclonic seizures, consciousness may be preserved or only mildly affected. A variable postictal hemiplegia is commonly seen. Clonic seizures occur only in young children with idiopathic generalized or symptomatic epilepsies or with febrile seizures.

Reference

Gastaut H, Broughton R. *Epileptic seizures, clinical and electrographic features, diagnosis and treatment.* Springfield: Charles C. Thomas, 1972.

• • • • • •
CLONIC-TONIC-CLONIC (SEIZURES)

Clonic-tonic-clonic seizures are generalized seizures beginning with massive bilateral myoclonic jerks occurring at seizure onset, before consciousness is lost. They are then followed by tonic-clonic seizures. These seizures are usually seen in juvenile myoclonic epilepsy.

Reference

Delgado-Escueta AV, Enrile-Bacsal G. Juvenile myoclonic epilepsy of Janz. *Neurology* 1984;34:285–94.

• • • • • •
CLORAZEPATE (TRANXENE®)

Clorazepate is a second-line AED used in chronic epilepsies (1–3). In Europe, intravenous administration has been used in status epilepticus.

References

1. Fujii T, Okuno T, Go T, Ochi J, Hattori H, Katoaka K, Mikawa H. Clorazepate therapy for intractable epilepsy. *Brain Dev* 1987;9:288–91.
2. Naidu S, Greuner G, Brazis P. Excellent results with clorazepate in recalcitrant childhood epilepsies. *Pediat Neurol* 1986;2:18–22.
3. Troupin AS, Friel P, Wilensky AJ, Moretti-Ojemann L, Levy RH, Freigl P. Evaluation of clorazepate (Tranxene) as an anticonvulsant: a pilot study. *Neurology* 1979;29:458–60.

• • • • • •
COCAINE

This central nervous system stimulant drug is a frequent substance of abuse. Even a single intake may precipitate seizures (1).

Reference

Baxter LR Jr, Schwartz JM, Phelps ME, et al. Localization of the neurochemical effects of cocaine and other stimulants in the human brain. *J Clin Psychiatry* 1988;49(Suppl 2):23–26.

• • • • • •
COGNITIVE (SEIZURES)

These partial seizures consist of:

• A dreamy state in which the patient is aware of an alteration in perception of real events or hallucinates because of mild confusion. Temporal epileptiform abnormalities have been reported;
• Forced thinking in which an unshakable perception is noted by the patient. Epileptic focus is often in the mesial or inferior frontal lobes.

Seizures with cognitive manifestations may evolve into complex partial seizures and may be seen in symptomatic or cryptogenic epilepsies.

● ● ● ● ● ●
COMMISSUROTOMIES

These provide palliative therapy in severe epilepsies with several seizure types, aimed at diminishing the frequency of the most debilitating seizures, i.e., drop attacks with atonic or tonic-clonic seizures. Partial or total section of the corpus callosum (see Callosotomy) as well as a section of the fornix, the anterior commissure, and the fields of Forel in the subthalamic region have been attempted. These procedures are less used at present.

Reference

Ramani SV, Yap JC, Gumnit RS. Stereotactic fields of Forel interruption for intractable epilepsy. *Appl Neurophysiol* 1980;43:104–108.

● ● ● ● ● ●
COMPLEX (PARTIAL SEIZURES) (1,2)

Complex partial seizures are the most prevalent seizure type in an unselected adult population of patients with epilepsy. These seizures present with simple partial seizures (auras) in 50% of cases, arrest of activity, staring, fumbling automatisms (automatisms are present in the majority), and blunting of awareness or recall (occurs in all cases, by definition). The term "complex" has changed in meaning with respect to epilepsy. In the International Classification of Epileptic Seizures of 1970, it represented involvement of cortical association areas responsible for memory with ideational, affective, and hallucinatory perturbation. In the 1981 classification, it indicates nongeneralized seizures associated with an alteration in the level of consciousness (see also Consciousness). Complex partial seizures do not necessarily arise from the temporal lobe.

References

1. Williamson PD, Spencer DD, Spencer SS, Novelly RA, Mattson RH. Complex partial seizures of frontal lobe origin. *Ann Neurol* 1985;18:497–504.
2. King DW, Ajmone MC. Clinical features and ictal patterns in epileptic patients with EEG temporal lobe foci. *Ann Neurol* 1977;2:138–47.

• • • • • •
COMPLIANCE

Compliance refers to the manner in which a patient follows a medical prescription, including the dosage and timing of medication intake. It is one
of the most important factors, if not the most imporant, in failure of AED
therapy. Noncompliance may consist of excessive intake, but more frequently involves decreased intake or the neglect of a variable number of
doses. Poor compliance creates problems in all chronic disorders where
daily or multiple daily doses of medication are required (1,2). To a certain
extent, compliance may be evaluated using serum drug levels or the count-
ing of remaining tablets in the bottle. Such verification is, however, subject to error (3). Compliance may be maximized by decreasing the numbers of times a day that medication must be taken or by arranging intake
to occur at convenient times. It largely depends on the care with which
doctors inform patients of the goals and means of treatment.

References

1. Schmidt D, Leppik I (eds.). Compliance in epilepsy. *Epilepsy Res* 1988;(Suppl
   1):1–182.
2. Leppik IE. Compliance during treatment of epilepsy. *Epilepsia* 1988;29 (Suppl
   2):S79–S84.
3. Cramer JA, Mattson RH, Prevey ML, Scheyer RD, Ouellette VL. How often is
   medication taken as prescribed? A novel assessment technique. *JAMA* 1989;
   261:3273–77.

• • • • • •
CONFUSION

A confusional state may be seen in patients with epilepsy for several reasons:

- During a seizure: A brief confusional state is frequently seen following complex partial seizures with temporal and frontal lobe foci
  (see these headings), and has been attributed to postictal discharges
  in the meso-limbic structures bilaterally. It has been seen after generalized seizures as a result of impairment of consciousness and may
  last from several hours to 1–2 days. It may be difficult to distinguish
  a postictal confusional state from the ictal confusional state seen in
  complex partial or generalized nonconvulsive status epilepticus
  without an EEG.
- Between seizures: These may occur because of interictal psychoses,
  adverse drug reactions (usually drug toxicity), and metabolic abnormalities (e.g., hyponatremia).

• • • • • •
CONSCIOUSNESS

In epileptology, consciousness is defined as the ability to react to an external stimulus (1) and to be able to remember events, internal or external, that have occurred during the seizure. Evaluation of the level of consciousness during a seizure is frequently difficult. Only complex tasks may reveal mild perturbations in consciousness or alertness. If total loss of consciousness is brief, patients may be unaware of the fact or deny it. The inability to speak during a seizure should not be confused with an alteration in the level of consciousness. The term "alteration in awareness" is preferred to "alteration in level of consciousness" (2).

During a seizure, consciousness may be:

- Preserved in simple partial seizures or myoclonic seizures;
- Impaired, at the start or secondarily: complex partial seizures, generalized seizures other than myoclonic.

References

1. Porter RJ. Recognizing and classifying epileptic seizures and epileptic syndromes. *Neurol Clin* 1986;4:495–508.
2. Geier S, Bancaud J, Talairach J, Bonis A, Szikia G, Enjelvin M. The seizures of frontal lobe epilepsy. A study of clinical manifestations. *Neurology* 1977; 27:951–58.

• • • • • •
CONTRACEPTIVES (ORAL)

Enzyme-inducing AEDs such as phenytoin, phenobarbital, primidone, and carbamazepine may decrease oral contraceptive effectiveness, especially in the case of low-dose estrogen preparations. Valproate (2), benzodiazepines, and ethosuximide have less influence on oral contraceptive effectiveness. Conversely, oral contraceptives can alter serum protein binding characteristics and change the efficacy of a given AED regimen.

References

1. Coulam CB, Annegers JF. Do anticonvulsants reduce the efficacy of oral contraceptives? *Epilepsia* 1979;20:519–26.
2. Crawford P, Chadwick D, Cleland P, Tjia J, Cowie A, Back DJ, Orme ML. The lack of effect of sodium valproate on the pharmacokinetics of oral contraceptive steroids. *Contraception* 1986;33:23–29.

• • • • • •
CONVULSIONS

The term "convulsion" refers to the sudden jerking movements or clonic movements seen during seizures. The term is used more loosely in pediatrics for all epileptic events (see Febrile convulsions; Neonatal (S)).

• • • • • •
CONVULSIVE SYNCOPE

Syncope due to cerebral hypoxia may be caused by cardiac dysrhythmias, orthostatic drops in blood pressure, emotional stimuli, coughing, Valsalva maneuvers, or micturition, to name some of the more common causes. Convulsive syncope describes the rapid, brief, and often asymmetric limb flexion that appears concurrently, shortly after the fall to the ground, and which may be confused for a brief tonic-clonic seizure. Distinguishing characteristics include the brief duration of convulsion, the infrequent urinary incontinence and tongue biting, and the brief period of subsequent confusion.

Reference

Gastaut H. Syncopes: generalized anoxic cerebral seizures. In: Magnus O, Lorentz de Haas AM (eds.). *The epilepsies* (*Handbook of Clinical Neurology*, Vol. 15). Amsterdam: North Holland, 1974:815–35.

• • • • • •
CORTICECTOMY

The aim of a corticectomy is to eradicate seizures by resecting the epileptic focus. Much of the early work was done by the group in Montreal (1–3).

INDICATIONS

Corticectomy is potentially indicated in partial epilepsies with a clearly defined epileptic focus in areas where resection does not place the patient at risk of deficit greater than that of the seizures themselves, and where AED therapy has failed (see Antiepileptic drugs (AEDs)).

TECHNIQUES

- The first step is confirmation of a diagnosis of epilepsy and identification of the seizure focus using EEG and clinical correlates or with electrocorticography, epidural or subdural grid recording, or stereo-electroencephalography (5).
- The seizure focus may be excised by:
  - ▪ A standard temporal lobectomy, anterior temporal lobectomy, or amygdalohippocampectomy (4).
  - ▪ Selective corticectomy guided by electrocorticography or after preoperative stereotactic evaluation using depth electrodes or subdural grids.

RESULTS (4–6)

Results depend on the precision of seizure localization and the nature of the population under study. With accurate localization, seizures may be eliminated in 50–80% of temporal lobe epilepsies, 40–60% of patients with extratemporal epilepsies, and a significant seizure reduction may be seen in approximately half the remainder.

References

1. Penfield W, Jasper H. *Epilepsy and the functional anatomy of the human brain.* Boston: Little, Brown and Co., 1954.
2. Fish DR, Andermann F, Oliver A. Complex partial seizures and posterior temporal or extratemporal lesions: surgical strategies. *Neurology* 1991;41:1781–84.
3. Cascino GD, Boon PAJM, Fish DR. Surgically remediable lesional syndromes. In: Engel J Jr (ed.). *Surgical treatment of the epilepsies,* 2nd edition. New York: Raven Press, 1993.
4. Dodrill CB, Wilkus RJ, Ojemann GA, Ward AA, Wyler AR, Van Belle G, Tamas L. Multidisciplinary prediction of seizure relief from cortical resection surgery. *Ann Neurol* 1986;20:2–12.
5. Talairach J, Bancaud J. Stereotaxic approach to epilepsy. Methodology of anatomofunctional stereotaxic investigations. *Prog Neurol Surg* 1973;5:297–354.
6. Wieser GH. Selective amygdalo-hippocampectomy for temporal lobe epilepsy. *Epilepsia* 1988;29 (Suppl 2):S100–S113.
7. Guldrog B, Loying Y, Hanglie-Hanssen E, Flood S, Bjornaes H. Surgical versus medical treatment for epilepsy. I. Outcome related to survival, seizures and neurologic deficit. *Epilepsia* 1991;32:375–88.

• • • • • •
CORTICOGRAPHY (1–3)

Corticography is the direct recording of cerebral rhythms at the cortex, usually during a craniotomy. This technique avoids artifact and signal decrement caused by intervening scalp, skull, and meninges. Electrodes are placed directly on the cortex; the area investigated is limited by the size of the skull flap. Operative recording can only be performed for limited periods, and may be further confounded by anesthetic agents.

References

1. Penfield W, Jasper H. *Epilepsy and the functional anatomy of the human brain.* Boston: Little, Brown and Co., 1954.
2. Stefan H, Quesney LF, Abou-Khalil B, Olivier A. Electrocorticography in temporal lobe epilepsy surgery. *Acta Neurol Scand* 1991;83:65–72.
3. Reid SA. Toward the ideal electrocorticography array. *Neurosurgery* 1989;25: 135–37.

• • • • • •
CRYPTOGENIC

The Commission on Classification Terminology of the International League Against Epilepsy reserves the term "cryptogenic epilepsy" for partial or generalized epilepsies in which neither the history, clinical examination, nor ancillary investigations reveal a lesion accounting for the seizures. An apparent cryptogenic epilepsy may become symptomatic, for example, when a normal head CT scan is followed by abnormalities seen on MRI. Cryptogenic epilepsies are thus based on negative criteria, whereas idiopathic epilepsies are defined by positive criteria.

Reference

Commission on Classification and Terminology of the International League Against Epilepsy. Proposal for classification of epilepsies and epileptic syndromes. *Epilepsia*1989;30:389–99.

• • • • • •
CURE

In epileptology, the use of the term "cure" is controversial because of the ever-present possibility of the reappearance of seizures after remission lasting 5, 10, or even 20 years off treatment. The term "remission" is preferred, especially when continued AEDs are required. All the same, the use of the term "cure" can be applied in pulmonary tuberculosis, for example, even though relapses are possible. The term "cure" has been used regarding certain epileptic syndromes: absence epilepsy of childhood, benign idiopathic partial epilepsy of childhood. These syndromes may be considered to have been "cured" even if other epilepsy syndromes later develop.

• • • • • •
CURSIVE (SEIZURES)

Cursive seizures are brief seizures characterized by ambulatory automatisms affecting the gait. The patient may walk or run into obstacles (1). These seizures are thought to be due to limbic foci and may be related to gelastic (laughing) seizures (2). Cursive seizures should be distinguished from the automatisms occurring during postictal or ictal confusional periods, during which patients ambulate in a more coordinated and purposeful fashion (see also Versive (S)).

References

1. Gastaut H. *Dictionary of epilepsy. Part 1: Definitions.* Geneva: World Health Organization, 1973.
2. Chen RC, Forster FM. Cursive epilepsy and gelastic epilepsy. *Neurology* 1973;23:1019–29.

•••••••
DACRYSTIC (SEIZURES) (1,2)

Dacrystic seizures are characterized by brief episodes of crying, with or without impairment of consciousness, and may occur postictally. Foci are frequently in the nondominant antero-mesial temporal, or mesial frontal regions. These seizures are types of symptomatic partial epilepsies.

References

1. Offen ML, Davidoff RA, Troost BT, Richey ET. Dacrystic epilepsy. *J Neurol Neurosurg Psychiatry* 1976;39:829–34.
2. Liciano D, Devinsky O, Perrine K. Crying seizures. *Neurology* 1993;43:2113–17.

•••••••
DELTA ACTIVITY

This EEG frequency band is under 4 Hz (see also EEG). In waking adult patients, this frequency is usually abnormal. Diffuse delta activity may be seen with diffuse cerebral dysfunctions such as toxic, metabolic, or infectious encephalopathies, frontal delta activity with midline tumors, hydrocephalus, hypoglycemia, diffuse encephalopathies, and dialysis dementia. Focal delta activity can overlie structural abnormalities such as tumors, intracranial bleeds, or strokes involving subcortical and cortical areas.

Occipital delta occurs with childhood absence epilepsy, posterior fossa, and deep midline dysfunctions. Pseudoperiodic lateralized epileptiform discharges (PLEDS) (see this heading) in the delta range occur frequently after seizures in patients with strokes, and more rarely with tubers, cysts, or cerebral abscesses.

Delta activity occurs physiologically during sleep and can be brought on by hyperventilation, especially with low blood glucose levels.

• • • • • •
DENDRITE

A dendrite is classically defined as the receiving end of a neuron, by which information flows from the axon to the dendrite. Interactions among axons and dendrites undoubtedly play large roles in generation of the EEG (1). Modern views of dendrites also allow for a wide variety of dendritic morphologies and functions, including dendro-dendritic interactions (2)

References

1. Llinas R, Sugimori M. Electrophysiological properties of in vitro Purkinje cells in cerebellar slices. *J Physiol* 1980;305:197–213.
2. Shepherd G. *The synaptic organization of the brain,* 3rd edition. New York: Oxford University Press, 1990.

• • • • • •
DENTATO-PALLIDO-RUBRO-LUYSIAN ATROPHY

Atrophy of this system is seen only in Japanese patients.

Typical presentation includes a progressive myoclonic epilepsy with chorea, ataxia, and dementia. Transmission is autosomal dominant.

Reference

Naito H, Oyangi S. Familial myoclonus epilepsy and choreoathetosis hereditary dentato-pallido-rubro-luysian atrophy. *Neurology* 1982;32:798–807.

• • • • • •
DEPAKENE® (VALPROIC ACID), DEPAKOTE® (DIVALPROEX SODIUM) (SEE VALPROATE)

Valproate is usually taken two to three times daily, by mouth. Per rectum administration has been used in the treatment of status epilepticus.

Syrup (1 ml = 250 mg)

Enteric-coated tablets: 125, 250, and 500 mg.

Depakene® 250 mg capsules; long-acting formulation 500 mg (valproate and valproic acid).

• • • • • • •
DIAGNOSIS

There are several steps in the diagnosis of seizures.

1. Recognition that an event is epileptic in nature.
    *   Clinical features: Epileptic seizures are generally brief events usually unwitnessed by medical personnel. They must be reconstructed like a puzzle, using pieces obtained from the history. The quality of the history obtained from patients, relatives, or witnesses may be extremely variable. New features may surface when the history is taken on several occasions. Miming of the seizure by witnesses may reveal typical clinical features of the seizure.
    *   EEG: Interictal EEG scalp recordings are standard. Recordings performed during a seizure may confirm a diagnosis; the absence of EEG abnormalities in the interictal period does not, however, exclude it.
2. Finding the underlying cause of the seizure. A seizure is a symptom, not a diagnosis (Hughlings Jackson). Determining the cause depends on the history and clinical examination, and on ancillary measures such as blood chemistry, underlying biological and metabolic abnormalities, EEG patterns, head CT, or MRI scans. Neuroimaging is an essential investigation for seizures without evident etiology. However, repeated CT scans are not indicated for most epilepsies.
3. Defining the seizure type and determining the seizure focus, if any.
    *   Clinical aspects: The history may be suggestive of particular seizure types.
    *   EEG: Interictal information may be nonlocalizing or misleading. The ultimate goal (often not feasable) is to capture a typical seizure. This may be attempted by routine, outpatient recordings using scalp electrodes or semi-invasive electrodes (e.g., sphenoidal), or if specifically indicated, inpatient prolonged video/EEG recording.
    *   Imaging: SPECT and PET scans may show zones of hypometabolism corresponding to epileptogenic zones.
    *   Magnetoencephalography (MEG) (see this heading).
4. Characterization of specific epilepsy syndromes: This may provide guidance for prognosis and management. The recognition of an epilepsy syndrome is usually easier than defining the seizure type.
    Epilepsy invariably has a clinical expression. There is no such thing as "latent epilepsy, subclinical epilepsy, or larval epilepsy." Whatever the EEG abnormality, a diagnosis of epilepsy cannot be made without seizures.

• • • • • •
DIAMOX® (SEE ACETAZOLAMIDE)

Tablets 125 mg and 250 mg scored; capsules 500 mg sustained-release.

• • • • • •
DIAZEPAM (VALIUM®)

Diazepam is one of the drugs of first choice in the treatment of status epilepticus, serial seizures, prolonged seizures, or febrile convulsions.

Mode of administration: direct slow IV infusion over 2–5 minutes because of the problems of precipitation within IV bags or tubes; rectal administration of the solution. It may be given repeatedly every 20–30 minutes until seizures stop; maximal dose in 24 hours: 100–120 mg. Decreasing doses (given orally) may be given over subsequent days.

Reference

Levy RH, Dreifuss FE, Mattson RH, Meldrum BS, Penry JK (eds.). *Antiepileptic drugs,* 3rd edition. New York: Raven Press, 1989.

• • • • • •
DILANTIN®; PHENYTOIN IV
(SEE ALSO PHENYTOIN)

Ampules of 250 mg/5 ml. Available in hospital pharmacies.

This parenteral form may be used in status epilepticus and eclampsia. The loading dose of 16–20 mg/kg is given by slow intravenous infusion at 25–50 mg/minute while monitoring blood pressure and ECG.

Reference

Ramsay RF. Pharmacokinetics and clinical use of parental phenytoin, phenobarbital and paraldehyde. *Epilepsia* 1989;30(Suppl 2): S1–S3.

• • • • • •
DIONES (OXAZOLINE-DIONES)

Diones were the first drugs used in the treatment of typical absence seizures. They have since been supplanted by ethosuximide and valproate.

• • • • • •
DISCHARGE (EPILEPTIC)

"A neuronal discharge resulting from the simultaneous activation of a large number of neurons" (1).

Marked neuronal depolarization in the epileptic focus spreads and depolarizes neighboring neurons by synaptic and extrasynaptic mechanisms. It is spread by axons to distant or nearby cortical structures via intracortical association pathways, commissures, cortico-thalamo-cortical or cortico-subcortical commissures (2). Inhibitory mechanisms mediate the end of the discharge.

- There is no absolute correlation between the seizure focus and the clinical correlate. If the focus resides in a cortically "silent" area, the initial discharge may be asymptomatic. The first signs or symptoms of a seizure will be those brought about by involvement of more distant areas.
- Although slow direct spread frequently occurs, more rapid involvement of distant structures via long pathways can occur.
- The propagation of the seizure discharge depends on the starting point. Frontal discharges spread more rapidly to the contralateral hemisphere than to the extrafrontal ones.
- A seizure is rarely the result of a single discharge with spread in one direction. Spread along multiple axes is more common. Depth recordings illustrate the variability of spread of the seizure discharge from seizure to seizure (3).
- The clinical features of the seizures may remain relatively stereotyped because of spread preferentially along certain pathways.
- There is no simple correlation between seizures and the surface EEG. Certain seizures localized on the internal or inferior aspects of the hemispheres may not reach the scalp (hence the need for semi-invasive electrodes, such as sphenoidal electrodes, or invasive electrodes, such as depth wires or grids); others have such a rapid spread that the first scalp EEG recordings show a widespread field of distribution.

References

1. Gastaut H. *Dictionary of epilepsy. Part I: Definitions.* Geneva: World Health Organization, 1973.
2. Spencer SS. Corpus callosum section and other disconnection procedures for medically intractable epilepsy. *Epilepsia* 1988;29(Suppl):S85–S99.
3. Talairach J, Bancaud J. Stereotaxic approach to epilepsy. Methodology of anatomo-functional stereotaxic investigations. *Prog Neurol Surg* 1973;5:297–354.

• • • • • •
DOWN (SYNDROME) (TRISOMY 21) (MONGOLISM)

In Down syndrome, seizures rarely occur in childhood (1–2%) (1), but may occur as infantile spasms (2). The treatment of hypotonia with 5–hydroxytryptophan is believed to be responsible for their appearance (3). Seizures are more frequent in adults (12%) (4).

References

1. Tatsuno M, Hayashi M, Yawamato H, Suzuki Y, Kuroki Y. Epilepsy in childhood. Down syndrome. *Brain Dev* 1984;6:37–44.
2. Pollack MA, Golden GS, Schmidt R, Davis JA, Leeds N. Infantile spasms in Down syndrome: a report of 5 cases and review of the literature. *Ann Neurol* 1978;3:406–408.
3. Coleman M. Infantile spasms associated with 5 hydroxytryptophan administration in patients with Down syndrome. *Neurology* 1971;21:911–19.
4. Veall RM. The prevalence of epilepsy among mongols related to age. *J Ment Defic Res* 1974;18:99–106.

• • • • • •
DRIVING

1. The potential danger of driving for patients with epilepsy:
    • Patients with epilepsy have a slightly higher risk for traffic accidents than the baseline population (1). From 9–17% of patients with epilepsy have had an accident (2); the relative risk is approximately twice baseline. In relative terms, many other factors, such as young age, old age, male sex, and alcohol consumption, exert more of a risk on the driving accident rate than does a history of seizures (3).
    • At greatest risk are:
        Patients with tonic-clonic seizures (2), complex partial seizures (4,5), and frequent seizures (5);
        Patients with poorly controlled seizures, noncompliant, depressed, or socially maladjusted patients.
    • Accidents are serious in 2.5% (5) to 10% (4) of cases.
2. The law:
    • Legal restrictions vary from state to state and country to country. The guiding principle has been that individuals likely to have seizures should not drive. The time elapsed since the last seizure has been used as an index of likelihood of subsequent seizures. In some places, the required seizure-free interval may

be as short as three months after the last seizure, and others may require indefinite suspension. Recent trends have developed in the direction of shorter seizure-free intervals, and individualized reviews of factors (exclusively nocturnal seizures, prolonged and consistent auras, non-recurring precipitants) that may permit safe driving. Commercial driver's licenses are usually regulated under stricter standards than are individual licences. In most areas, it is the obligation of the patient, rather than the physician, to inform the Bureau of Motor Vehicles, but a few states in the United States still require physician reporting (1).

3. Reporting requirements:
   - Reporting compliance is a major problem; 86% of patients with epilepsy who drive and have had an accident did not inform the Bureau of Motor Vehicles of their illness when taking the driver's test (5). If seizures are in remission, a driver's permit may be obtained.
   - Advice given on driving depends on prognosis, which in turn is dependent on the underlying cause of seizures, their frequency, whether they involve alteration of consciousness, compliance, and the patient's occupation (6).
   - An open and frank discussion between patients and doctors may be of greater value than merely filling out a questionnaire at the time of application for driver's license (6,7). Physicians should in all cases inform patients of the risks of driving with seizures, and document their discussions in the medical record. The ethical dilemmas in epilepsy and driving involve the interests of the patient and the interest of society (8).

References

1. Grattan E, Jeffcoate GO. Medical factors and road accidents. *Br Med J* 1968;1:75.
2. Hormia A. Does epilepsy mean higher susceptibility to traffic accidents? *Acta Psychiat Scand* 1961;36 (Suppl 150):210–12.
3. Krumholz A, Fisher RS, Lesser RP, Hauser WA. Driving and epilepsy: a review and reappraisal. *JAMA* 1991;265:622–26.
4. Gastaut H, Zifkin BG. The risk of automobile accidents with seizures occurring while driving: relation to seizure type. *Neurology* 1987;37:1613–19.
5. Van Der Lugt PJM. Is an application form useful to select patients with epilepsy who may drive? *Epilepsia* 1975;16:743–46.
6. Jones MW, Bruni J. A cross Canada survey of neurologists on controversial issues in epilepsy management. *Can J Neurol Sci* 1989;16:365.
7. Harvey P, Hopkins A. Views of British neurologists on epilepsy, driving and the law. *Lancet* 1983;401–404.
8. Ozund J. Ethical dilemmas in epilepsy and driving. *J Epilepsy* 1993;6:185–88.

• • • • • • •
DROP ATTACKS; FALLS (EPILEPTIC)

Falls are frequent during generalized tonic-clonic seizures, myoclonic seizures, atonic and tonic seizures (1). Occasionally, falls are seen during absence seizures (see Absence). Falls may also be seen in partial seizures arising from the temporal lobe (2) or frontal lobe (see Frontal (S,E); Temporal lobe (S,E)).

(See also Atonic (S); Arrhythmia; Autonomic (S).)

References

1. Egli M, Mothersill I, O'Kane M, O'Kane F. The axial spasm. The predominant type of drop seizure in patients with secondary generalized epilepsy. *Epilepsia* 1985;26:401–25.
2. Jacome DE. Temporal lobe syncope: clinical variants. *Clin EEG* 1989;20:58–65.

• • • • • • •
DUPUYTREN'S (DISEASE)

Dupuytren's disease consists of fibrosis and contraction of the palmar aponeurosis; it is occasionally associated with long-term phenobarbital treatment. The contracture may improve with discontinuation of the AED. It may coexist with other connective tissue diseases: plantar fibromas (Ledderhosen sydrome), juxtarticular nodules, Peyronie's disease, scapulo-humeral peri-arthritis.

Reference

Mattson RH, Cramer JA, McCutchen CB, and the Veterans Administration Epilepsy Cooperative Study Group. Barbiturate-related connective tissue disorders. *Arch Intern Med* 1989;149:911–14

• • • • • • •
DYSKINESIAS

Dyskinesias may be seen with phenytoin (1,2) and occasionally with carbamazepine (3) or phenobarbital (4). They consist predominantly of buccofacial dyskinesias with choreic, athetotic, or ballistic movements of the limbs appearing either uni- or bilaterally. There may also be dystonic movements of the trunk and limbs with asterixis. Typically, the abnormal movements persist from several hours to several days and may be intermittent or (rarely) permanent. They appear most frequently in patients with encephalopathy when high AED levels are reached, but may also be seen in the so-called therapeutic range.

References

1. Dravet C, Dalla-Bernadina B, Mesdjian E, Galland MC, Roger J. Dyskinésies paroxystiques au cours des traitements par la diphénylhydantöine. *Rev Neurol* (Paris) 1980;136:1–14.
2. Roulet E, Koskas P, Mahieux F, Marteau R. Dyskinésies aigues récidivantes seules manifestations d'un surdosage en phenytöine. *Rev Neurol* (Paris) 1987;143:836–38.
3. Joyce RP, Gunderson CH. Carbamazepine-induced orofacial dyskinesia. *Neurology* 1972;26:78–84.
4. Wiznitzer M, Younkin D. Phenobarbital-induced dyskinesia in a neurologically-impaired child. *Neurology* 1984;34:1600–1601.

●●●●●●
DYSMNESTIC (SEIZURES)

These partial seizures produce distortions of perception and memory. This may induce the feeling that on-going events have already been seen (déjà vu), already heard (déjà entendu), or, more frequently, already lived (déjà vecu).

- There is a fleeting sensation of disorientation, strangeness, or a new experience previously unseen, unheard of, or unlived.
- There may be "panoramic" vision in which the patient experiences episodes in his or her life in rapid succession (1).
- Ecmnestic hallucinations occur in which the patient re-experiences minutiae of previous experiences (1).

According to some authors, these features are due to the simultaneous ictal involvement of Ammon's horn and the external temporal cortex (2) and may be regarded as hallucinatory, ideational, dysmnestic illusions. Some seizures consist of recurrent episodes of anterograde amnesia, somewhat resembling transient global amnesia (3).

References

1. Gastaut H, Broughton R. *Epileptic seizures, clinical and electrographic features, diagnosis and treatment.* Springfield: Charles C. Thomas, 1972.
2. Bancaud J. Sémiologie clinique des crises épileptiques d'origine temporale. *Rev Neurol* (Paris) 1987;143:392–400.
3. Pritchard PB, Holmstrom VL, Roitzsch JC, Giacinto BS. Epileptic amnesia attacks: benefit from antiepileptic drugs. *Neurology* 1985;35:1188–89.

• • • • • • •
DYSPHASIC (SEIZURES)

Dysphasic seizures involve the impairment of language function due to epileptic discharges in the region of the inferior frontal lobe (expressive aphasia), or the temporoparietal region of the dominant hemisphere (1,2). Accurate determination of aphasia in partial seizures is difficult: (a) because of its brevity; (b) because ictal involvement of other cortical regions may bring about speech arrest or vocalization that are not truly aphasic in nature; (c) because expressive and comprehensive difficulties may be due to impairment of consciousness. Postictal dysphasia is easier to determine (3) and the coexistence of other features of temporal lobe disturbance is helpful in diagnosis (4).

References

1. Ardila A, Lopez MV. Paroxysmal aphasias. *Epilepsia* 1988;29:630–34.
2. Koerner M, Laxer KD. Ictal speech, postical language dysfunction, and seizure lateralization. *Neurology* 1988;38:634–36.
3. Gabr M, Lüders H, Dinner D, Morris H, Wyllie E. Speech manifestations in lateralization of temporal lobe seizures. *Ann Neurol* 1989;25:82–87.
4. Kanemoto K, Janz D. The temporal sequence of aura-sensations in patients with complex focal seizures with particular attention to ictal aphasia. *J Neurol Neurosurg Psychiatry* 1989:52:52–56.

$\mathcal{E}$

••••••
ECLAMPSIA

Eclampsia is characterized by the appearance of seizures or coma in a pregnant woman (usually after the 20th week), without coincident neurological disease such as epilepsy. Seizures usually occur with preeclampsia, which includes one or more of the following: proteinuria (at least 5 g/24 hours); widespread peripheral and facial edema; persistent hypertension above baseline (at least 20 mm Hg systolic, or 10 mm Hg diastolic for more than 4 hours). Typically, single seizures, repeated seizures, or status epilepticus appear after the 28th week of pregnancy, during labor, or in the 24 hours after delivery. The pathophysiology is unknown, but a hypertensive encephalopathy, cerebral edema, cerebral vasospasm. and loss of cerebrovascular autoregulation are clinical features. Therapy is aimed at:

- Delivery of the baby;
- Prevention of arterial hypertension during pregnancy, especially near delivery, e.g., with hydralazine;
- The control and prophylaxis of seizures, typically using rapidly acting AEDs such as intravenous benzodiazepines and/or phenytoin.

In the United States, magnesium sulfate is widely used by obstetricians for preeclampsia and eclampsia (1), although obstetricians and neurologists worldwide and neurologists in the United States do not clearly endorse its use for the seizure control (2–4). Eclampsia is no more frequent in epileptics than in nonepileptics and does not increase the risk of developing epilepsy.

References

1. Pritchard JA, Cunningham FG, Pritchard SA. The Parkland Memorial Hospital protocol for treatment of eclampsia: evaluation of 245 cases. *Am J Obstet Gynecol* 1984;148:951–63.
2. Dommisse J. Phenytoin sodium and magnesium sulphate in the management of eclampsia. *Br J Obstet Gynaecol* 1990;97:104–107.
3. Kaplan PW, Lesser RP, Fisher RS, Repke JT, Hanley DF. No, magnesium sulfate should not be used in treating eclamptic seizures. Controversies in neurology. *Arch Neurol* 1988;45:1361–64.
4. Kaplan PW, Lesser RP, Fisher RS, Repke JT, Hanley DF. Magnesium sulfate in the treatment of eclamptic seizures. *Arch Neurol* 1990;47:1031–32.

• • • • • • •
EEG (ELECTROENCEPHALOGRAPHY)

Electroencephalography consists of the analog display (traditionally on paper; more recently on a video monitor) of an amplified electrical signal derived from cerebral neuronal activity.

EEG rhythms have been divided into different frequency bands: Delta frequency band (under 4 Hz); theta frequency band (4 to under 8 Hz); alpha frequency band (8 to 13 Hz); and beta frequency band (over 13 Hz). These divisions are somewhat arbitrary as most EEGs contain mixtures of frequencies spanning these categories. Classification into these bands facilitates the determination of normal and abnormal waves in the clinical EEG, since frequency provides one of the important criteria for evaluation of normality (1): waves above 13 Hz are fast waves and are usually normal; waves under 8 Hz are slow waves and may be abnormal.

EEG recordings are of prime importance in epileptology, providing information used in the diagnosis, classification, prognosis, and management of patients with epilepsy.

Standard scalp EEG recordings are subject to a number of shortcomings:

- they record signals at a point distant from the source, leading to signal distortion;
- a deep focus may not reach the scalp;
- recording time is limited and might miss events under investigation;
- interpretation of the tracing is subjective and generally nonspecific.

Some of these problems may be minimized by:

- repeated, more prolonged recordings;
- the use of ambulatory EEG;
- activation techniques to bring out abnormal or epileptic events (hyperventilation, intermittent photic stimulation, sleep, or sleep deprivation).

For children under three to four years of age, a sleep recording is essential as it may show paroxysmal abnormalities not seen during wakefulness. The recording of a period of sleep may be the only means of reaching a diagnosis (e.g., spike and slow wave abnormalities during slow-wave sleep in ESES syndrome);

To minimize the subjective aspect of EEG interpretation, a widely accepted standardization has been developed, and quantitative measurements are now available. Topographical mapping is visually attractive, but is not yet accepted for diagnostic purposes and remains a research tool.

Reference

Spehlman R. *EEG primer.* New York: Elsevier Biomedical Press, 1985.

• • • • • •

ELDERLY, LATE-LIFE ONSET (EPILEPSY)

Most epilepsy begins in childhood or adolescence. Epidemiological studies of epilepsies beginning after 17 (1), 25 (2), or 45 (3) years show these groups of epilepsies to be heterogeneous. Common etiologies in this group include trauma and alcoholism in adults younger than 50 years, and cerebrovascular accidents in those older than 50 years.

Any epilepsy beginning after the age of 60 years may be considered epilepsy of late-life onset. The incidence of seizures beginning after 60 years of age has probably been underestimated. Recent estimates suggest rates as high as 104–127/100,000/year (4,5). Seizures are single in 60% of cases and recurrent in 34% of cases (5). Thus, the incidence of recurrence after a first late-life onset seizure is similar to the recurrence rate in a younger population.

Seizures of late-life onset are more frequent in males and in the 70–79 year age group (4,5). Partial seizures predominate, particularly motor. The cause of seizures is unknown in 25–50% (6). Spike wave stupor is not rare (7); generalized seizures during sleep are common, representing about 20% of the epilepsies in the elderly. Seizures, in general, are mild, infrequent, or even isolated events (4).

Because of altered metabolism in the aged, therapy must be modified. The physician should prescribe smaller doses of AEDs and provide more frequent reevaluation. Aged patients are subject to the problems of polypharmacy and drug interactions (8).

References

1. Forsgren L. Prospective incidence study and clinical characterization of seizures in newly referred adults. *Epilepsia* 1990;31:292–301.
2. Mouritzen Dam A, Fuglsang-Frederiksen A, Svarre-Olsen O, Dam M. Late-onset epilepsy: etiologies, types of seizure, and value of clinical investigation. EEG, and computerized tomography scan. *Epilepsia* 1985;26:227–31.
3. Hyllested K, Pakenberg H. Prognosis in epilepsy of late onset. *Neurology* 1963;13:641–44.
4. Lühdorf K, Jensen LK, Plesner AM. Epilepsy in the elderly: incidence, social function and disability. *Epilepsia* 1986;27:135–41.
5. Loiseau J, Loiseau P, Duché B, Guyot M, Dartigues JF, Aublet B. A survey of epileptic disorders in Southwest France: seizures in elderly patients. *Ann Neurol* 1990;28:232–37.

6.   Lühdorf K, Jensen LK, Plesner AM. Etiology of seizures in the elderly. *Epilepsia* 1986;27:458–63.
7.   Thomas P, Beaumanoir A, Genton P, Dolisi C, Chatel M. 'De novo' absence status of late onset: report of 11 cases. *Neurology* 1992;42:104–10.
8.   Lühdorf K, Jensen LK, Plesner AM. Epilepsy in the elderly: prognosis. *Acta Neurol Scand* 1986;74:409–15.

● ● ● ● ● ● ●

ELECTROCONVULSIVE THERAPY

Electroconvulsive therapy is a controversial, but medically accepted, procedure for treatment of severe depression (1). ECT overlaps the subject of epilepsy in several ways. First, electroconvulsive therapy is a model of generalized tonic-clonic epileptic seizures. Some phenomena that occur after seizures can more conveniently be studied after ECT. Increases of serum prolactin, for example, have been evaluated after ECT (2).

ECT is also particularly difficult to induce in individuals who are being treated for epilepsy. Many of these individuals are on anticonvulsant medications. Pharmaceutical companies screen AEDs in an electroshock animal model of epilepsy (3). It, therefore, may be necessary to reduce or withhold seizure medications for a day or two prior to ECT in order to obtain a satisfactory electroconvulsive response.

Some investigators have considered the influence of ECT on underlying tendency for epilepsy. A few have suggested that ECT exerts a chronic antiepileptic effect (4,5). Other investigators have considered that the incidence of epilepsy might increase after ECT (6) or that status epilepticus might result from a treatment (7). A more recent study of the incidence of epilepsy following ECT by Blackwood and colleagues (8) found no significant increase in seizures for the year after receiving ECT in 166 patients. Therefore, it appears that precipitation of seizures by ECT is a rare event.

In summary, ECT is a psychiatric modality of treatment for depression that involves intentional induction of an electrographic seizure. It may be difficult to induce such seizures in patients taking anticonvulsant medications. The role of ECT in decreasing or increasing seizures has been raised anecdotally, but no evidence for such a relationship has yet been established.

References

1.   Crowe RR. Electroconvulsive therapy—current therapy. *N Engl J Med* 1984;311:163–67.
2.   Aroto M, Erdosa, Kurka M, et al. Studies on the prolactin response induced by electroconvulsive therapy in schizophrenics. *Acta Psychiatr Scand* 1980;61:239–44.

3. Fisher RS. Animal models of the epilepsies. *Brain Res Rev* 1989;14:25–78.
4. Wolff GE. Electro-convulsive treatment—a help for epileptics. *Med Prac Dig Treat* 1956;7:1791–93.
5. Post RM, Putnam F, Uhde TW, Weiss SRB. Electroconvulsive therapy as an anti-convulsant: implications for its mechanism of action in affective illness. *Ann NY Acad Sci* 1986;462:376–88.
6. Blumenthal IJ. Spontaneous seizures and related electroencephalographic findings following shock therapy. *J Nerv Ment Dis* 1955;122:581–88.
7. Roith AI. Status epilepticus as a complication of ECT. *Brit J Clin Pract* 1959;13:711–12.
8. Blackwood DHR, Cull RE, Freeman CPL, Evans JI, Modsley C. A study of the incidence of epilepsy following ECT. *J Neurol Neurosurg Psychiatry* 1980; 43:1098–1102.

● ● ● ● ● ●

ELECTRODES, SUBDURAL (EPIDURAL)

Subdural electrodes are used to localize an epileptic focus prior to surgery for seizures and to localize normal areas of cortical function in a given patient (1–4). A grid of electrodes is placed over areas of cortex thought to contain the seizure focus. Placement of a grid enables uninterrupted EEG recording for several days and can be used to provide information about normal cortical activities (e.g., language, motor function) by means of cortical stimulation while these functions are tested. Depending on the requirements of a particular patient, a certain number of electrodes, grids, or electrode strips may be passed through a bone flap or burr hole and placed over one lobe, one hemisphere, or on several lobes of both hemispheres (3,4).

The results obtained are superior to scalp EEG, allowing precise evaluation of hemispheric convexities and some areas in cerebral fissures. In expert hands, there are few complications (e.g., infections, bleeding). In some cases, certain epileptic foci (within the amygdala and hippocampus) are less accessible. Thus, EEGs with depth electrodes may still be required; both methods may be used together.

References

1. Goldring S, Gregoric EM. Surgical management of epilepsy using epidural recordings to localize the seizure focus. *J Neurosurg* 1984;60:457–66.
2. Wyllie E, Lüders H, Morris HH, Lesser RP, Dinner DS, Rothner AD, Erenberg G, Cruse R, Friedman D. Subdural electrodes in the evaluation for epilepsy surgery in children and adults. *Neuropediatrics* 1988;19:80–86.
3. Kaplan PW, Lesser RP. Long-term EEG monitoring. In: Daly DD, Pedley TA (eds.). *Current practice of clinical electroencephalography,* 2nd edition. New York: Raven Press, 1990.

4. Kaplan PW, Lesser RP. Prolonged extracranial and intracranial in-patient monitoring. In: Wada JA, Ellingson RJ (eds.). *Clinical neurophysiology handbook of epilepsy, EEG handbook* (Revised series, Vol. 4) Part II, 121–54. Amsterdam: Elsevier Science Publishers, 1990.

● ● ● ● ● ● ●

EMPLOYMENT

Employment statistics for patients with epilepsy have shown that 27% are professionals or in business; 28% are skilled workers or office workers; 20% are salesmen; 25% are unskilled laborers; taxi, automobile, and truck drivers constitute 4% (1). Despite problems during schooling, patients with epilepsy in childhood may have normal professional development (2), although scholastic success usually determines the ultimate level of employment (3).

Seventy-three to eighty percent of patients with epilepsy work full-time (1–3), but in 40% of patients, the level of skill required at the job is often less than the patient's potential. There are frequent, recurrent job changes requiring decreasing levels of skill and job terminations because of the occurrence of seizures in the work-place. Reasons include seizures, subnormal IQ, poor neuropsychological test results, lack of self-confidence, diminished motivation at work, social ostracism, behavioral problems, and lack of initial professional qualifications (3). Adaptation may thus be difficult (4–8).

Accidents in the work-place are no more frequent in patients with epilepsy than in persons without epilepsy (7,10).

To promote the appropriate occupational match, patients should be individually evaluated for particular employment opportunities using psychological, aptitude, and work-place assessments. A scale for occupational levels of risk has been developed by Goodglass et al. (4):

- Low risk situations: risks must be kept at a minimum, possibly with work at home, or in a protected environment away from machines or moving parts. There should be immediate access to care when seizures arise. Work should be under conditions in which brief pauses due to seizures do not affect productivity.
- Moderate level of risks allowed: jobs requiring interactions with the public. Patients may have a supervisory responsibility as long as continuous surveillance is not an integral part of the work
- Large risks permitted: for work at heights, involving a driver's permit (never for an airplane, bus, or other means of public transport), and for jobs requiring responsibility for the security and well-being of others.

References

1. Lennox WG, Cobb S. Employment of epileptics. *Indust Med Surg* 1942;2:571–75.
2. Schneider JW, Conrad P. In the closet with illness: epilepsy, stigma potential and information control. *Social Problems* 1980;28:32–44.
3. Rodin EP, Lennick P, Dendrill Y, Lin Y. Vocational and educational problems of epileptic patients. *Epilepsia* 1972;13:149–60.
4. Goodglass H, Morgan M, Folsom AT, Quadfasel FA. Epileptic seizures. Psychological factors and occupational adjustment. *Epilepsia* 1963;4:322–41.
5. Hull RP, Haerer AT. Follow-up of epileptic outpatients. *Southern Med* 1973;66:292–96.
6. Lennox WG, Markham GH. Sociopsychological treatment of epilepsy. *JAMA* 1953;152:1690–95.
7. Levin R, Banks S, Berg B. Psychosocial dimensions of epilepsy: a review of the literature. *Epilepsia* 1988;29:805–16.
8. Pond DA, Bidwell BH. A survey of epilepsy in fourteen general practices. II: Social and psychological aspects. *Epilepsia* 1959;1:285–95.
9. Wilson WP, Stewart LF, Parker JB. A study of the socio-economic effects of epilepsy. *Epilepsia* 1959;1:300–15.
10. Lione JG. Convulsive disorders in a working population. *J Occup Med* 1961; 3:369–73.

• • • • • •

ENCEPHALITIS/ENCEPHALITIDES

ACUTE ENCEPHALITIDES

Viral encephalitis may cause seizures in two clinical contexts:

• in the acute phase of the illness, regardless of age or virus involved;
• after a variable latent period. Viral encephalitis is reported to account for 1–13% of childhood epilepsies and 3–5% of adult epilepsies (1). Epilepsy appears somewhere along the course of 10–20% of encephalitides (2); the risk of epileptic sequelae is twofold if seizures supervene in the acute phase (2). Epilepsy generally follows directly after the illness (2), but occasionally months or as much as 5 years may pass before the onset of seizures. Seizures are usually partial.

CHRONIC VIRAL INFECTIONS

These include:

• latent viral infections with acute exacerbations in which the virus often can not be isolated (herpes); chronic infections in which the virus is invariably present (CMV, Epstein-Barr, hepatitis B, measles, and chicken pox) (3);

- slow virus infections, responsible for progressive deterioration as seen in subacute sclerosing panencephalitis and unusual agents (prions).

References

1. Pedersen E. Postencephalitic epilepsy. *Epilepsia* 1964;5:43–50.
2. Annegers JF, Hauser WA, Beghi E, Nicolosi A, Kurland LT. The risk of unprovoked seizures after encephalitis and meningitis. *Neurology* 1988;38:1407–10.
3. Russell J, Fisher M, Zivin JA, Sullivan J, Drachman DA. Status epilepticus and Epstein-Barr virus encephalopathy. *Arch Neurol* 1985;42;789–92.

● ● ● ● ● ●
ENCEPHALOPATHIES

This general term refers to diffuse cerebral abnormalities that are mostly noninfective in nature: anoxic, metabolic, toxic, degenerative encephalopathies, etc.

Seizures may appear during the course of these disorders, usually in the early stages. These symptomatic epilepsies are mostly caused by the underlying encephalopathic process.

Chronic epilepsies may result from progressive or static encephalopathies. The encephalopathic process may dominate the clinical picture to such an extent that the term "epileptic encephalopathy" has been used to refer to the West and Lennox-Gastaut syndromes.

● ● ● ● ● ●
EPIDEMIOLOGY OF THE EPILEPSIES

Descriptive epidemiological studies have provided information regarding frequency, clinical expression, and distribution, as well as the incidence, prevalence, and mortality rate of the epilepsies. These studies enable assessment of the susceptibility of an individual to the disease and lead to possible hypotheses regarding risk factors.

Analytic epidemiology is used to confirm hypotheses based on results obtained from descriptive epidemiology. It enables the determination of risk factors for the appearance of epilepsy.

Further strategies can then be developed for cost-benefit assessment, evaluation of the effects of therapy, research, patient and family education, teaching, etc.

Disparate results obtained in different studies of epilepsy may be due to the inherent bias involved in all epidemiological studies; more specifically, those related to epilepsy: e.g., the exact definition of the disorder, the means by which seizures were identified, the source of case ascertainment (e.g., community vs. medical centers), and the case identification of seizure disorders (febrile or afebrile seizures or both; symptomatic and/or cryptogenic epilepsies; both isolated and recurrent seizures or recurrent seizures only; acute symptomatic seizures and unprovoked seizures, or unprovoked seizures only).

Reference

Hauser WA, Hesdorffer, DC. *Epilepsy: frequency, causes, and consequences.* New York: Demos Publications, 1990.

• • • • • •
EPIGASTRIC (SEIZURES)

The seizures consist of a rising epigastric discomfort. They often precede complex partial seizures and have been correlated to a mesial temporal focus. (see also Abdominal (E); Amygdala)

• • • • • •
EPILEPSY

"A chronic brain disorder of various etiologies characterized by recurrent seizures due to excessive discharge of cerebral neurons, associated with a variety of clinical and laboratory manifestations. A single epileptic seizure and occasional epileptic seizures therefore do not constitute epilepsy, nor does the more or less frequent repetition of epileptic seizures during an acute illness."

Epilepsy is thus defined as a disorder in which repeated seizures arise spontaneously in the same patient. This definition, however, is unclear with regard to certain situations, e.g., patients with one seizure who receive AED therapy; patients with seizures 10 to 20 years apart; and patients without seizures for a number of years.

Reference

Gastaut H. *Dictionary of epilepsy. Part 1: Definitions.* Geneva: World Health Organization, 1973.

• • • • • •

EPILEPSY WITH CONTINUOUS SPIKES AND WAVES DURING SLOW SLEEP/ESES (ELECTRICAL STATUS EPILEPTICUS DURING SLOW SLEEP)

This rare syndrome, described in 1971 (1), occurs only in children around 4–14 years of age and is associated with continuous runs of bilateral synchronous spike and slow wave discharges during slow wave sleep. Multiple seizure types may occur (2).

Spike and slow wave discharges occur typically as bilaterally synchronous and symmetrical 2.5 per second high amplitude discharges in prolonged runs. Spike and slow wave discharges should be seen during 85% of slow wave sleep (2). Epileptiform activity disappears during rapid eye movement (REM) sleep. Aside from the striking seizure discharges, normal electroencephalographic sleep patterns are preserved.

Seizures that are associated with this syndrome are of several types (2): unilateral seizures, partial motor seizures arising from sleep, tonic-clonic generalized seizures, myoclonic seizures, atonic seizures with falls, or absence seizures. Seizures remit between the ages of 10 and 15 years, and spike and slow wave discharges disappear between 8 and 13 years. Marked neuropsychological abnormalities with language problems have been noted, especially with a previous history of psychomotor retardation.

Differential Diagnosis: The differential diagnosis includes benign partial epilepsies of childhood, especially when centrotemporal spike and slow wave discharges increase during slow wave sleep. Atypical forms of benign partial epilepsy without cognitive impairment (3) are difficult to distinguish from this syndrome.

The Lennox-Gastaut syndrome may have similar features, particularly when atonic seizures and psychomotor problems are present. The Landau-Kleffner syndrome of acquired epileptic aphasia (4–6) can present with copious spike-wave discharges during sleep and overlap the clinical EEG picture of ESES (see also Aphasia, epileptic).

None of the standard AEDs are consistently effective in ESES. ACTH has been reported to diminish spike and slow wave activity and improve language functions.

References

1. Patry G, Lyagoubi S, Tassinari CA. Subclinical "electrical status epilepticus" induced by sleep in children. *Arch Neurol* 1971;24:242–52.
2. Tassinari CA, Bureau M, Dravet C, Dalla-Bernardina B, Roger J. Epilepsy with continuous spikes and waves during slow sleep. In: Roger J, Dravet C, Bureau M, Dreifuss FE, Perret A, Wolf P (eds.). *Epileptic syndromes in infancy, childhood and adolescence,* 2nd edition. London: John Libbey Eurotext, 1992:245–56.

3. Aicardi J, Chevrie JJ. Atypical benign partial epilepsy of childhood. *Dev Med Child Neurol* 1983;24:281–92.
4. Beaumanoir A. The Landau-Kleffner syndrome. In: Roger J, Dravet C, Bureau M, Dreifuss FE, Perret A, Wolf P (eds.). *Epileptic syndromes in infancy, childhood and adolescence,* 2nd edition. London: John Libbey Eurotext, 1992:231–43.
5. Kellerman K. Recurrent aphasia with subclinical bioelectric status epilepticus during sleep. *Eur J Pediatr* 1978:128:207–12.
6. Hirsch E, Marescaux C, Maguet P, et al. Landau-Kleffner syndrome: a clinical and EEG study of five cases. *Epilepsia* 1990:31;756–67.

• • • • • • •
EPILEPTIC ENCEPHALOPATHY

"Epileptic encephalopathy" is a term that has been used in reference to two conditions:

1. Certain cryptogenic or symptomatic generalized epilepsies, e.g., West syndrome and Lennox-Gastaut syndrome (in which the seizures are but one manifestation of severe neurological impairment).
2. A dementia-like picture seen in some patients taking certain AEDs (1–4).

References

1. Vallarta JM, Bell DB, Reichert A, Wash B. Progressive encephalopathy due to chronic hydantoin intoxication. *Am J Dis Child* 1974;128:27–34.
2. Meistrup-Larsen KI, Hermann S, Permin H. Chronic diphenyl-hydantoin encephalopathy in mentally retarded children and adolescent with severe epilepsy. *Acta Neurol Scand* 1979;60:50–55.
3. Ambrosetto G, Tassinari CA, Baruzzi A, Lugaresi E. Phenytoin encephalopathy as probable idiosyncratic reaction: case report. *Epilepsia* 1977;18:405–408.
4. Zaret BS, Cohen RA. Reversible valproic acid-induced dementia: a case report. *Epilepsia* 1986;27:234–40.

• • • • • •
EPILEPTIC EQUIVALENT

This term is no longer used; previously it represented episodic disturbances in patients with generalized tonic-clonic seizures believed to be "equivalents" of those seizures. Among them were:

• clearly epileptic phenomena such as partial seizures;
• nonepileptic phenomena such as migraines, asthma, anger;
• enuresis which may be epileptic or nonepileptic.

● ● ● ● ● ● ●
EPILEPTIC (SEIZURES)

"A seizure can be defined as a paroxysmal disorder of the central nervous system (CNS) characterized by abnormal cerebral neuronal discharge with or without a loss of consciousness" (1). "An epileptic seizure may be defined as a paroxysmal discharge of cerebral neurones sufficient to cause clinically detectable events that are apparent either to the subject or to an observer" (2).

A seizure is always a clinical event. Paroxysmal EEG abnormalities without a clinical correlate are not seizures. All the same, isolated paroxysms seen interictally may be recorded with scalp EEG and may resemble those seen during seizures. There is no clear distinction between epileptiform discharges and electrographic seizures. The final determination depends on how the EEG and clinical manifestations are viewed. During neuropsychological testing, it has been shown that bursts of epileptiform discharges (recorded on EEG) may disrupt cognitive functions (3–5).

The first international classification of epileptic seizures was initially proposed in 1970 and further modified in 1981. Certain terms changed meaning. Most partial seizures consist of a succession of signs and symptoms. Current practice is to apply to the seizure the name of the first sign or symptom or principal presenting feature of the disorder.

Seizures may also be characterized according to:

- Frequency: whether they are isolated phenomena or are recurrent;
- Etiology: symptomatic, cryptogenic, or idiopathic. Symptomatic seizures are those with a demonstrable etiology. These may be further subdivided according to the temporal relationship between the seizure and the cause (6).

Some seizures may be directly correlated with an acute cerebral insult; either direct (trauma, CVA, infection) or systemic (toxic or metabolic abnormalities, septicemia, fever). These seizures are related to concurrent circumstances: situation-related (7), or acute symptomatic (1), also referred to as occasional seizures (8).

Others appear to be unrelated to the insult, representing delayed symptomatic seizures.

References

1. Hauser WA, Kurland LT. The epidemiology of epilepsy in Rochester, Minnesota, 1935 through 1967. *Epilepsia* 1975;16:1–66.
2. Hopkins A. Definitions and epidemiology of epilepsy. In: Hopkins A (ed.). *Epilepsy.* New York: Demos Publications, 1987.
3. Mirsky AF, Ducan CC, Myslobodsky MS. Petit Mal epilepsy: a review and integration of recent information. *J Clin Neurophysiol* 1986;3:179–208,

4. Rausch R, Lieb JP, Crandall PH. Neuropsychologic correlates of depth spike activity in epileptic patients. *Arch Neurol* 1978;35:699–705.
5. Kasteleijn-Nolst Trenite DGA, Bakker DJ, Binnie CD, Buerman A, Van Raaij M. Psychological effects of subclinical epileptiform EEG discharges. I: Scholastic skills. *Epilepsy Res* 1988;2:111–16.
6. Hauser WA, Anderson VE, Loewenson RB, McRoberts SM. Seizure recurrence after a first unprovoked seizure. *N Engl J Med* 1981;307:522–28.
7. Commission on Classification and Terminology of the International League Against Epilepsy. Proposal for classification of epilepsies and epileptic syndromes. *Epilepsia* 1989;30:389–99.
8. Gastaut H. *Dictionary of epilepsy. Part 1: Definitions.* Geneva: World Health Organization, 1973.

• • • • • •
EPILEPTOGENESIS (SECONDARY)

The hypothesis underlying this concept involves the repeated bombardment of normal cortex by discharges from a focal epileptogenic lesion or primary focus which eventually produces a secondary epileptic focus—this, in turn, becomes independent.

In favor of this hypothesis are:

• the finding of mirror foci in certain animal models with a frontal focus;
• the experimental epilepsy model of kindling (see under this heading);
• in man, the appearance of secondary bilateral synchrony on the EEG.

Some arguments in favor of secondary epileptogenesis in man have been reported (1,2).

The concern regarding possible secondary epileptogenesis underlies the urge for more prompt surgical treatment of AED-resistant focal epilepsy before it becomes established in the contralateral hemisphere. The frequency with which secondary foci might be generated is unknown.

References

1. Morrell F. Varieties of human secondary epileptogenesis. *J Clin Neurophysiol* 1989;6:227–79.
2. Morrell F. Secondary epileptogenesis in man. *Arch Neurol* 1985;42:318–35.

• • • • • •
ESSENTIAL EPILEPSY

A term now in disuse, it was used to "designate any form of epilepsy not depending upon an apparent organic cerebral cause or a recognized metabolic disturbance. It was believed to represent 'true' epilepsy."

Epilepsies subsumed under the label "essential" included idiopathic and cryptogenic epilepsies or seizures (see these headings).

Reference

Gastaut H, Broughton R. *Epileptic seizures, clinical and electrographic features, diagnosis and treatment.* Springfield: Charles C. Thomas, 1972.

• • • • • •
ETHOSUXIMIDE (ZARONTIN®)

Capsules of 250 mg.
Syrup: 250 mg/5 ml (1 teaspoon)

Ethosuximide is a first-line AED used in the treatment of absence seizures and may enable complete seizure control in 80% of cases (1,2). It has little or no activity in other types of seizures. In animal models, it is more effective against pentylenetetrazol-induced seizures than maximal electroshock seizures. Its antiepileptic mechanism is unknown.

PHARMACOKINETICS (3)

Bioavailability is 96–100%. Peak plasma levels are obtained in 3–7 hours after oral administration. The drug is not significantly bound to plasma proteins. The half-life of ethosuximide is 60 hours in adults and 30 hours in children. Despite this long half-life, the drug is often given in divided doses to minimize gastrointestinal side effects but can be given once a day (4). Steady-state levels are achieved in 4–8 days. The volume of distribution (Vd) is 0.7. The drug causes very little hepatic enzyme induction.

Therapeutic drug levels are 40–80 mg/l (300–600 µmol/l).

Side effects include:

- dose-dependent gastrointestinal problems;
- headaches, dizziness, fatigue, irritability, confusion;
- tonic seizures, occasionally occurring in clusters;
- eosinophilia and neutropenia—frequently seen, usually of minimal clinical significance; occasional pancytopenia;
- acute psychotic episodes—rare, and only in adults.

There are only occasional drug interactions with valproic acid (5) and isoniazid. Carbamazepine and possibly phenytoin, phenobarbital, and primidone may reduce serum ethosuximide levels (6).

References

1. Berkovic SF, Andermann F, Andermann E, Gloor P. Concepts of absence epilepsies: discrete syndromes or biological continuum? *Neurology* 1987;37:993–1000.
2. Brown TR, Dreifuss FE, Dyken PR, et al. Ethosuximide in the treatment of absence (petit mal) seizures. *Neurology* 1975;25:515–24.
3. Levy RH, Dreifuss FE, Mattson RH, Meldrum BS, Penry JK (eds.). *Antiepileptic drugs,* 3rd edition. New York: Raven Press, 1989
4. Dooley JM, Camfield PR, Camfield CS, Fraser AD. Once-daily ethosuximide in the treatment of absence epilepsy. *Pediatr Neurol* 1990;6:38–39.
5. Wallace SJ. Use of ethosuximide and valproate in the treatment of epilepsy. *Neurol Clin* 1986;4:601–16.
6. Warren JW, Benmaman JD, Braxton B, Wannamaker BB, Levy RH. Kinetics of a carbamazepine-ethosuximide interaction. *Clin Pharmacol Ther* 1980;28:646–51.

• • • • • • •

ETIOLOGY

Genetic (see also Genetics) and acquired factors both contribute to the tendency to have seizures. Genetically determined seizures appear at particular ages and are not associated with cerebral pathology. Nevertheless, even in genetically transmitted epilepsies, previous cerebral injury favors clinical expression. Acquired epilepsies (for example, perinatal injury (1) or posttraumatic epilepsy) and symptomatic seizures (such as alcohol withdrawal seizures) may be more likely to occur in genetically predisposed individuals. The risk of seizures in the offspring of patients with epilepsy is three times the baseline risk (2–4).

Acquired factors that predispose to epilepsy include any cerebral insult, as well as a large number of systemic disorders. Clinicians must determine the contribution of a possible predisposing factor to the epilepsy, although many cases may be multifactorial. A few etiologic factors for epilepsy are listed below, but the list is far from exhaustive. In all age groups, the etiology of epilepsy often remains undetermined.

- *Neonatal:* Perinatal injury, hypoxia, hypoglycemia, hypocalcemia, pyridoxine deficiency, intraventricular, parenchymal, or subdural hemorrhage.
- *Children:* Perinatal injury, developmental malformation, febrile seizures, cerebral vascular accidents, vascular malformations, head injury, infections, parasites, tumors, amino acid disorders, urea cycle disorders, gray matter storage diseases.
- *Adults:* Trauma, tumor, alcohol, drug abuse or drug withdrawal (alcohol, benzodiazepines, barbiturates, anticonvulsants), drug reactions (stimulants, antihistamines, tricyclics, phenothiazines,

butyrophenones, certain antibiotics, aminophylline), CNS infections (parasitic, bacterial, fungal, viral, tubercular), stroke, brain hemorrhage, vascular malformations, metabolic derangements (hypoxia, hypoglycemia, hyponatremia, hypocalcemia, hypomagnesemia). With new-onset seizures in the middle years, there is a high risk for neoplasm, and in the group over 65 years for underlying cerebrovascular disease as a cause.

The International Classification of Epileptic Syndromes distinguishes between:

- idiopathic epilepsies, whether with partial or generalized seizures, associated with certain characteristic EEG abnormalities; primarily genetic epilepsies (either presumed or established);
- symptomatic epilepsies, either partial or generalized, resulting from progressive CNS problems or a sequela of previous cerebral insult;
- cryptogenic epilepsies, either partial or generalized, without a demonstrable genetic or acquired cause;
- seizures resulting from a particular epileptogenic context.

A diagnosis of idiopathic epilepsy is based on particular electroclinical characteristics. If a patient does not fit this picture and does not have a clear history of previous cerebral insult, a CT scan or MRI scan may reveal a potentially epileptogenic lesion. If none is found, the epilepsy is referred to as "cryptogenic." If the seizures are seen in a particular context, the history, clinical examination, and investigation for toxic or metabolic disturbances will help clarify the situation. There is a subtle, but important distinction between idiopathic epilepsies and seizures believed to be secondary to a lesion not yet identified.

References

1. Deymeer F, Leviton A. Perinatal factors and seizure disorders: an epidemiologic review. *Epilepsia* 1985;26:287–98.
2. Commission for the Control of Epilepsy and Its Consequences. Vol. II, Part 1, Sections 1–V1. DHEW Publication N CNIHJ 78–276. Bethesda: National Institutes of Health, 1978:235–38.
3. Ottman R. Genetics of epilepsy: a review. *Epilepsia* 1989;30:107–10.
4. Ottman R, Annegers JF, Hauser WA, Kurland LT. Seizure risk in offspring of parents with generalized versus partial epilepsy. *Epilepsia* 1989;30:157–61.

• • • • • •
EVOKED POTENTIALS

In progressive myoclonic epilepsies, somatosensory evoked potentials show an increase in evoked potential amplitude (particularly of the N25–P33 waves) recorded in the central regions after contralateral median nerve stimulation (1). Somatosensory evoked potentials with amplitudes greater than 100 microvolts may predict risk for epilepsy in children (2), but the incidence of false positives and negatives of this test has not been established. An amplitude increase in the negative phase of visual evoked potential wave forms has been described in photosensitive epilepsies (3).

Therapeutic doses of AEDs do not alter evoked potential latencies.

References

1. Shibasaki H, Yamashita Y, Neshige R, Tobeimatsu S, Fukui R. Pathogenesis of giant somatosensory evoked potentials in progressive myoclonic epilepsy. *Brain* 1985;108:225–40.
2. De Marco P, Tassinari CA. Extreme somatosensory evoked potentials (ESEP): an EEG sign forecasting the possible occurrences of seizure in children. *Epilepsia* 1981;22:569–75.
3. Harding GFA, Dimitrakoudi M. The visual evoked potentials in photosensitive epilepsy. In: Desmedt JE (ed.). *Visual evoked potentials in man. New developments.* Oxford: Clarendon Press, 1977:509–13.

• • • • • •
EVOLUTION (OF EPILEPSY)

The evolution or progression of epilepsy in a particular individual is highly variable and difficult to predict. Several patterns can be identified:

1. Certain seizures, either symptomatic or age-dependent, will remain as isolated events.
2. Certain epileptic syndromes have been clearly identified as benign (see Benign epilepsies). Idiopathic partial epilepsies of childhood and, to a lesser extent, absence epilepsy of childhood remit or are "cured" by the end of puberty in most cases.
3. Some untreated patients have normal lives despite persisting seizures: 3–35% (1–3) of patients in population-based epidemiological surveys (1–3).
4. Seizures may remit with AED treatment and not reappear when treatment is stopped (see Remission; Prognosis).
5. Seizures may respond to AED therapy but reappear when therapy is stopped (e.g., juvenile myoclonic epilepsy).

6. Seizures may persist despite aggressive AED treatment. Approximately 20% of epilepsies may represent a group of AED-resistant or medically intractable epilepsies.

References

1. Gudmundsson G. Epilepsy in Iceland. *Acta Neurol Scand* 1966;43 (Suppl 25):1–14.
2. Haerer AF, Anderson DW, Schoenberg BS. Prevalence and clinical features of epilepsy in a biracial United States population. *Epilepsia* 1986;27:66–75.
3. Zielinski JJ. Epileptics not in treatment. *Epilepsia* 1974;15:203–10.

FAMOUS PEOPLE WITH EPILEPSY

Epilepsy is not necessarily an impediment to achievement of a high station in life. Many famous people have suffered from epileptic seizures. The following list is largely extracted from Temkin: Napoleon Bonaparte, Julius Caesar, King Charles V, Dostoevski, Flaubert, Handel, President William McKinley, Molière, St. Paul, Peter the Great, Petrarch, Jonathan Swift. Each of these individuals performed his or her historic functions prior to the availability of effective and nontoxic antiepileptic medication.

Reference

Temkin O. *The falling sickness: the history of epilepsy from the Greeks to the beginnings of modern neurology,* 2nd edition. Baltimore: Johns Hopkins Press, 1971.

······

FEBRILE CONVULSIONS/SEIZURES

Febrile convulsions are seizures occurring with fever, seen only in children under the age of five, usually under the age of two. The prevalence of febrile convulsions is 2–4% of the normal pediatric population (1); the incidence is slightly higher in boys, but seizures occur at an earlier age; they are more severe in girls. Family history is positive for febrile convulsions in 10–50% of cases (2). An autosomal dominant transmission with variable penetrance or polygenic mechanisms has been suggested.

CAUSES

Febrile seizures may occur with any childhood febrile illness, but especially with viral upper respiratory tract infections; childhood exanthems, e.g., measles, mumps, chickenpox, German measles; or following a vaccination (especially mumps). By definition, meningitis and encephalitis are excluded. With fever, the temperature usually rises above 38° centigrade. The rate of rise of the temperature has been implicated.

CLINICAL FEATURES

Febrile convulsions are usually predominantly clonic convulsions, more rarely tonic, atonic, or tonic-clonic. They generalize from the start.

- Simple febrile convulsions are brief, are seen in normal children, are generalized, and have no postictal deficit.
- Severe febrile convulsions are prolonged, occasionally repeated, frequently focal, and are occasionally followed by postictal neurological deficit. Severe febrile convulsions are frequently seen in children with abnormal neurological development or a family history of febrile convulsions or seizures. They may provoke mesial temporal sclerosis. The ictal EEG shows bilateral posterior slow waves or focal slow waves with focal seizures.

PROGNOSIS

Recurrent febrile convulsions may be seen in 25–31% of cases (4–6) if the patient is younger than one year old at the time of the first seizure, if there is a family history of febrile convulsions and with severe focal febrile convulsions. With each recurrent seizure, there is increased chance of recurrence (7). Severe neurological sequelae such as hemiconvulsions-hemiplegia-epilepsy syndrome (HHE) (see this heading) are rare even after prolonged seizures.

Recurrent seizures not associated with fever (epilepsy) are seen in 3–9% of cases (8). Febrile convulsions are associated with mesial temporal sclerosis and thus to complex partial seizures, but a causal connection has been difficult to document.

TREATMENT

With simple febrile convulsions, AEDs are not necessary. Treatment of fever and the underlying illness suffices. With prolonged or frequently recurrent febrile convulsions, intravenous diazepam or per rectum diazepam (available in Europe) is the treatment of choice (9). Prophylactic therapy is aimed at diminishing the chance of recurrence and subsequent epilepsy. Prophylaxis using phenobarbital (10) or sodium valproate (11) may be used to the age of five. Indications for prophylaxis include a focal febrile seizure or prolonged febrile seizure; neurological abnormalities; nonfebrile convulsions in a near relative; multiple seizures in a 24-hour period in patients under a year old. Meta-analysis of published series suggests that most children do not require treatment even with one of the above risk factors (12). When fever appears, diazepam may be given when the temperature exceeds 38.5° C (9,13,14).

References

1. Hauser WA, Kurland FT. The epidemiology of epilepsy in Rochester, Minnesota, 1935 through 1967. *Epilepsia* 1975;16:1–66.
2. Lennox-Buchthal MA. Febrile convulsions. A reappraisal. *Electroencephalogr clin Neurophysiol* 1973;32 (Suppl):1–132.
3. Chevrie JJ, Aicardi J. Duration and lateralization of febrile convulsions. Etiological factors. *Epilepsia* 1975;16:781–89.
4. Annegers JF, Blackley SA, Hauser WA, Kurland LT. Recurrence of febrile convulsions in a population-based cohort. *Epilepsy Res* 1990;5:209–16.
5. Nelson KB, Ellenberg JH. Prognosis in children with febrile seizures. *Pediatrics* 1978;61:720–27.
6. Verity CM, Butler NR, Goldring J. Febrile convulsions in a national cohort followed from birth. I. Prevalence and recurrence in the first five years of life. *Br Med J* 1985;290:1307–10.
7. Viani F, Beghi E, Romeo A, Van Lierde A. Infantile febrile status epilepticus: risk factors and outcome. *Dev Med Child Neurol* 1987;29:495–501.
8. Falconer MA, Serafetidines EA, Corsellis JAN. Etiology and pathogenesis of temporal lobe epilepsy. *Arch Neurol* 1964;19:353–61.
9. Lombroso C. Intermittent home treatment of status and clusters of seizures. *Epilepsia* 1989;30 (Suppl 2):11–14.
10. Wolf SM, Carr A, Davis DC, et al. The value of phenobarbital in the child who has had a single febrile seizure: a controlled prospective study. *Pediatrics* 1977;59:378–85.
11. Ngwane E, Bower E. Continuous sodium valproate or phenobarbitone in the prevention of "simple" febrile convulsions. *Arch Dis Child* 1980;55:171–74.
12. Berg AT, Shinnar S, Hauser WA, Leventhal JM. Predictors of recurrent febrile seizures: a meta-analytic review. *J Pediatr* 1990;116:329–37.
13. Knudsen FU. Vestermak S. Prophylactic diazepam or phenobarbitone in febrile convulsions: a prospective controlled study. *Arch Dis Child* 1978;53:660–63.
14. Freeman JM. Febrile seizures: a consensus of their significance, evaluation, and treatment. *Pediatrics* 1980;66:1009

• • • • • • •
FELBAMATE (FELBATOL®)

Tablets 400 mg, 600 mg; oral suspension 600 mg/5 mL.

Felbamate is an AED chemically characterized as 2–phenyl-1,3–propanediol dicarbamate. It is thought to act as a glycine antagonist. Felbamate has efficacy in animal models against both electroshock and pentylenetetrazol seizures. It has a substantial therapeutic to toxic ratio and a good profile of safety (1,2). Initial studies suggest safety and efficacy for felbamate in the treatment of partial seizures and secondarily generalized tonic-clonic seizures, either as add-on or as monotherapy (3–4). It is also effective in Lennox-Gastaut syndrome (5). Side effects include mild, transient nausea and vomiting, insomnia, anorexia, and weight loss.

Absorption is over 90% with a Tmax of 1–4 hrs, Vd is 0.7–0.8 L/kg with 24% protein binding. Elimination is mostly hepatic with a T1/2 of 20 hrs as monotherapy and 11–16 hrs when used with CBZ or PHT. As of this writing, the FDA in conjunction with Carter-Wallace, Inc. have recommended that Felbatol® remain as a second-line therapy for refractory epilepsy patients with a warning of the risks of aplastic anemia and liver failure. The company recommends a complete discussion of the risks followed by written informed consent.

References

1. Wagner ML, Graves NM, Marienau K, Holmes GB, Remmel RP, Leppik IE. Discontinuation of phenytoin and carbamazepine in patients receiving felbamate. *Epilepsia* 1991;32:398–406.
2. Theodore WH, Raubertas RF, Porter RJ, et al. Felbamate: a clinical trial for complex partial seizures. *Epilepsia* 1991;32:392–97.
3. Sachdeo R, Kramer LD, Rosenberg A, Sachdeo S. Felbamate monotherapy: controlled trial in patients with partial onset seizures. *Ann Neurol* 1992;32:386–92.
4. Faught E, Sachdeo RC, Remler MP, et al. Felbamate monotherapy for partial-onset seizures: an active-control trial. *Neurology* 1993;43:688–92.
5. Ritter FJ, Leppik IE, Dreifuss FE, et al. Efficacy of felbamate in childhood epileptic encephalopathy (Lennox-Gastaut syndrome). *N Engl J Med* 1993; 328:29–33.

• • • • • •
FERTILITY

Patients with epilepsy—particularly an early onset partial epilepsy (1)—have fewer children (2,3). This may be due to fewer marriages, shorter marriages, or later marriages, as well as the effect of AEDs on sexuality (3), a fall in testosterone level, or hypogonadism (4).

References

1. Dansky LV, Andermann E, Andermann F. Marriage and fertility in epileptic patients. *Epilepsia* 1980;21:261–71.
2. Webber MP, Hauser WA, Ottman R, Annegers JF. Fertility in persons with epilepsy, 1935–1974. *Epilepsia* 1986;27:746–52.
3. Alstrom CH. A study of epilepsy in its clinical, social and genetic aspects. *Acta Psychiat Neurol Scand* 1950;63 (Suppl):75–90.
4. Herzog AG, Seibel MM, Schomer DL, Vaitukaitis JL, Geschwind N. Reproductive endocrine disorders in men with partial seizure of temporal origin. *Arch Neurol* 1986;43:347–50.

• • • • • •
FIRST AID FOR EPILEPSY

There are various suggested regimens for first aid treatment of an individual with epilepsy. Such first aid depends on the nature of the seizures and the circumstances in which they occur. As a general guideline, the following are suggested for first aid for individuals having a generalized tonic-clonic seizure. Onlookers and assistants should remain calm. They should refrain from inserting anything into the convulsing individual's mouth because of risk of breaking teeth or incurring bites. Clothing should be loosened around the neck to facilitate breathing, and the head or body turned to the side. The patient should be kept away from sharp corners or edges. A soft object such as a pillow or rolled up coat may be placed under the person's head.

There is an unwarranted fear that individuals having a seizure may "swallow their tongue." Although gagging and respiratory movements become irregular during a seizure, it is impossible to swallow the tongue. Nothing can be done on site to shorten the duration of the seizure. If continual jerking persists for longer than five to ten minutes, then arrangements should be made to immediately transport the patient to a medical facility for further evaluation. After the seizure, the subject should be protected and reassured as he or she returns to normal awareness.

In cases of complex partial seizures, the most important feature of first aid is steering individuals having such seizures out of harm's way, such that they avoid steps, edges, traffic, or other dangerous circumstances. It is best to do this without physically restraining an individual, since this may cause them to become alarmed and strike out or struggle. Onlookers should be aware that complex partial seizures may become secondarily generalized tonic-clonic seizures which may then cause falls.

• • • • • •
FIRST SEIZURE

The incidence of all seizures, whether spontaneous or provoked (excluding febrile convulsions), is approximately 71–77/100,000 population/year (1,2). This specific incidence varies according to age, with a biphasic distribution: more than 100/100,000 in children and in the aged, fewer in middle years. The commonest cause of seizures in the elderly is stroke, accounting for over 50% (3). Symptomatic seizures resulting from an acute cerebral insult should be considered distinct from idiopathic first seizures, since the prognosis and therapy of symptomatic seizures depends largely on the underlying cause. With the first seizure, the risk of recurrence must be evaluated.

RISK OF RECURRENCE

The risk of recurrence after a first seizure varies among different studies, in part because of differences in definition of a first seizure (for example, should prior unobserved losses of consciousness be counted?), differences in time elapsed between seizure and evaluation, variations in testing and treatment strategies, and in clinical judgments by the investigators (4,5). The following summarizes conclusions from various studies of recurrence rates after a first seizure.

1. Grouping all ages and seizure types, the risk at 1 year is 36%, at 3 years 48%, at 5 years 56% (6); other studies show a risk of 49% at 1 year and 52% at 3 years (7); or 16% at 1 year, 21% at 2 years, and 27% at 3 years (8).
2. For adults, taking into account all seizure types, the recurrence rate is 52% at 3 years (9).
3. Among adults, generalized seizures (not all idiopathic) recur 62% of the time by 1 year, 71% by 3 years (10).
4. Among children, recurrence rate has been found to be 62% at 3 years (11), 52% at 5 years (12), 48.6% at 2 years (13), and 37.7% at 8 years (14).
5. A second seizure occurs within 1 month in one-third of cases, within 6 months in 58% of cases (14), within 1 year in 70–87% of cases (12,14,15), and within 2 years in 90% of cases. The second seizure, therefore, may occur soon after the first, introducing a selection bias in those studies where a certain time lag separates the first seizure from therapeutic intervention. This leads to underestimation of the recurrence rate.

RISK FACTORS

1. The period between the first and second seizure is a predictor of further recurrence. If there has been no second seizure within the first year, the recurrence rate at five years is 26% for idiopathic epilepsies and 49% for symptomatic epilepsies. If no seizure occurs within four years, the risk in the fifth year is low.
2. Neurologic deficits markedly increase the risk of recurrence (6,11,12).
3. With symptomatic seizures, the risk of recurrence is twice as high.
4. Seizure type has been claimed to have both no effect on recurrence rate (8,9) and a marked effect (6,11).
5. Age at time of the seizure appears to have no effect on recurrence risk in adults and children (6,8,9,14), with the exception of brain-damaged infants.

6. EEG can be an important factor in predicting recurrence. The presence of spike and slow wave EEG discharges, whether focal or bilateral, increases the risk of recurrence, either slightly (6) or twofold (8,12,13).

7. A family history of epilepsy may (8) or may not (11,14) increase the risk of recurrence.

TREATMENT

Most authorities advise against AED therapy after a first seizure. In several reports, however, 11–68% of patients were treated after the first seizure (6,9,11–15). Some studies show a reduction in seizure relapse with AEDs after a first unprovoked seizure (16,17). An argument against treatment is the relatively low risk of recurrence and the significant incidence (30%) of AED side effects in those treated (18). A (controversial) argument in favor of treatment is that early AED therapy might forestall the worsening of epilepsy (3) (see also Bilateral synchrony). The evaluation of risk factors is essential for the proper assessment of the risk/benefit ratio for AED treatment after a single seizure. The patient's profession, his or her attitude with respect to seizures, and the certainty of diagnosis are all relevant factors (19).

Most epilepsy specialists recommend treatment after a second seizure, since further seizures are likely.

References

1. Hauser WA, Kurland KT. The epidemiology of epilepsy in Rochester, Minnesota, 1935 through 1967. *Epilepsia* 1975;16;1–66.

2. Loiseau J, Loiseau P, Guyot M, Duché B, Dartigues JF, Aublet B. Survey of seizure disorders in the French Southwest. I. Incidence of epileptic syndromes. *Epilepsia* 1990;31:391–96.

3. Ettinger AB, Shinnar S. New onset seizures in an elderly hospitalized population. *Neurology* 1993;43:489–92.

4. Van Donselaar CA, Geerts AT, Meulstee J, Habbema JDF, Staal A. Reliability of the diagnosis of a first seizure. *Neurology* 1989;39:267–71.

5. Fisher RS. First seizure management reconsidered. *Arch Neurol* 1987; 44:1189–90.

6. Annegers JF, Shirts SB, Hauser WA, Kurland LT. Risk of recurrence after an initial unprovoked seizure. *Epilepsia* 1986;27:43–50.

7. Collaborative Group for the Study of Epilepsy. Principal investigators: Beghi E, Tognoni G. Prognosis of epilepsy in newly referred patients: a multi-center prospective study. *Epilepsia* 1988;29:236–43.

8. Hauser WA, Anderson VZ, Loewenson RB, McRoberts SM. Seizure recurrence after a first unprovoked seizure. *N Engl J Med* 1982;307:522–28.

9. Hopkins A, Garman A, Clarke C. The first seizure in adult life. Value of clinical features, electroencephalography, and computerized tomographic scanning in prediction of seizure recurrence. *Lancet* 1988;i:721–26.

10. Elwes RDC, Chesterman P, Reynolds EH. Prognosis after a first untreated tonic-clonic seizure. *Lancet* 1985;ii:752–53.

11. Blom S, Heijbel J, Bergfors PG. Incidence of epilepsy in children: a follow-up study three years after the first seizure. *Epilepsia* 1978;19:343–50.

12. Camfield PR, Camfield CS, Dooley JM, Tibbles JAR, Fung T, Garner B. Epilepsy after a first unprovoked seizure in childhood. *Neurology* 1985;35:1657–60.

13. Shinnar S, Berg AT, Moshe S, Eckstein A, Goldensohn E, Hauser WA. Recurrence risk after a first unprovoked seizure in childhood. *Ann Neurol* 1988;24:315.

14. Boulloche J, Leloup P, Mallet E, Parain D, Tron P. Risk of recurrence after a single unprovoked, generalized tonic-clonic seizure. *Dev Med Child Neurol* 1989;31:626–29.

15. Hirtz DG, Ellenberg JH, Nelson KB. The risk of recurrence of nonfebrile seizures in children. *Neurology* 1984;34:637–41.

16. Camfield P, Camfield C, Dooley J, Smith E, Garner B. A randomized study of carbamazepine versus no medication after a first unprovoked seizure in childhood. *Neurology* 1989;39:851–52.

17. FIR.S.T. GROUP. Randomized clinical trial on the efficiency of antiepileptic drugs in reducing the risk of relapse after a first unprovoked tonic-clonic seizure. *Neurology* 1993;43:478–83.

18. Hauser WA. Should people be treated after a first seizure? *Arch Neurol* 1986;43:1287–88.

19. Hachinski V. Management of a first seizure. *Arch Neurol* 1986;43:1290.

• • • • • •
FLUNARIZINE (1)

Flunarizine is a fluorinated derivative of piperazine, used in the treatment of migraine and vertigo (2). Animal studies show an antiepileptic property. The suspected mechanism of action is via the sodium channels or by blockade of calcium channels (see Calcium channel blockers). In man, it has inconsistent antiepileptic properties (3,4), often at doses that may lead to side effects, such as sedation or extrapyramidal symptoms.

References

1. Levy RH, Dreifuss FE, Mattson RH, Meldrum BS, Penry JK (eds.). *Antiepileptic drugs,* 3rd edition. New York: Raven Press, 1989.

2. Holmes B, Brogden RN, Heel RC, Speight TM, Avery GS. Flunarizine. A review of its pharmacodynamic and pharmacokinetic properties and therapeutic use. *Drugs* 1984;27:6–44.

3. Binnie CD, de Beukelaar F, Meijer JWA, Meinardi H, Overweg J, Wauquier A, Van Wieringen A. Open dose-ranging trial of flunarizine as add-on therapy in epilepsy. *Epilepsia* 1985;26:424–28.
4. Froscher W, Bulau P, Burr W. Double-blind placebo-controlled trial with flunarizine in therapy-resistant epileptic patients. *Clin Neuropharmacol* 1988;11:232–40.

• • • • • •
FOCAL (SEIZURES)

Focal or partial seizures (see also Partial (S), seizures with focal onset) may affect sensory, motor, psychic, or autonomic modalities without affecting consciousness (i.e., simple partial seizures), impair consciousness (complex partial seizures), and/or secondarily generalize (with convulsive or nonconvulsive features). Frequent causes include structural abnormalities such as trauma and vascular malformations in younger age groups; cerebral infarction, hemorrhage, and tumors in the elderly. An underlying cause may not be determined (cryptogenic) (see also Cerebrovascular accidents and seizures; Cryptogenic (S,E); Tumors).

• • • • • •
FOCUS (EPILEPTOGENIC)

The epileptogenic focus is the site from which epileptic discharges arise (see Discharge, epileptic). Excitatory and inhibitory influences interplay among neurons in the focus and in surrounding cortex. A particular lesion and an epileptic focus may not necessarily be congruent; thus the distinction between an "epileptic zone" (1) and an "irritant or irritative zone" (1–3). The epileptic zone is the region from which seizure discharges arise. The irritant zone is the brain region from which interictal discharges may be recorded at the scalp, at the cortical surface, or with depth recordings. Discharge foci may vary in time and space. Interictal discharges may be due to entirely different cellular mechanisms from ictal discharges, although clearly sites of interictal and ictal discharges are often correlated (4).

References

1. Engel J Jr. Terminology and classifications. In: *Seizures and epilepsy.* Philadelphia: F.A. Davis, 1989:8,9.
2. Talairach J, Bancaud J. Stereotaxic approach to epilepsy. Methodology of anatomofunctional stereotaxic investigations. *Prog Neurol Surg* 1973;5:297–354.

3. Talairach J, Bancaud J. Lesion, "irritative" zone and epileptogenic focus. *Confin Neurol* 1966;27:91–94.
4. Jensen MS, Yaari Y. The relationship between interictal and ictal paroxysms in an in vitro model of focal hippocampal epilepsy. *Ann Neurol* 1988; 24:591–98.

• • • • • • •
FOCUS, LESION-RELATED

In partial epilepsies arising from a particular lesion, the lesion itself evinces no ictal activity (1,2). Seizures arise in an epileptogenic zone at the border of the lesion, or sometimes at a distance from the lesion.

References

1. Engel J Jr. Terminology and classifications. In: *Seizures and epilepsy.* Philadelphia: F.A. Davis, 1989:8,9.
2. Talairach J, Bancaud J. Stereotaxic approach to epilepsy. Methodology of anatomofunctional stereotaxic investigations. *Prog Neurol Surg* 1973;5:297–354.

• • • • • •
FOLATE

Folates are enzymatic co-factors of DNA synthesis essential for the normal metabolism and maturation of the central nervous system. AEDs interfere with folate metabolism (1,2), producing a fall in serum and CSF folate levels in 50% of patients on long-term AED therapy (particularly with phenytoin). Folate deficiency may lead to macrocytosis, megaloblastic anemia, and altered mental status (see also Anemia). Pregnancy may lead to a fall in serum folate, thereby increasing the risk of fetal malformations (3,4).

Folic acid is a convulsant in animals (2), but does not appear to cause seizures in humans (1). Because of a postulated relationship between folate levels and neural tube defects, folate supplementation up to 4 mg/day has been recommended for pregnant women even though vitamin supplementation has not been shown to decrease the incidence of neural tube defects (5).

References

1. Reynolds EH. Chronic antiepileptic toxicity: a review. *Epilepsia* 1975;16:319–52.
2. Mauguière F, Quoex C, Bello S. Epileptogenic properties of folic acid and N5 methyltetrahydrofolate in cat. *Epilepsia* 1975;16:535–41.
3. Dansky LV, Andermann E, Rosenblatt D, Sherwin AL, Andermann F. Anticonvulsants, folate levels and pregnancy outcome: a prospective study. *Ann Neurol* 1987;21:176–82.

4. Engelsen B, Strandjord R, Gjerde IO, Markestad T, Ulstein M, Evyen OK.
    Folate concentrations in pregnancy in women on antiepileptic drug therapy.
    Acta Neurol Scand 1984;69 (Suppl 98):83–84.
5. Mills JL, Rhoads GG, Simpson JL, et al. The absence of a relation between the
    peri-conceptional use of vitamins and neural-tube defects. *N Engl J Med*
    1989;321:430–35.

• • • • • •
FRAGILE-X SYNDROME

Fragile-X syndrome is the commonest cause of moderate mental retardation and is occasionally associated with epilepsy. It is characterized additionally by macro-orchidism, a prominent jaw, large ears, and peculiar
speech. The EEG is normal (1). Abnormal cyclic adenosine monophos-
phate production has been found in multiple tissues from patients with
this disorder (2).

References

1. DeArce MA, Kearns A. The fragile X syndrome: the patients and their chro-
    mosome. *J Med Genet* 1984;21:84–91.
2. Berry-Kravis E, Hodges C. Demonstration of abnormal cyclic adenosine
    monophosphate production in multiple tissue from individuals with fragile X
    syndrome. *Ann Neurol* 1991;30:450A.

• • • • • •
FRONTAL PAROXYSMS, IN BENIGN PARTIAL
EPILEPSIES IN CHILDHOOD

A tentative delineation of a new type of idiopathic partial epilepsy in childhood, this rather rare syndrome begins at 4 to 8 years of age (1,2). Seizures
present with obtundation, autonomic problems, facial flushing, forced deviation of the head and eyes, and sometimes gyration. The EEG shows rhythmic spike and slow waves involving the frontal areas contralateral to the
direction of head deviation, followed by generalization. Frontal discharges
are not rare in children with multiple functional foci. Seizures and EEG
discharges remit between the ages of 8 and 13. Seizures may reappear after
treatment has been terminated, even when the EEG is normal.

References

1. Beaumanoir A, Nahory A. Les épilepsies bénignes partielles: 11 cas d'épilepsie partielle frontale a evolution favorable. *Rev EEG Neurophysiol Clin* 1983;13:207–11.
2. Dalla Bernardina B, Sgrō V, Fontana E, Colamaria V, LaSelva L.. Idiopathic partial epilepsies in childhood. In: Roger J, Bureau M, Dravet C, Dreifuss FE, Perret A, Wolf P (eds.). *Epileptic syndromes in infancy, childhood and adolescence.* London: John Libbey Eurotext, 1992:173–88.

· · · · · ·

FRONTAL SEIZURES, EPILEPSIES (1)

Frontal epilepsy syndromes are characterized by simple or complex partial seizures, secondary generalized seizures, or a combination. Seizures frequently occur several times a day, frequently during sleep, and are easily mistaken for psychogenic seizures (2). Frontal seizures are seen with cryptogenic or symptomatic partial epilepsies and in benign frontal epilepsies of childhood (see this heading). Frontal lobe origin of status epilepticus is not rare. Frontal seizures are characterized by:

*   short duration;
*   partial seizures with little or no postictal confusion;
*   rapid secondary generalization;
*   predominantly motor manifestations;
*   frequent complex gestural automatisms at the beginning of the seizure;
*   frequent falls with bilateral discharges (3).

With frontal foci, interictal scalp EEG recordings may show:

*   no abnormalities;
*   background asymmetries;
*   spikes, sharp waves, unilateral frontal spike and slow waves, bilateral frontal spike and slow waves, or multiple unilateral discharges.

EEG findings at the beginning of the seizure may vary. They may precede clinical signs of the seizure and are then of localizing value:

*   low amplitude, high frequency spikes, spike and slow waves, or rhythmic slow waves may appear in the frontal regions or other areas, frequently bilaterally;
*   high-voltage sharp waves which can then be followed by diffuse suppression.

Although rapid cortical spread of seizure activity may affect several frontal regions, making seizure onset identification problematic (4), particular presentations have been characterized:

- Supplementary motor area seizures may cause tonic elevation of an upper extremity with abduction, followed by head and eye deviation to the same side (fencing posture), vocalization, and speech arrest. Contralateral head turning is more common than ipsilateral; however, ipsilateral turning is not rare.
- Cingulate seizures may cause partial seizures with simple motor activities at the onset, leading to elaborate gestural automatisms (5).
- Mesial frontal foci may cause vocalization, laughter, respiratory difficulties, or hand, foot, and trunk movement (6).
- Fronto-polar seizures may induce forced thinking or early impairment in vigilance, adversive movement of the head and eyes followed by controversive movements, clonic trunk movements, falls, or changes in affect. Secondary generalization is frequent.
- Orbito-frontal seizures may cause partial complex seizures with early gestural automatisms, hallucinations, and olfactory illusions (see Olfactory seizures), and changes in affect.
- Opercular seizures (see Oropharyngeal seizures).
- Motor cortex seizures: Simple somato-motor seizures that correlate with the site of the seizure focus:
  - Basal pre-Rolandic area discharges lead to speech arrest, vocalization or aphasia, contralateral hemifacial tonic-clonic movements, or swallowing automatisms. Generalization is frequent;
  - Rolandic region seizures present as partial motor seizures with or without a jacksonian march (see Jacksonian march);
  - Paracentral lobule discharges result in clonic movements of the contralateral leg, and occasional tonic contraction of the ipsilateral foot;
  - Kojewnikow's syndrome (see this heading) is a synonym for "epilepsia partialis continua."

In effect, ictal activity can rapidly propagate in several directions and thus affect cortical areas situated at quite a distance from the seizure origin, particularly the temporal lobe (7). Frontal seizures occur in cryptogenic or symptomatic partial epilepsies, and benign frontal epilepsy of childhood (see Benign epilepsies). An autosomal dominant frontal epilepsy with brief motor attacks may be confused with a sleep disorder (8).

References

1. Commission on Classification and Terminology of the International League Against Epilepsy. Proposal for classification of epilepsies and epileptic syndromes. *Epilepsia* 1989;30:389–99.

2. Williamson PD, Spencer DD, Spencer SS, Novelly RA, Mattson RH. Complex partial seizures of frontal lobe origin. *Ann Neurol* 1985;18:497–504.

3. Geier S, Bancaud J, Talairach J, Bonis A, Szikla G, Enjelvin M. The seizures of frontal lobe epilepsy. A study of clinical manifestations. *Neurology* 1977; 27:951–58.

4. Quesney LF. Electroencephalographic and clinical manifestations of frontal and temporal lobe epilepsy. *Clin Neurol Neurosurg* 1987;89:41–42.

5. Talairach J, Bancaud J, Geier S, Bordas-Ferer M, Bonis A, Szikla G, Rusu M. The cingulate gyrus and human behavior. *Electroenceph clin Neurophysiol* 1973;34:45–52.

6. Waterman K, Purves SJ, Kozaka B, Strauss E, Wada JA. An epileptic syndrome caused by mesial frontal lobe seizure foci. *Neurology* 1987;37:577–82.

7. Quesney LF, Constain M, Fish DR, Rasmussen R. The clinical differentiation of seizures arising in the parasagittal and anterolaterodorsal frontal convexities. *Arch Neurol* 1990;47:677–79.

8. Scheffer IE, Bhation KP, Lopes-Cendes I, et al. Autosomal dominant frontal epilepsy misdiagnosed as sleep disorder. *Lancet* 1994;343:515–17.

· · · · · ·

FUGUE (EPILEPTIC)

An epileptic fugue consists of aimless wandering by the patient, of which he or she has no memory. It usually lasts several hours and appears during nonconvulsive status epilepticus or as a postictal phenomenon. More prolonged fugue states or states in which complex "intelligent" activities are accomplished are more likely to be hysterical in nature (factitious).

· · · · · ·

FUNCTIONAL EPILEPSY

This term, no longer widely used, referred to epilepsies in which no organic epileptogenic lesions are evident and which are thought to result from a genetically transmitted cerebral disturbance or some acquired metabolic disorder. Frequently generalized at onset, unilateral or partial seizures are seen in childhood.

Reference

Gastaut H, Broughton R. *Epileptic seizures, clinical and electrographic features, diagnosis and treatment.* Springfield: Charles C. Thomas, 1972.

FUNCTIONAL FOCI (1–3)

A functional focus is an EEG discharge focus unrelated to an underlying cortical pathology.

COMMON CHARACTERISTICS

- Functional foci are usually seen in children between the ages of 5 and 10 years, occasionally age 2–3 years or as late as puberty. Such foci remit with age;
- The EEG tracing shows high-voltage sharp waves followed by slow waves, either appearing in isolation or pseudo-periodically;
- The background EEG activity is normal;
- EEG discharges are increased by drowsiness and sleep;
- Foci are ephemeral and may appear to shift in different recordings from one region or hemisphere to the other;
- Functional foci are characteristic of certain epileptic syndromes, such as idiopathic partial epilepsies and patients with known cerebral insult presenting during childhood with seizures resembling benign partial epilepsies. They may also be found as EEG abnormalities in patients with cortical damage, but without epilepsy; in children with psychomotor or learning difficulties; and in normal children.

CHARACTERISTICS

The characteristics of functional foci are topographically related:

- a centrotemporal or centroparietal focus is usually associated with benign focal epilepsy of childhood or Rolandic epilepsy (see these headings);
- occipital foci are often related to partial epilepsy of childhood with occipital spike waves; occipital blindness; or epilepsy-migraine overlap syndromes;
- temporal foci may be associated with a higher incidence of behavioral problems;
- frontal foci have been linked to benign partial epilepsy.

Several foci may exist in the same patient and may change localization with age. A hereditary abnormality of cerebral maturation may underlie these functional foci (1,4).

References

1. Niedermeyer E. Focal spikes in childhood and the concept of "functional" spike activity. *Neurology* 1980;30:1122–25.
2. Drury I. Epileptiform patterns of children. *J Clin Neurophysiol* 1989;6:1–39.
3. Lerman P, Kivity ES. Focal epileptic EEG discharges in children not suffering from clinical epilepsy: etiology, clinical significance and management. *Epilepsia* 1981;22:551–58.
4. Doose M, Baier WK. Benign partial epilepsy and related conditions: multi-factorial pathogenesis with hereditary impairment of brain maturation. *Eur J Pediat* 1989;149:152–58.

G

· · · · · ·
GABA

GABA (gamma-aminobutyric acid) is the most important inhibitory neurotransmitter of the central nervous system (1). GABA is a 4–carbon dicarboxylic acid formed by decarboxylation of glutamic acid, under the control of the enzyme glutamic acid decarboxylase (GAD). GABA is metabolized sequentially by the mitochondrial enzymes, GABA transaminase and succinic acid dehydrogenase. A substantial fraction of brain synapses, from 30 to 50%, are GABAergic. GABA inhibits neurons by several mechanisms (2), the most important of which is the opening of chloride channels, resulting in chloride anion influx into the neuron, hyperpolarization of the membrane potential, and lowered cell membrane resistance because of the opened channels (thereby making excitatory potentials less effective).

GABA interacts with neurons via a $GABA_A$ receptor complex (3). The GABA receptor is a macromolecular structure with a chloride channel, binding sites for GABA, and for several modulatory compounds, including benzodiazepines, barbiturates, beta-carbolines, picrotoxin, penicillin, and zinc (4). The classic GABA receptor is referred to as the $GABA_A$ receptor. Antagonists at the $GABA_A$ receptor include picrotoxin, penicillin, and bicuculline (5). A second GABA receptor, $GABA_B$, is involved in postsynaptic inhibition in certain pathways of the CNS, and presynaptic inhibition in the spinal cord (6). The antispastic drug baclofen is an agonist for the $GABA_B$ receptor.

Numerous investigators have manipulated the GABA system for therapeutic purposes. GABA may be increased by inhibiting GABA uptake at the synapse, with agents such as tiagabine (7), an analog of nipecotic acid (8), or by interfering with its metabolism, as with vigabatrin (8,9), which is marketed in several countries. Use of putative GABA pro-drugs, such as progabide (10), has so far met with limited success.

The GABA theory of epilepsy is supported by a number of experimental findings (see Basic mechanisms of the epilepsies). Convulsions may be produced by agents that selectively modify GABAergic transmission; GABA agonists can play a protective role against seizures. Some human

124

epilepsies have been shown to involve abnormal GABAergic states (11,12). Nevertheless, GABAergic function is increased in some models of epilepsy (see Basic mechanisms of the epilepsies), and GABA clearly is not the only important neurotransmitter in this multifactorial disorder.

References

1. Roberts E, Chase TN, Tower DB (eds). *GABA in nervous system function.* New York: Raven Press, 1976.
2. Fariello RG. Action of inhibitory amino acids on acute epileptic foci: an electrographic study. *Exp Neurol* 1979;66:55–63.
3. Costa E, DiChiara G, Gessa GL (eds.). *GABA and benzodiazepine receptors.* New York: Raven Press,1981.
4. Westbrook GL, Mayer ML. Micromolar concentrations of Zn^{2+} antagonize NMDA and GABA responses of hippocampal neurons. *Nature* 1987;328:640–43.
5. Fariello RG, Forchetti CM, Fisher RS. GABAergic function in relation to seizure phenomena. In: Fisher RS, JT Coyle. *Neurotransmitters and epilepsy.* New York, Wiley-Liss, Inc., 1991:77–93.
6. Bowery NG, Hill DR, Hudson AL, Doble A, Middlemiss DN, Shaw J, Turnbull M. Baclofen decreases neurotransmitter release in the mammalian CNS by an action at a novel GABA receptor. *Nature* 1980; 283:92–94.
7. Pierce MVV, Suzdak PD, Gustavson LE, Mengel BH, McKelvy JV, Mant T. Tiagabine. *Epilepsy Res* 1991;3(Suppl):157–60.
8. Krogsgaard-Larson P. Inhibitors of the GABA uptake system. *Mol Cell Pharmacol* 1980;35:105–21.
9. Loiseau P, Hardenberg JP, Pestre M, Guyot M, Schechter PJ, Tell GP. Double-blind, placebo-controlled study of vigabatrin (gamma-vinyl GABA) in drug-resistant epilepsy. *Epilepsia* 1986;27:115–20.
10. Schechter PJ. Clinical pharmacology of vigabatrin. *Br J Clin Pharmacol* 1989;27(Suppl 1):S19–S22.
11. Loiseau P, Bossi L, Guyot M, Orofiamma B, Morselli PL. Double-blind crossover trial of progabide versus placebo in severe epilepsies. *Epilepsia* 1983;24:703–15.
12. Jones EG. Neurotransmitters in the cerebral cortex. *J Neurosurg* 1986;65:135–53.
13. Meldrum BS. GABAergic mechanisms in the pathogenesis and treatment of epilepsy. *Br J Clin Pharmacol* 1989;27:35–115.

• • • • • •
GABAPENTIN (NEURONTIN®)

This GABA analog was developed and used as an AED based on the GABAergic theory of epileptogenesis, but has no known interaction with the GABA receptor and is thought to act on a gabapentin-specific receptor. Gabapentin is not protein-bound, Vd 0.6–0.8 L/kg, is 100% renally excreted unchanged, does not alter other AED levels, and is not metabolized. The half-life is 5–7 hours, Tmax is 2–4 hrs, and absorption is dose-dependent: 60% at 300–400 mg.

Clinical trials so far have been as an add-on AED in refractory partial epilepsies (1,2), and hence the efficacy of gabapentin as a primary agent is difficult to determine. It appears to be effective in partial seizures and generalized tonic-clonic seizures (3) with up to 26% achieving at least a 50% reduction in seizure frequency (4). There are few side effects: somnolence, ataxia, dizziness. As of this writing, the drug is in clinical use in the United States and the United Kingdom.

References

1. UK Gabapentin Study Group. Gabapentin in partial epilepsy. *Lancet* 1990;335:1114–17.
2. Sivenius J, Kalviainen A, Ylinen A, Riekkinen P. Double-blind study of gabapentin in the treatment of partial seizures. *Epilepsia* 1991;32:539–42.
3. Crawford P, Ghadiali E, Lane R, Blumhardt L, Chadwick D. Gabapentin as an antiepileptic drug in man. *J Neurol Neurosurg Psychiatry* 1987;50:682–86.
4. The US Gabapentin Study Group. Gabapentin as add-on therapy in refractory partial epilepsy: a double-blind, placebo-controlled, parallel group study. *Neurology* 1993;43:2292–98.

• • • • • •
GABRENE® (PROGABIDE)

Not available in the United States. See Progabide.

• • • • • •
GAMMA-GLUTAMYLTRANSFERASE (GGT)

GGT is an enzyme involved in the transport of substances across the cell membrane. An increase in the serum level of GGT may be seen with enzyme-inducing AEDs. An elevation of GGT alone is of little concern and may merely indicate chronic compliance with AED drug therapy.

Reference

Rosalki SB, Tarlow D, Rau D. Plasma gamma-glutaryl transpeptidase elevation in patients receiving enzyme-inducing drugs. *Lancet* 1971;ii:376.

• • • • • •
GANGLIOSIDOSIS

Gangliosidosis is a sphingolipidosis (see this heading) caused by an inborn error of metabolism that leads to multi-organ deposition of gangliosides. Two typical forms exist:

- GM1 (Landing disease)
- GM2 (Tay-Sachs disease) (see this heading)

The clinical picture of a gangliosidosis is that of a severe, symptomatic, generalized epilepsy associated with typical dysmorphic features and mental retardation. The diagnosis is made by demonstrating the specific enzyme deficiency.

Reference

Johnson WG. The clinical spectrum of hexosaminidase deficiency diseases. *Neurology* 1981;31:1453–56.

• • • • • •
GAUCHER'S (DISEASE)

Gaucher's disease is a sphingolipidosis (see also this heading) belonging to the group of glycosyl-ceramidoses. In its juvenile form (type III), Gaucher's disease may present as a progressive, myoclonic epilepsy. Onset is at age 6 to 8 years. Neuropsychiatric features include ataxia, pyramidal signs, supranuclear palsy, progressive retardation, and generalized tonic-clonic and myoclonic seizures (1).

Early EEG abnormalities consist of widespread synchronous bursts of slow waves predominantly in the posterior regions, abnormal response to photic stimulation, and slowing of the background frequencies (1,2). Death commonly ensues within 3 to 10 years of onset. The diagnosis is made by demonstrating diminished leukocyte beta-glucocerebrosidase activity (2).

References

1. King JO. Progressive myoclonic epilepsy due to Gaucher's disease in an adult. *J Neurol Neurosurg Psychiatry* 1975;38:849–54.
2. Winkelman MD, Banker BQ, Victor M, Moser HW. Non-infantile neuronopathic Gaucher's disease: a clinico-pathologic study. *Neurology* 1983;33:994–1008.

• • • • • •
GELASTIC (SEIZURES)

Gelastic seizures present with inappropriate laughter (1). A distinction must be made between true gelastic seizures and seizures with laughter from embarrassment or pleasure. The laughter of gelastic seizures often sounds forced, braying, and close to crying. Gelastic seizures are partial seizures associated with ictal activity in the central regions (forced laughter due to facial muscle contraction without emotional context) or the mesial temporal and cingulate regions (laughter accompanied by other behavioral manifestations of joy or pleasure). Gelastic features also occur in symptomatic generalized epilepsies. Some gelastic seizures result from lesions in the floor of the third ventricle or the temporal lobes (2). Cursive seizures may have gelastic components. (see also Cursive (S))

A syndrome of "hypothalamic hamartomas and ictal laughter" (3) consists of early onset, brief gelastic seizures that may pass unnoticed in previously normal children. Onset is around age 4 to 10 years, with progression to more prolonged gelastic seizures, other seizure types, cognitive and behavior problems. This clinical picture is suggestive of a hypothalamic hamartoma, and confirmation may be obtained with an MRI head scan. Ictal subdural recording has revealed seizures arising from the left anterior cingulate gyrus; electrical stimulation of the fusiform gyrus and parahippocampal gyrus produced laughter (4). Prognosis for seizure control and social adaptation is poor.

References

1. Loiseau P, Cohadon F, Cohadon S. Gelastic epilepsy. A review and report of five cases. *Epilepsia* 1971;12:313–28.
2. Gascon GG, Lombroso CT. Epileptic (gelastic) laughter. *Epilepsia* 1971;12:63–76.
3. Berkovic SF, Andermann F, Melanson D, Ethier RE, Feindel W, Gloor P. Hypothalamic hamartomas and ictal laughter: evolution of a characteristic epileptic syndrome and diagnostic value of magnetic resonance imaging. *Ann Neurol* 1988;23:429–39.
4. Arroyo S, Lesser RP, Gordon B, Uematsu S, Hart J, Schwerdt P, Andreasson K, Fisher RS. Mirth, laughter and gelastic seizures. *Brain* 1993;116:757–80.

• • • • • •
GENERALIZED (EPILEPSIES)

Generalized epilepsies and epileptic syndromes present as generalized convulsive or nonconvulsive seizures involving both hemispheres simultaneously.

According to the International Classification of Epileptic Syndromes, there are several types:

- idiopathic generalized epileptic syndromes (see this heading) classified according to age of onset;
- cryptogenic and symptomatic generalized epileptic syndromes classified according to etiology (see these headings).

• • • • • •
GENERALIZED (SEIZURES)
(OR BILATERAL AND SYMMETRIC SEIZURES)

Primary generalized seizures are those in which the clinical characteristics give no indication of anatomical localization. These seizures may involve motor manifestations (tonic-clonic, tonic, clonic, myoclonic, atonic) or alterations in consciousness (tonic-clonic, absence). Motor signs may be bilateral or generalized, and are symmetric. Ictal and interictal EEG findings show bilateral synchronous and symmetric spikes, polyspikes, sharp waves, and slow waves over both hemispheres. Seizures that are generalized from the onset are seen in the symptomatic or idiopathic generalized epilepsies, epilepsies of indeterminate nature, and in certain special syndromes (febrile convulsions, seizures due to toxic or metabolic disturbances, isolated seizures).

Secondarily generalized seizures are discussed elsewhere (see Partial seizures).

• • • • • •
GENERIC DRUGS

Generic drugs, including generic AEDs, have an advantage of being less expensive. In general, generic drugs should be used, provided that the reliability and efficacy are equal or nearly equal to those of proprietary medication. Unfortunately, this has not always been the case in the United States for AEDs. Occasional batches of poorly absorbable carbamazepine have generated recalls of medication in Canada and the United States. A few studies found increased seizure frequency with generic medications such as primidone (1) and increased side effects with generic carbamazepine (2).

Because of the variability and absorption of AEDs, the decision to use brand name or generic medications should be individualized between physician and patient.

References

1. Wyllie E, Pippenger CE, Roth AD. Increased seizure frequency with generic primidone. *JAMA* 1987;258:1216–17.
2. Hartley R, Aleksandrowitz J, Ng PC, McLain B, Bowmer CJ, Forsythe WI. Breakthrough seizures with generic carbamazepine: a consequence of poor bioavailability? *Brit J Clin Pract* 1990;44:270–73.

• • • • • •
GENETICS

Genetics play a role in epilepsy because proclivity toward seizures may be transmitted genetically, and also because seizures may be but one sign of a genetically determined neurological or generalized disease. Examples include tuberous sclerosis (Bourneville's disease), neurofibromatosis, amino acidopathy, Lafora body disease, etc. (see also Etiology)

The probability of disease transmission is multifactorial, depending on the epileptic syndrome, the degree of consanguinity, the degree of genetic penetrance, and environmental factors. Studies involving monozygotic twins (1,2) and the study of genetic markers (3) have contributed to our understanding of these issues.

Genetic factors are particularly involved in:

* idiopathic partial epilepsies with a specific age of onset: partial epilepsy with centro-temporal spikes, (4,5), benign childhood epilepsy with occipital spikes (6);
* idiopathic generalized epilepsies: childhood absence epilepsy (7), juvenile myoclonic epilepsy (8), generalized epilepsy on awakening.

Genetic markers have been identified in benign familial neonatal convulsions (9) and juvenile myoclonic epilepsy (10) (see these headings).

Genetic factors may be involved with febrile convulsions (11), symptomatic partial epilepsies (12,13), or symptomatic epilepsies due to metabolic or other disturbances, but the genetic contribution in these instances is less clear.

References

1. Lennox WG. The heredity of epilepsy as told by relatives and twins. *JAMA* 1951;146:529–36.

2. Metrakos K, Metrakos JD. Genetics of convulsive disorders. II. Genetic and electroencephalographic studies in centrencephalic epilepsy. *Neurology* 1961; 11:474–83.

3. Leppert MF. Gene mapping and other tools for discovery. *Epilepsia* 1990;31(Suppl 3):S11–S18.

4. Bray PF, Wiser WC. Hereditary characteristics of familial temporal central focal epilepsy. *Pediatrics* 1965;36:207–11.

5. Heijbel J, Blom S, Rasmusson M. Benign epilepsy of childhood with centro-temporal EEG foci: a genetic study. *Epilepsia* 1975;16:285–93.

6. Gastaut H. Benign epilepsy of childhood with occipital paroxysms. In: Roger J, Bureau M, Dravet C, Dreifuss FE, Perret A, Wolf P (eds.). *Epileptic syndromes in infancy, childhood and adolescence,* 2nd edition. London: John Libbey Eurotext, 1992:201–17.

7. Currier RD, Kooi A, Sandman LJ. Prognosis of pure petit mal: follow-up study. *Neurology* 1963;13:959–67.

8. Tsuboi T, Christian W. On the genetics of the primary generalized epilepsy with sporadic myoclonias of impulsive petit mal type. *Hum Genet* 1973;19:155–82.

9. Leppert M, Anderson VE, Quatterlbaum T, et al. Benign familial neonatal con-vulsions linked to genetic markers on chromosome 20. *Nature* 1989;337:647–48.

10. Delgado-Escueta AV, Serratosa JM, Liv A, et al. Progress in mapping human epilepsy genes. *Epilepsia* 1994;35(Suppl 1):529–40.

11. Tsuboi T. Genetic aspects of febrile convulsions. *Hum Genet* 1977, 38:169–73.

12. Ottman R. Genetics of the partial epilepsies, a review. *Epilepsia* 1989;30:107–11.

13. Ottman R, Annegers JF, Hauser HA, Kurland LT. Seizure risk in offspring of parents with generalized versus partial epilepsy. *Epilepsia* 1989;30:157–61.

● ● ● ● ● ●
GLUTAMATE-ASPARTATE

Glutamate and aspartate are primary excitatory neurotransmitters in the CNS, as well as having other metabolic functions (1–3) (see also Aspar-tate). Three distinct receptors are involved: quisqualic acid receptors, kainic acid receptors, and N-methyl-D-aspartate (NMDA) receptors. These recep-tors have different pharmacological specificities and are associated with different ionic channels. Their antagonists, in particular the antagonist of the NMDA receptor, can be anticonvulsant in animal model systems (4). Excessive amounts of aspartic, glutamic, and aspartic aminotransferase acids have been found in epileptic cortex (5).

Glutamate is also an excitotoxin which, when in excess, brings about neuronal death, e.g., during status epilepticus.

References

1. Fonnum F. Glutamate: a neurotransmitter in mammalian brain. *J Neurochem* 1984;42:1–11.
2. Greenamyre JT. The role of glutamate in neurotransmission and in neurologic disease. *Arch Neurol* 1986;43:1058–63.
3. Engelsen B. Neurotransmitter glutamate: its clinical importance. *Acta Neurol Scand* 1986;74:337–55.
4. Meldrum BS. Possible therapeutic applications of antagonists of excitatory amino acid neurotransmitters. *Clin Sci* 1985; 68:113–22.
5. Kish SJ, Dixon LM, Sherwin AL. Aspartic acid aminotransferase activity is increased in actively spiking compared with non-spiking human epileptic cortex. *J Neurol Neurosurg Psychiatry* 1988;51:552–56.

• • • • • • •
GRAND MAL (SEIZURES AND EPILEPSIES)

Grand mal seizures are primary generalized tonic-clonic seizures, although colloquial usage often refers to any tonic-clonic seizure as a grand mal seizure. This usage blurs the important distinction between partial and generalized seizures, each with separate etiologies and treatments. Literature regarding grand mal epilepsy is similarly confounded by the difficulty, in many cases, of determining from history alone whether the event is a primary or secondarily generalized seizure.

Grand mal seizures occur in several epileptic syndromes: idiopathic generalized epilepsies, symptomatic generalized epilepsies, and epilepsies of uncertain localization. Some idiopathic generalized epilepsies present only as grand mal seizures or with grand mal seizures and other types of seizures, including absence and myoclonic generalized seizures. These constitute clear electroclinical syndromes with etiologic, therapeutic, and prognostic implications.

The general characteristics of idiopathic generalized epilepsies presenting with grand mal epilepsies are:

- an age of onset in late childhood, adolescence, or early adulthood;
- an increased incidence of a primary generalized epilepsy in a family member;
- frequent co-existence with absence or myoclonic seizures;
- seizures triggered by sleep deprivation, excess alcohol intake, fatigue, menses, or photic stimuli (see also Induced (S));
- an interictal EEG showing bilateral, synchronous, symmetric spike, polyspike and slow wave discharges at 2.5 to 4 Hertz with a normal background frequency. Photoconvulsive electrographic respons-

es are common. In patients with infrequent seizures, the EEG is often normal, but repeated EEG recordings or recordings with sleep deprivation and activation may disclose abnormalities;

- typically, there is an excellent response to AEDs. However, relapses are not infrequent after stopping medication, even after several years seizure-free;
- the International Classification of Epilepsies lists epilepsy with grand mal seizures on awakening, as described by Janz (1–2), but other idiopathic, generalized forms of epilepsy may be unrelated to awakening (2,3);
- in patients with grand mal epilepsy, typically there is an excellent response to AEDs.

References

1. Janz D. The Grand Mal epilepsy and the sleeping-waking cycle. *Epilepsia* 1962;3:69–109
2. Wolf P. Epilepsy with Grand Mal on awakening. In: Roger J, Bureau M, Dravet C, Dreifuss FE, Perret A, Wolf P (eds.). *Epileptic syndromes in infancy, childhood and adolescence.* London: John Libbey Eurotext, 1992:329–41.
3. Billiard M. Epilepsies and the sleep-wake cycle. In: Sterman MB, Shouse MN, Passouant P (eds.). *Sleep and epilepsy.* New York: Academic Press, 1983:269–86.

● ● ● ● ● ●
GUSTATORY (SEIZURES)

Seizures with gustatory manifestations include:

- illusions: increase in the sense of taste (hypergeusia);
- hallucinations: the perception of taste without objective cause: bitterness, acidity, metallic taste.

Gustatory seizures have been associated with foci in the supra-insular cortex, operculum, Rolandic or parietal and extratemporal cortex.

An abnormal taste in the mouth may persist for several hours after the seizure.

Reference

Hauser-Hauw C, Bancaud J. Gustatory hallucinations in epileptic seizures. *Brain* 1987:110:339–59.

••••••
GYRATORY (SEIZURES, EPILEPSY)
(SEE ALSO VERSIVE (S))

A rare form of epilepsy consisting of turning of the entire body in the vertical axis for 180° or more, occasionally in a "ballet-like" manner at the start of the seizure. It may be associated with 3 per second spike and slow wave discharges (1) and generalized seizures. Seizures may occur secondary to frontotemporal or thalamic lesions (2,3).

References

1. Gastaut H, Aguglia V, Tinuper P. Benign versive or circling epilepsy with bilateral 3–cps spikes-and-wave discharges in late childhood. *Ann Neurol* 1986;19:301–303.
2. Donalson I. Volvular epilepsy: a distinctive and underreported seizure type. *Arch Neurol* 1986;43:260–62.
3. Leiguarda R, Nogués M, Berthier M. Gyratory epilepsy in a patient with a thalamic neoplasm. *Epilepsia* 1992;33:826–28.

HALLERVORDEN-SPATZ (SYNDROME)

Hallervorden-Spatz syndrome is a heredodegenerative disease of the central nervous system occasionally presenting with a progressive myoclonic epilepsy (see this heading).

Reference

Dooling EC, Schoene WC, Richardon EP. Hallervorden-Spatz syndrome. *Arch Neurol* 1974;30:70–83.

HALLUCINATORY (SEIZURES)

Hallucinatory seizures are a form of simple partial seizures characterized by a stereotyped visual, auditory, gustatory, olfactory, or somatic (see these headings) hallucination. Symptoms usually present as pseudo-hallucinations, in that subjects recognize the perceptions to be false. Simple partial seizures with hallucinations may progress to complex partial seizures, as may any simple partial seizure.

HAMARTOMAS

Hamartomas are developmental abnormalities in which histologically normal tissue resides in an abnormal location. These malformations appear macroscopically as cerebral tumors, either stable over time or slow-growing. They have different clinical presentations because of their variable anatomical localization. Hamartomas may be associated with seizures that originate in the area around the hamartoma (see also Arteriovenous malformation; Gelastic seizures).

• • • • • • •
HEADACHES

Several types of headaches are typically associated with seizures (see also Migraines):

- prodromal headaches: occurring 1–2 days before the seizure, generally associated with a feeling of malaise, fatigue, and moodiness;
- ictal headaches: sudden brief and severe—attributed to hippocampal or amygdalar onset (1). Headaches occasionally may be the first symptom of seizures (2);
- postictal headaches are seen in half of those patients with generalized seizures; less frequently after partial seizures. Headaches are severe, unilateral or bilateral, and may be associated with vomiting, photophobia, and worsened by sudden movement (3). They may result from the sudden increase in cerebral and cranial blood flow associated with tonic-clonic seizures.

In benign epilepsy with occipital spike waves (BEOSW) (4), there may be an "interictal" migraine or postictal headache as part of the syndrome which may be hemicranial or diffuse, and may be associated with nausea or vomiting.

References
1. Andermann F. Migraine-epilepsy relationship. *Epilepsy Res* 1987;1:213–16.
2. Young GB, Blume WT. Painful epileptic seizures. *Brain* 1983;106:537–54.
3. Schon F, Blau JN. Post-epileptic headache and migraine. *J Neurol Neurosurg Psychiatry* 1987;50:1148–52.
4. Gastaut H. Benign epilepsy of childhood with occipital paroxysms. In: Roger J, Dravet C, Bureau M, Dreifuss FE, Perret A, Wolf P (eds.). *Epileptic syndromes in infancy, childhood and adolescence*, 2nd edition. London: John Libbey Eurotext, 1992:201–17.

• • • • • • •
HEMATOMA, INTRACEREBRAL NONTRAUMATIC

Bleeding may occur in one or more of several intracranial compartments including the epidural, subdural, and subarachnoid "spaces"; and intracerebrally in one or more lobes, the thalamus, basal ganglia, brain stem, and the ventricles. In adults, seizures are frequently seen with nontraumatic bleeding after aneurysmal and vascular malformation rupture and neoplasms; they are somewhat less common when spontaneous or due to hypertension. Lobar hemorrhage in the frontal (1), parietal, and temporal regions (1,2) are most commonly associated with seizures. (See also Cerebrovascular accidents (S,E)).

Seizure incidence ranges from 6% to 25% (1–4) for both early and late-onset seizures and is about 16% in the early post-hemorrhage period (4,5), usually within 12 hours of hemorrhage.

Subarachnoid hemorrhage results in seizures in 26–35% (4,6) of patients.

Prophylactic AED therapy has been advocated in patients with hemorrhage involving the cerebral cortex.

References

1. Weisberg LA, Shamsnia M, Elliott D. Seizures caused by nontraumatic parenchymal brain hemorrhages. *Neurology* 1991;41:1197–99.
2. Faught E, Peters D, Bartolucci A, Moore L, Miller PC. Seizures after primary intracerebral hemorrhage. *Neurology* 1989;39:1089–93.
3. Mohr JP, Caplan LR, Melski JW, Goldstein RJ, Duncan GW, Kistler JP, Pessin MS, Bleich HC. The Harvard cooperative stroke registry: a prospective registry. *Neurology* 1978; 28:754–62.
4. Lewis RF, Kaplan PW. Intracranial hemorrhage and early seizures. *Epilepsia* 1989;30:684.
5. Berger AR, Lipton RB, Lesser ML, Lantos G, Porteney RK. Early seizures following intracerebral hemorrhage: implications for therapy. *Neurology* 1988;38:1363–65.
6. Hart RG, Byer JA, Slaughter JR, Hewett JE, Easton JD. Occurrence and implications of seizures in subarachnoid hemorrhage due to ruptured intracranial aneurysms. *Neurosurgery* 1981;8:417–21.

• • • • • •

HEMICONVULSION-HEMIPLEGIA-EPILEPSY (HHE) SYNDROME

HHE is an electroclinical syndrome described by Gastaut in 1957 (1). The syndrome appears in 2 stages:

- HH syndrome. A unilateral convulsion or unilateral status epilepticus in early infancy followed by transitory or fixed hemiplegia (2). This syndrome has multiple etiologies, including vascular lesions and encephalitis, or the etiology may be unknown. Fever is an essential triggering factor.
- In about half of the cases experiencing HH syndrome, partial or generalized epilepsy may appear, usually with a latency of 2–6

years. HHE syndrome has become less frequent, possibly because of improved management for febrile convulsions and status epilepticus.

References

1. Gastaut H, Poirier F, Payan H, Salamon G, Toga M, Vigouroux M. H.H.E. syndrome. Hemiconvulsions, hemiplegia, epilepsy. *Epilepsia* 1960;1:418–47.
2. Gastaut H. *Dictionary of epilepsy. Part 1: Definitions.* Geneva: World Health Organization, 1973.

• • • • • •
HEMINEVRIN® (CHLORMETHIAZOLE)

Chlormethiazole is a hypnotic and sedative agent, given intravenously, used in the United Kingdom, Central Europe, Asia, and Africa as an AED for the control of status epilepticus and in the treatment of eclampsia. It is not presently available in the United States.

• • • • • •
HEMIPLEGIA, POSTICTAL (TODD'S PARALYSIS)

After partial motor seizures or hemiclonic seizures, especially in children, focal weakness of the involved body part may persist for minutes to a few days. Clinical judgment may be required to distinguish a Todd's hemiplegia from a primary vascular event with an accompanying seizure.

Reference

Yarnell PR. Todd's paralysis: a cerebrovascular phenomenon? *Stroke* 1975;6:301–303.

• • • • • •
HEMISPHERECTOMY

Hemispherectomy comprises removal of the major portion of a hemisphere for intractable unilateral seizures. Since hemiplegia, hemihypesthesia, and homonymous hemianopsia result, the procedure is rarely performed, and when performed is usually done on children with preexisting focal deficits or clearly progressive lesions. Specific indications include infantile hemiplegia with refractory seizures, hemimegalencephaly, Rasmussen's encephalitis, Sturge-Weber syndrome in young children, or extensive neoplasm. After hemispherectomy, children can recover to a condition of mild hemiparesis with independent gait and a clumsy, but useful hand. Surgical techniques have improved (1,2) and have reduced the incidence of late complications due to cerebral hemosiderosis. Early operation may forestall some intellectual decline that accompanies continued seizures and their treatment (3). Hemispherectomy is effective in improving seizure control and interictal behavioral problems in 70–90% of cases.

References

1. Rasmussen T. Hemispherectomy for seizures revisited. *Can J Neurol Sci* 1983;10:71–78.
2. Tinuper P, Andermann F, Villeneuve JG, Rasmussen TB, Quesney LF. Functional hemispherectomy for treatment of epilepsy associated with hemiplegia: rationale, indications, results and comparison with callosotomy. *Ann Neurol* 1988;24:27–34.
3. Vining EPG, Freeman JM, Brandt J, Carson BS, Uematsu S. Progressive unilateral encephalopathy of childhood (Rasmussen's syndrome): a reappraisal. *Epilepsia* 1993;34:639–50.

• • • • • •
HEPATITIS (DRUG-INDUCED)

In evaluating hepatic function in a patient on AEDs, the physician should distinguish between:

- mild changes in hepatic function, reflected by increase in gamma-glutamyltransferase, alkaline phosphatase, lactate dehydrogenase, and a slight, frequently transient, increase in AST and ALT, indicating hepatic enzyme induction. These changes are usually without clear pathological significance (1,2);
- acute or subacute hepatitis. This condition is rare, with an estimated overall incidence of 0.1% for valproic acid and phenytoin, less for phenobarbital and carbamazepine, and approximately 1% for progabide. In the case of valproic acid (3) and possibly other AEDs as well, hepatotoxicity is more frequent in children under the age of 10 years who are taking multiple medications. Hepatitis usually appears during the first 3 months of treatment. The microscopic picture of AED-related hepatotoxicity is one of acute hepatocellular or mixed hepatitis with cholestasis and necrosis. More recently, liver failure has been reported with felbamate (see Felbamate (Felbatol®)).

Two mechanisms of acute AED-related hepatotoxicity have been suggested:

- hypersensitivity syndromes with skin rashes, lymphadenopathy, hepatosplenomegaly, arthralgias, renal insufficiency, and fever; seen with phenytoin (4,5) and barbiturates (6,7).
- specific drug toxicity found in particularly predisposed patients (progabide) or the elaboration of metabolites because of rarely used degradation pathways (valproate).

The course of acute AED-related hepatitis is variable. Immediate discontinuation of the offending AED may avoid morbidity and mortality. Other causes of hepatitis must be excluded.

The question of a chronic, insidious hepatotoxicity is less clear. In some patients, chronic AED therapy might be the cause of significant hepatocellular damage (8).

References

1. Verma N, Haidukewych D. Differential but infrequent alterations of hepatic enzyme levels and thyroid hormone levels by anticonvulsant drugs. *Arch Neurol* 1994;51:381–84.
2. Rosalki SB, Tarlow D, Rau D. Plasma gamma-glutamyl transferase elevation in patients receiving enzyme-inducing drugs. *Lancet* 1971;ii:376.
3. Dreifuss FE, Santilli N, Langer DH, Sweeney KP, Moline KA, Menander KB. Valproic acid hepatic fatalities: a retrospective review. *Neurology* 1987;37:379–85.
4. Parker WA, Shearer CA. Phenytoin hepatotoxicity: a case report and review. *Neurology* 1979;2:175–78.
5. Smythe MA, Umstead GS. Phenytoin hepatotoxicity: a review of the literature. *DICP* 1989;23:13–18.
6. Shapiro PA, Antonioli DA, Peppercorn MA. Barbiturate-induced submassive hepatic necrosis. *Am J Gastroenterol* 1980;74:270–73.
7. Jeavons PM. Hepatotoxicity of antiepileptic drugs. In: Oxley J, Janz D, Meinardi H (eds.). *Antiepileptic therapy: chronic toxicity of antiepileptic drugs.* New York: Raven Press, 1983:1–45.
8. Foster GR, Goldin RD, Freeth CJ, Nieman E, Oliviera DBG. Liver damage in long-term anticonvulsant therapy: a serological and histological study. *Quart J Med* 1991;79:315–22.

• • • • • •

HERPES SIMPLEX ENCEPHALITIS (SEE ALSO ENCEPHALITIS/ENCEPHALITIDES)

Herpes simplex type I encephalitis may cause seizures in adults; herpes simplex type II may do so in neonates. This infection accounts for 5–10% of the annual encephalitis cases in the United States. Infection is characterized by headache, fever, seizures, confusion, obtundation, and coma with an aseptic, but often hemorrhagic cerebrospinal fluid. Olfactory hallucinations, anosmia, aphasia, and paresis occur in addition to psychosis, correlating with the predilection of the virus for temporal and frontal lobes. Untreated or treated late, the mortality is 30%–70%, with marked residua among the survivors: severe seizures, dementia, and aphasia. The clinical signs and symptoms, CSF findings, CT or MRI scans showing frontal and temporal involvement, and EEG showing focal slowing, periodic lateralizing epileptiform discharges (PLEDs) or focal seizures suggest the diagnosis. Fluorescent antibody investigation, viral culture, and the finding of microscopic inclusion bodies from biopsied cerebral tissue may be obtained to confirm the diagnosis. Treatment with acyclovir (1,2) early in the course of the illness has been reported to lower the mortality to about 17% (2).

References

1. Whitley RJ, Alford CA, Hirsh MS, et al. Vidarabine vs acyclovir therapy in herpes simplex encephalitis. *N Engl J Med* 1986;314:144–49.
2. Hanley DF, Johnson RT, Whitley RJ. Yes, brain biopsy should be a prerequisite for herpes simplex encephalitis treatment. *Arch Neurol* 1987;44:1289–90.

● ● ● ● ● ●
HIPPOCAMPUS

The hippocampus is part of the limbic system and is believed to be the most seizure-prone region of the brain. It occupies the internal aspect of the temporal lobe and includes the hippocampus proper (Ammon's horn), the dentate gyrus, and the subiculum. The hippocampus is divided regionally into four fields: CA1, CA2, CA3, CA4, with "CA" an abbreviation of "Cornu Ammonis."

Repeated status epilepticus during the neonatal period or childhood may bring about ischemic lesions and sclerosis of the hippocampus (1), predominantly involving areas CA1, CA3, and the dentate gyrus (see also Mesial temporal sclerosis). Hippocampus is a favored target for surgery to treat complex partial epilepsy of temporal origin (2).

References

1. Meldrum BS. Physiological changes during prolonged seizures and epileptic brain damage. *Neuropaediatrie* 1978;9:203–12.
2. Wieser HG, Yasargil MC. Selective amygdalohippocampectomy as a surgical treatment of mesiobasal limbic epilepsy. *Surg Neurol* 1982;17:445–57.

• • • • • •
HIRSUTISM

Hirsutism, or excessive facial and body hair, is a relatively frequently seen side effect with phenytoin. This side effect is especially troublesome in young females.

Reference

Eadie MJ. Anticonvulsant drugs. An update. *Drugs* 1984;27:328–63.

• • • • • •
HIV (HUMAN IMMUNODEFICIENCY VIRUS)/ ACQUIRED IMMUNODEFICIENCY SYNDROME (AIDS)

Human immunodeficiency virus is one of a group of retroviruses that cause an almost universally fatal disorder, acquired immunodeficiency syndrome (AIDS). Direct nervous system invasion by the HIV group of viruses as well as by opportunistic infection with AIDS result in neurological complications in most cases by the time of demise (1–3). Primary CNS lymphoma or other neoplasms may also occur. Each of these mechanisms can lead to seizures.

Seizures frequency is about 7–11% (4,5) in seropositive patients, patients with AIDS-related complex (ARC), or patients with AIDS. Seizures are more frequently seen (32–54% of cases) with toxoplasmosis or lymphoma, more rarely with encephalopathy or meningitis (6). Seizures may also represent an early sign of the AIDS-dementia complex in about 10% of such cases (4–5). Seizures occur in approximately one-third of cases of AIDS and are usually of a partial complex or simple type, often with secondary generalization. AED therapy is often problematic as patients may develop hypersensitivity reactions (14%), breakthrough seizures with therapeutic AED levels, or more rarely drug fever, reversible leukopenia, or Stevens-Johnson syndrome (5)

References

1. Kieburtz K, Schiffer RB, Neurologic manifestations of human immunodeficiency virus infections. *Neurol Clin* 1989;7:447–68
2. Janssen RS, Cornblath DR, Epstein LG, McArthur J, Price RW. Human immunodeficiency virus (HIV) infection and the nervous system: report from the American Academy of Neurology AIDS task force. *Neurology* 1989;39:119–22.
3. McArthur JC. Neurologic manifestations of AIDS. *Medicine* 1987;66:407–37.

4. Wong MC, Suite NDA, Labar DR. Seizures in human immunodeficiency virus infection. *Arch Neurol* 1990;47:640–42.

5. Holtzman DM, Kaku DA, So YT. New-onset seizures associated with human immunodeficiency virus infection: causation and clinical features in 100 cases. *Am J Med* 1989; 87:173–77.

• • • • • • •
HORMONES

Hormones influence epilepsy and seizures affect the endocrine system.

1. *The effect of hormones on epilepsy (1,2):*
    Animal experiments and clinical observations have shown that estrogens decrease seizure threshold and increase seizure frequency, while progesterone-related agents have the reverse effect (see Catamenial (S)). Much more marked changes in the estrogen-progesterone status occur during pregnancy, frequently without having any effect on seizure frequency.

2. *The effect of seizures on hormones (1):*
    Seizures that spread to the limbic system and hypothalamus may increase release of prolactin into the systemic circulation (see also Prolactin). There may also be alterations in release of melatonin, luteinizing hormone (LH), and follicle stimulating hormone (FSH). These transient increases appear to have no long-term consequence. Basal circulating hormone levels and pituitary stimulation-induced changes are the same for untreated patients with epilepsy and for normal subjects (3).

3. *The effect of AEDs on hormones:*
    AED-induced enzyme induction may bring about increased hormone metabolism, thus changing blood levels and the feedback through the hypothalamic-pituitary axis. Some AEDs appear to act directly on this axis. Although changes in endocrine function are common, they rarely have any clinical significance, a concept that must be kept in mind when interpreting hormone levels in patients with epilepsy (4).

HYPOTHALAMIC-PITUITARY AXIS

• Antidiuretic hormone (ADH): Inhibited by phenytoin (without clinical significance). Increased by carbamazepine (possibly responsible for water intoxication and hyponatremia);

• Prolactin: Inhibited by certain GABAergic and dopaminergic drugs, but not valproic acid. Increased by carbamazepine (3);

- Human growth hormone (HgH): Increased by the GABAergic and dopaminergic drugs.
- Corticotrophin releasing factor (CRF): Inhibited by valproic acid.

THYROID (5)

T3 and T4 levels are decreased by phenytoin and carbamazepine, whereas TSH is unchanged. Hypothyroidism has been reported (6). There is a less prominent effect on thyroid by valproic acid (7). Clinically significant effects are rare (8).

ADRENAL

- Free cortisol levels are decreased by phenytoin and carbamazepine via peripheral inhibition and hypothalamic inhibition, and by increased metabolism as well as hepatic enzyme induction.
- Secretion of 17–ketosteroids are decreased and other metabolites, increased by phenytoin and carbamazepine.

INSULIN

Phenytoin decreases the glucose-induced insulin response, but does not affect glucose tolerance. This action is probably due to an inhibition of insulin secretion associated with increased sensitivity to insulin (9).

SEX HORMONES (1,2)

- Phenytoin, carbamazepine, phenobarbital, and primidone, but not valproic acid (3) increase specific sex hormone binding globulins (SHBG) that serve as transport proteins. This may result in an increase in total testosterone, a decrease in free testosterone, and an increase in pituitary LH secretion.
- Testosterone homeostasis is altered by AEDs, with the decreased excretion of androsterone and ethiocholanolone.

ORAL CONTRACEPTIVES

Decreased effectiveness of oral contraceptives has been reported in patients taking phenobarbital, primidone, carbamazepine, and phenytoin, but not valproic acid and benzodiazepines (10,11).

References

1. Mattson RH, Cramer JA. Epilepsy, sex hormones, and antiepileptic drugs. *Epilepsia* 1985;26 (Suppl 1):S40–S51.
2. Schachter SC. Hormonal considerations in women with seizures. *Arch Neurol* 1988;45:1267–70.
3. Macphee GJA, Larkin JG, Butler E, Beastall GH, Brodie MJ. Circulating hormones and pituitary responsiveness in young epileptic men receiving long-term antiepileptic medication. *Epilepsia* 1988;29:468–75.

4. Luhdorf K. Endocrine function and antiepileptic treatment. *Acta Neurol Scand* 1983;94 (Suppl):15–19.

5. Jung RT. Anticonvulsants, thyroid and other endocrine functions. In: D Chadwick (ed.). Fourth International Symposium on Sodium Valproate and Epilepsy, 1989, Royal Society of Medicine Services International Congress and Symposium. Series No152, published by Royal Society of Medicine Services Ltd., 1169–73.

6. Aanderud S, Strandjord RE. Hypothyroidism induced by antiepileptic drugs. *Acta Neurol Scand* 1980;61:330–32.

7. Connacher AA, Borsey DR, Browning MCK, Davidson DLW, Jung RT. The effective evaluation of thyroid status in patients on phenytoin, carbamazepine or sodium valproate attending an epilepsy clinic. *Postgrad Med J* 1987;63:841–45.

8. Verma N, Haidukewych D. Differentiated but infrequent alterations of hepatic enzyme levels and thyroid hornome levels by anticonvulsant drugs. *Arch Neurol* 1994;51:381–84.

9. Perry-Keene DA, Larkins RG, Heyma P, Peter CT, Ross D, Sloman JG. The effect of long-term diphenylhydantoin therapy on glucose tolerance and insulin secretion. *Clin Endocrinol* 1980;12:575–80.

10. Coulam CB, Annegers JG. Do anticonvulsants reduce the efficacy of oral contraceptives? *Epilepsia* 1979;20:519 26.

11. Back DJ, Bates M, Bowden A, et al. The interaction of phenobarbital and other anticonvulsants with oral contraceptive steroid therapy. *Contraception* 1980;22:495–503.

●●●●●●

HUNTINGTON'S CHOREA (DISEASE)

Seizures occur with early onset Huntington's chorea (1). There are no specific EEG or clinical features of seizures in Huntington's chorea, although low-voltage EEGs and abnormal evoked potentials are common associations and myoclonic seizures have been reported (2).

References

1. Green JB, Dickinson, ES, Gunderman JR. Epilepsy in Huntington chorea: clinical and neurophysiological studies. In: Barbeau A, Chase TN, Paulson GW (eds.). *Advances in Neurology,* Volume 1. New York: Raven Press, 1973;105–13.

2. Vogel CM, Drury I, Terry LC, Young AB. Myoclonus in adult Huntington's disease. *Ann Neurol* 1991;29:213–15.

• • • • • •
HYDANTOINS

Following Merritt and Putnam's discovery of the anticonvulsant effects of phenytoin, several hydantoins were marketed, including mephentoin and ethotoin. At present, phenytoin is the most widely used.

• • • • • •
HYDROCEPHALUS

Seizures occur in 30% of patients with hydrocephalus, either with obstructive or nonobstructive types of hydrocephalus. Hydrocephalic seizures are more common in children, but also occur in adults with secondary hydrocephalus (e.g., from intracranial hemorrhage or infection) (1). Atrial-ventricular or ventriculo-peritoneal shunts may increase seizure tendency for up to 4 years after placement (2,3).

Several seizure types are seen, including hemiconvulsions in children (from cortical scarring at surgery), generalized tonic-clonic seizures, and complex partial seizures. Epilepsy is severe in approximately one-third of cases (3). A critical clinical distinction must be made between seizures in association with hydrocephalus and tonic activity from brainstem compression associated with acute rises in intracranial pressure.

References

1. Dan NG, Wade HS. The incidence of epilepsy after ventricular shunting procedures. *J Neurosurg* 1986;65:19–21.
2. Graebner RW, Celesia GG. EEG findings in hydrocephalus and their relation to shunting procedures. *Electroencephalogr clin Neurophysiol* 1973;35:517–20.
3. Varfis G, Berney J, Beaumanoir A. Electro-clinical follow-up of shunted hydrocephalic children. *Child's Brain* 1977;3:129–39.

• • • • • •
HYPEREKPLEXIA
(PATHOLOGICAL STARTLE RESPONSE) (1–3)

Hyperekplexia is a stereotyped response to unexpected stimuli. To a certain degree, it is a normal reaction, but it becomes pathologic because of increased frequency or decreased threshold (1,2). The differential diagnosis includes:

- myoclonic seizures or sudden drop attacks;
- startle epilepsy;
- infantile spasms.

References

1. Saenz-Lope E, Herranz-Tanarro FJ, Masdeu JC, Chacon Pena JR. Hyperekplexia: a syndrome of pathological startle responses. *Ann Neurol* 1984;15:36–41.
2. Andermann F, Andermann E. Startle disease or hyperekplexia. *Ann Neurol* 1984;16:367–68.
3. Vigevano F, Di Capua M, Dalla-Bernardina B. Startle disease: an avoidable cause of sudden infant death. *Lancet* 1989;i:216.

● ● ● ● ● ●
HYPERGLYCEMIA (1–3)

Nonketotic hyperglycemia and other hyperosmolar conditions may precipitate spontaneous or movement-induced focal motor status epilepticus. Underlying focal cortical abnormalities may be present. Seizures usually remit with correction of the underlying metabolic disturbance. (See also Kojewnikow's syndrome; Movement, seizures induced by).

References

1. Singh BM, Gupta DR, Strobos RJ. Non-ketotic hyperglycemia and epilepsia partialis continua. *Arch Neurol* 1973;29:187–90.
2. Brick JF, Gutrecht JA, Ringel RA. Reflex epilepsy and nonketotic hyperglycemia in the elderly: a specific neuroendocrine syndrome. *Neurology* 1989;39:394–99.
3. Hennis A, Corbin D, Fraser H. Focal seizures and non-ketotic hyperglycaemia. *J Neurol Neurosurg Psychiat* 1992;55:195–97.

● ● ● ● ● ●
HYPERVENTILATION

Hyperventilation or overbreathing incommensurate with physical effort may induce clinical absence seizures and bilateral synchronous 3 per second spike and slow discharges on EEG in some patients with idiopathic epilepsy and absence seizures (see also this heading). Diffuse slowing of the EEG pattern, especially with low blood glucose levels, frequently occurs in normal individuals. Focal slowing is abnormal and may occur with structural abnormalities including ischemic and mass lesions.

Reference

Kellaway P. An orderly approach to visual analysis: characteristics of the normal EEG of adults and children. In: Daly DD, Pedley TA (eds.). *Current practice of clinical electroencephalography,* 2nd edition. New York: Raven Press.

• • • • • •
HYPONATREMIA

Hyponatremia is one of the metabolic disturbances that may precipitate seizures in susceptible individuals. It is not infrequently seen as a side effect of carbamazepine in adults (1–3), with an increasing risk (6–31%) with age and blood carbamazepine level.

References

1. Soelberg Sorensen P, Hammer M. Effects of long-term carbamazepine treatment on water metabolism and plasma vasopressin concentration. *Eur J Clin Pharmacol* 1984;26:719–22.
2. Lahr MB. Hyponatremia during carbamazepine therapy. *Clin Pharmacol Ther* 1985;37:693–96.
3. Perucca E, Garratt A, Hebdige S, Richens A. Water intoxication in epileptic patients receiving carbamazepine. *J Neurol Neurosurg Psychiatry* 1978;41:713–18.

• • • • • •
HYPOXIA

Severe diffuse hyoxia in the pre- and perinatal period may cause secondary generalized epilepsy (see also Mesial temporal sclerosis); in adults, severe acute hypoxia may result in partial seizures (see also Kojewnikow's syndrome) or myoclonus, usually with poor prognosis. Posthypoxic action myoclonus, a chronic condition, may be seen after cardiorespiratory arrest (Lance-Adams syndrome) and responds to valproate or clonazepam. Brief hypoxia may cause convulsive syncope (see also this heading). (See also Anoxia/hypoxia).

Reference

Krumholtz A, Stern BJ, Weiss HD. Outcome from coma after cardiopulmonary resuscitation: relation to seizures and myoclonus. *Neurology* 1988;38:401–405.

• • • • • •
HYPSARRHYTHMIA

This pattern, initially reported by Gibbs and Gibbs, is a constantly abnormal pattern with asynchronous and synchronous, high-voltage slow waves with shifting multifocal spikes and sharp waves constituting a "chaotic" pattern. The greatest abnormality usually occurs during sleep. In addition to hypsarrhythmic patterns, electrodecremental periods of EEG suppression are seen during infantile spasms with West syndrome (see also this heading). Hypsarrhythmia usually occurs in infants under the age of one year.

Reference

Gibbs FA, Gibbs EL. *Atlas of electroencephalography, Vol. 2. Epilepsy.* Cambridge, MA: Addison-Wesley, 1952.

I

• • • • • •
ICTAL

"Ictal" refers to events occurring during an epileptic seizure. This includes clinical seizure manifestations, EEG changes, cardiovascular and metabolic alterations. It is often difficult to make a clear distinction between ictal, postictal, and interictal events. It is occasionally difficult to distinguish between ictal and postictal automatism, interictal and postictal alteration of consciousness (1), and postictal and interictal CT head scan (2) or MRI (3) changes. Furthermore, so-called "subclinical" epileptiform discharges may alter cognition (4,5).

References

1. Theodore WH, Porter RJ, Penry JK. Complex partial seizures: clinical characteristics and differential diagnosis. *Neurology* 1983;33:1115–21.
2. Feinstein A, Ron M, Wessely S. Disappearing brain lesions, psychosis and epilepsy: a report of two cases. *J Neurol Neurosurg Psychiatry* 1990;53:244–46.
3. Riela AR, Sires BP, Penry JK. Transient magnetic resonance imaging abnormalities during partial status epilepticus. *J Child Neurol* 1991;6:143–45.
4. Rausch R, Lieb JP, Crandall PH. Neuropsychologic correlates of depth spike activity in epileptic patients. *Arch Neurol* 1978;35:699–705.
5. Kasteleijn-Nolst Trenite DG, Bakken DJ, Binnie CD, Buerman A, Van Raazz M. Psychological effects of subclinical epileptiform EEG discharges. I. Scholastic skills. *Epilepsy Res* 1988;2:111–16.

• • • • • •
IDIOPATHIC (SEIZURES, EPILEPSY)

Idiopathic is a term once used in reference to any seizure or epilepsy without obvious cause. The Commission on Classification and Terminology of the International League Against Epilepsy reserves its use for certain partial and generalized epileptic syndromes with particular electroclinical characteristics seen predominantly in normal patients without cerebral abnormalities. Presence of epilepsy is believed to be due to a lowered seizure threshold with a genetic basis, whether a family history of seizures is present or not. Not all hereditary epilepsies are idiopathic (e.g., Lafora body disease). Idiopathic epilepsies should be distinguished from cryptogenic epilepsies (see Cryptogenic).

Reference

Commission on Classification and Terminology of International League Against Epilepsy. Proposal for classification of epilepsies and epileptic syndromes. *Epilepsia* 1989;30:389–99.

• • • • • •
IDIOSYNCRATIC REACTIONS

Idiosyncratic reactions are unexpected side effects of medication seen in patients. Patients experiencing such reactions often have abnormal drug metabolic pathways. Idiosyncratic reactions to AEDs are rare, are frequently serious, and occasionally lead to death. They are, by definition, unpredictable (see Antiepileptic drugs (AEDs)).

Reference

Booker HE. Idiosyncratic reactions to the antiepileptic drugs. *Epilepsia* 1975; 16:171–81.

• • • • • •
ILLUSIONAL (SEIZURES)

Illusional seizures are simple partial seizures whose principal symptom is that of abnormal perception in the form of an illusion—defined as the misperception of real objects. These seizures may be visual, auditory, gustatory, olfactory, or somatosensory (see these headings). Simple partial illusional seizures may evolve to complex partial or tonic-clonic seizures.

• • • • • •
IMMUNOSUPPRESSION

Prolonged AED intake may lead to changes in the immune system (1,2). Phenytoin has been implicated, perhaps because of its widespread use, but other AEDs may also have immunological side effects. Cell-mediated immunity and humoral immunity are decreased by:

- changes in immunoglobulin levels, usually decreased. This affects especially IgA levels (17–23% of patients with PHT, 11% with CBZ). There is less effect on IgG and IgM levels;

- decreased T lymphocyte function;
- antinuclear, antimuscle, and antimitochondrial antibodies in 25% of patients. These changes are apparently involved in idiosyncratic reactions: lupus, more rarely periarteritis nodosa, myasthenia, or thyroiditis. Benign transient lymphadenopathies (seen with hypersensitivity syndromes) or malignant lymphomas (3) rarely occur.

References

1. Booker HE. Idiosyncratic reactions to the antiepileptic drugs. *Epilepsia* 1975;16:171–81.
2. Andersen P, Mosekilde L. Immunoglobulin levels and autoantibodies in epileptics on long-term anticonvulsant therapy. *Acta Med Scand* 1977;201:69–74.
3. Anthony JJ. Malignant lymphoma associated with hydantoin drugs. *Arch Neurol* 1970;22:450–54.

••••••
INCIDENCE

The number of new cases of a particular disease arising in a given population over a given time is expressed as the incidence of that disease. Incidence is calculated most often as an annual rate per population, e.g., per 100,000 inhabitants/year. The numbers of cases seen depends on the reliability of the information collected and the accurate definition of the disease under study.

The worldwide incidence of epilepsy varies between 17.3/100,000 to 73/100,000, depending on the inclusion criteria: isolated seizures, febrile convulsions, or only recurrent seizures (1). The incidence rate of "active" epilepsy with at least 2 seizures in the preceding year is 48.7/100,000 (2). The incidence of first seizures (representing both acute symptomatic seizures as well as seizures heralding an epileptic syndrome) has been estimated at 73.1/100,000 (3). The age distribution curve of epilepsy incidence is bimodal, children younger than 10 years old (121/100,000/year) and patients over 60 years old (122/100,000/year). The incidence increases with age and decreases with younger children (2).

The incidence is raised in males and in blacks when studied in a multiracial population (see Race). The distribution varies with the type of seizure studied giving variable and frequently conflicting results (1,2).

References

1. Jallon P, Dartigues JF. Epidémiologie descriptive des épilepsies. *Rev Neurol* (Paris) 1987;143:341–50.

2. Hauser WA, Kurland LT. The epidemiology of epilepsy in Rochester, Minnesota, 1935 through 1977. *Epilepsia* 1975;16:1–66

3. Loiseau J, Loiseau P, Guyot M, Duche B, Dartigues JF, Aublet B. Survey of seizure disorders in the French Southwest. I: Incidence of epileptic syndromes. *Epilepsia* 1990;31:319–96.

• • • • • •
INCONTINENCE (URINARY)

With generalized tonic-clonic seizures, urinary incontinence is a frequent, but not a constant finding; it is not pathognomonic of seizures in the setting of abrupt loss of function or consciousness since it may be seen during syncope or cerebrovascular compromise. Incontinence was previously, but incorrectly, believed to be an epileptic equivalent. Some children are enuretic and have incidental seizures. When seizures occur during sleep, other signs of seizures are usually apparent.

- Incontinence may occur in certain absence seizures (see this heading);
- Incomplete incontinence sometimes occurs with partial seizures with or without loss of consciousness.

• • • • • •
INDUCED (SEIZURES)

Several factors can induce, precipitate, trigger, or provoke seizures. Seizure induction may be immediate (1), such as with intermittent photic stimulation. Seizure-inducing factors include (1):

1. *Alteration in the level of consciousness:* drowsiness or sleep, nocturnal sleep, daytime naps, relaxation, or inactivity. Sudden awakening, sleep deprivation, or sustained concentration.
2. *Physical activity:* fatigue, strenuous physical activity (see Sports).
3. *Emotional stress:* emotions, conflict, anxiety, tension, depression, and other psychosomatic aspects of epilepsy (2,3).
4. *Hormonal changes:* menses, pregnancy.
5. *Acid-base disequilibrium:* alkalosis.
6. *Hypoxia.*
7. *Fever, particularly in infants and young children.*
8. *Metabolic disturbances:* water intoxication, hypoglycemia, hypocalcemia.

9. **Renal or hepatic insufficiency:** either directly or by changing drug metabolism.
10. **Drugs:**
    • Either by lowering the seizure threshold: many classes of pharmacological agents have been implicated, including antidepressants, neuroleptics, hypoglycemic agents, penicillins, aminophylline, and a wide variety of other drugs.
    • Abrupt withdrawal seizures when anticonvulsants are stopped, particularly with barbiturates or benzodiazepines (4-6).
11. **Toxic,** especially alcohol. Tea and coffee in moderation are not epileptogenic.

References

1. Aird RB. The importance of seizure-inducing factors in the control of refractory forms of epilepsy. *Epilepsia* 1983;24:567–83.
2. Temkin NR, Davis GR. Stress as a risk factor for seizures among adults with epilepsy. *Epilepsia* 1984;25:450–56.
3. Trimble MR. Psychosomatic aspects of epilepsy. *Adv Psychosom Med* 1985; 13:133–50.
4. Messing RO, Closson RG, Simon RP. Drug-induced seizures: a 10-year experience. *Neurology* 1984;34:1582–86.
5. Cold JA, Wells BG, Froemming JH. Seizure activity associated with antipsychotic therapy. *DICP* 1990;24:601–606.
6. Zaccara G, Muscas GC, Messori A. Clinical features, pathogenesis and management of drug-induced seizures. *Drug Safety* 1990;5:109–51.

• • • • • • •
INHIBITORY (SEIZURES)

Focal limb weakness simulating transient ischemic attacks may be produced by somatic inhibitory seizures (1–3). The presumed mechanism is inhibition of motor function by seizure activity in the somatomotor areas. Surface EEGs have shown rhythmic delta activity (2) or phase-reversing spikes over the motor strip (3). A precipitating cause for the seizure may not be found (2), but subclinical ischemia reversed by carotid endarterectomy has been reported (3).

A differential diagnostic consideration is Todd's paralysis.

References

1. Globus M, Lavi E, Alexander F, Oded A. Ictal hemiparesis. *Eur Neurol* 1982;21:165–68.

2. Lee H, Lerner A. Transient inhibitory seizures mimicking crescendo TIAs. *Neurology* 1990;40:165–66.
3. Kaplan PW. Focal seizures resembling transient ischemic attacks due to subclinical ischemia. *Cerebrovasc Dis* 1993;3:241–43.

• • • • • •
ISOLATED (SEIZURES)

The first or only seizure occurring spontaneously, i.e., without clear cause. This concept is of great importance as the isolated seizure does not label a patient as being epileptic with its subsequent medical and social consequences.

Unfortunately, a first seizure in the context of what may be a subsequent epileptic condition is by definition isolated until the second seizure arises. This produces initial difficulties in providing prognostic and therapeutic reliability. The chance of seizure recurrence depends on a number of factors (see First seizure).

Absence seizures are never isolated events. Repeated partial seizures may occur before they are recognized as epilepsy. The time interval between isolated seizures depends, in part, on the timing of the use of AED therapy.

Reference

Shorvon SD. The temporal aspect of prognosis in epilepsy. *J Neurol Neurosurg Psychiatry* 1984;47:1157–65.

JACKSONIAN (SEIZURES)

Jacksonian seizures are partial seizures characterized by a progressive spread (march) from one part of the body to another, without perturbation of consciousness. Subsequent secondary generalization may occur. Jacksonian seizures may be:

- purely motor: tonic contraction of the thumb or big toe followed by the hand or the foot, then clonic involvement of the hand, forearm, arm or foot, leg, and thigh;
- purely sensory: ascending paresthesias;
- both sensory and motor.

Jacksonian seizures result from a progressive spread of electrical excitation in the Rolandic cortical region. Propensity to affect certain body parts parallels the area of cortical representation for that body part. Perioral and hand involvement are therefore most common. Jacksonian seizures are rare, especially in children, and their causes are multifactorial.

JANSKY-BIELCHOWSKY (DISEASE)

Jansky-Bielchowsky disease is a late infantile form of the ceroid-lipofuscinoses, seen especially in Finland (1,2). The disease is associated with autosomal recessive transmission. Onset is at age 2–4 years. Seizures are usually myoclonic in type, triggered by sensory stimuli; generalized tonic-clonic seizures, atonic seizures, atypical absences, or combinations of these seizure types may also occur. Patients with Jansky-Bielchowsky disease suffer rapid and progressive psychomotor retardation, involvement of the cerebellum, blindness, and spasticity. Death usually occurs within 5 years of onset.

EEG in Jansky-Bielchowsky disease shows multiple abnormalities, including occipital epileptiform activity in bursts or continuously, as well as polyphasic complexes with photic stimulation.

Histologic studies are consistent with the ceroid-lipofuscinoses (3)(see also Ceroid-lipofuscinoses).

References

1. Jansky J, Dosud neposany pripod familiarni amauroticke idiotie kompliko-vane hyprophasii moseckovou. *Sb Lek* 1908;13:165–96.
2. Bielchowski M. Uber spät-infantile familiare amaurotischen idiotic mit Klein-hirnsymptomen. *Dtsch Z Nervenheilk* 1913;50:7–29.
3. Dyken PR. The neuronal ceroid lipofuscinoses. *J Child Neurol* 1989;4:165–74.

● ● ● ● ● ●
JUVENILE MYOCLONIC EPILEPSY

Juvenile myoclonic epilepsy (JME) was first described by Janz (1), and subsequently by Delgado-Escueta and associates (11). The syndrome is sometimes referred to as "myoclonic epilepsy of Janz" or "benign juvenile myoclonic epilepsy"(1). Terms now in disuse include "myoclonic petit mal" and "impulsive petit mal" (1,2).

One of the best described epileptic syndromes, JME belongs to the group of idiopathic generalized seizures (3). JME is familial in more than 40% of cases (4,5), and recent results suggest genetic heterogeneity (6,7). JMR represents 4–12% of the epilepsies (1,4), with an incidence of 0.55/100,000 people (8). It occurs more frequently in females and usual-ly begins during adolescence. Patients with JME have a normal neurolog-ic examination.

JME is characterized by brief, irregular episodes of limb myoclonus often with clinical and EEG asymmetries that can lead to misdiagnosis (9,10,11). Consciousness is not disturbed. Myoclonus usually occurs soon after morning awakening. Myoclonus is increased by sleep deprivation, early rising, intermittent stimulation, emotional stress, and alcohol (1,2,11).

EEG findings in JME consist predominantly of polyspike-wave pat-terns, pathognomonic for JME when they occur ictally, corresponding to the myoclonic jerks. The discharge consists of a bilateral, more or less syn-chronous discharge of 5–20 negative spikes with a frequency of 12–15 Hz, and with increasing amplitude, sometimes reaching 150–300 microvolts. The spikes are followed by slow waves of changing frequency, but are at about 3.5 Hz. The duration of the discharge ranges from 3–5 seconds. Inter-ictal discharges are shorter, with fewer spikes. Other less specific spike-wave types are not rare (1,4,5). Background activity is normal (4,12). Seizure discharges on the EEG are increased by hyperventilation, sleep deprivation, and intermittent photic stimulation (13). Tonic-clonic seizures are seen in 58–90% of cases (4,5); absence seizures 15–20% of cases (1,12).

Seizures and myoclonus associated with JME usually respond well to sodium valproate (14,15) or primidone, but there is a high rate of recur-rence if treatment is discontinued (16).

References

1. Janz D. Epilepsy with impulsive Petit Mal (Juvenile Myoclonic Epilepsy). *Acta Neurol Scand* 1985;72:449–59.
2. Janz D, Christian W. Impulsive Petit Mal. *Dtsch Z Nervenheilk* 1957;176:346–86.
3. Dreifuss FE. Juvenile myoclonic epilepsy: characteristics of primary generalized epilepsy. *Epilepsia* 1989;30(Suppl 4):S1–S7.
4. Asconape J, Penry JK. Some clinical and EEG aspects of benign juvenile myoclonic epilepsy. *Epilepsia* 1984;25:108–14.
5. Obeid T, Panayiotopoulos CP. Juvenile myoclonic epilepsy: a study in Saudi Arabia. *Epilepsia* 1988;29:280–82.
6. Panayiotopoulos CP, Obeid T. Juvenile myoclonic epilepsy: an autosomal recessive disease. *Ann Neurol* 1989;25:440–43.
7. Delgado-Escueta AV, Serratosa JM, Liv A, et al. Progress in mapping human epilepsy genes. *Epilepsia* 1994;35(Suppl 1):529–40.
8. Tsuboi T. *Primary generalized epilepsy with sporadic myoclonias of myoclonic Petit Mal type.* Stuggart: Thieme, 1977.
9. Lancman ME, Asconapé JJ, Penry JK. Clinical and EEG asymmetries in Juvenile Myoclonic Epilepsy. *Epilepsia* 1994;35:302–306.
10. Loiseau P, Duché B. Juvenile myoclonic epilepsy. *Progress in Clin Neurosc* 1990;6:79–88.
11. Delgado-Escueta AV, Enrile-Bacsal F. Juvenile myoclonic epilepsy. *Neurology* 1984;34:285–94.
12. Panayiotopoulos CP, Obeid T, Waheed G. Absences in juvenile myoclonic epilepsy: a clinical and video-electroencephalographic study. *Ann Neurol* 1989;25:391–97.
13. Wolf P, Juvenile myoclonus epilepsy. In: Roger J, Bureau M, Dravet C, Dreifuss FE, Perret A, Wolf P (eds.). *Epileptic syndromes in infancy, childhood and adolescence,* 2nd edition. London: John Libbey & Co. Ltd., 1992:313–27.
14. Jeavons PM, Clerk JC, Maheshwari MC. Treatment of generalized epilepsies of childhood and adolescence with sodium valproate (Epilim). *Dev Med Child Neurol* 1977;19:9–25.
15. Wolf P, Inoue Y. Therapeutic response of absence seizures in patients of an epilepsy clinic for adolescents and adults. *J Neurol* 1984; 231:225–29.
16. Penry JK, Riela AR. Juvenile myoclonic epilepsy: long term response to therapy. *Epilepsia* 1989;30(Suppl 4):S19–S23.

• • • • • •
JUVENILE NEUROAXONAL DYSTROPHY (SEITELBERGER'S DISEASE)

A rare syndrome that, when presenting young, appears as a progressive myoclonic epilepsy with chorea, ataxia, dementia, and peripheral neuropathy. The diagnosis is made on the biopsy findings of spheroid axonal terminations of the autonomic nervous system.

Reference

Dorfmann LJ, Pedley TA, Tharp BR, Scheithauer TA. Juvenile neuroaxonal dystrophy: clinical, electrophysiological and neuropathological features. *Ann Neurol* 1978;3:419–28.

KETOGENIC DIET

The ketogenic diet was introduced in 1921 by Wilder based on observations that fasting decreased seizure frequency. It has been used in certain refractory epilepsies of childhood, including absence, akinetic, atonic, and myoclonic seizures, infantile spasms, and Lennox-Gastaut syndrome. The diet is low in proteins and carbohydrates, but high in fats, resulting in ketosis, a factor believed to be partly responsible for a raised seizure threshold. A typical "4/1" diet consists of 4 calories from fats for every 1 from proteins and carbohydrates, with a total caloric intake of 75 calories/kg of body weight. Medium chain triglycerides (1) or vegetable oils (2) may also be used. Short-term benefit has been obtained (3,4), but most patients have difficulty with compliance. Additionally, the diet becomes less effective around the time of puberty. The exact mechanism of the antiepileptic action of the ketogenic diet is unclear (1).

References

1. Schwartz RM, Boyes S, Aynsley-Green A. Metabolic effects of three ketogenic diets in the treatment of severe epilepsy. *Dev Med Child Neurol* 1989;31:152–60.
2. Woody RC, Brodie M, Hampton DK, Fiser RH. Corn oil ketogenic diet for children with intractable seizures. *J Child Neurol* 1988;3:21–24.
3. Schwartz RM, Eaton J, Bower BD, Aynsley-Green A. Ketogenic diets in the treatment of epilepsy: short term clinical effects. *Dev Med Child Neurol* 1989;31:145–51.
4. Kisman FL, Vining EP, Quaskey SA, Mellits D, Freeman JM. Efficacy of the ketogenic diet for intractable seizure disorders: review of 58 cases. *Epilepsia* 1992;33:132–36.

KINDLING (PHENOMENON)

Daily electrical stimulation (usually in animals) of certain cerebral structures (anterior neocortex, amygdala, hippocampus) using a small pulse, insufficient itself to cause seizures, eventually brings about remote discharges, which in turn cause focal and then generalized seizures. Kindling takes place after a variable period of time depending on the stimulus, the animal species, and the brain region. An isolated stimulus causes a single seizure and kindling persists long after repeated stimulation ceases. Three stages are described:

- the dependent stage: appearance of a secondary focus, which does not induce seizures and disappears with excision of the primary focus;
- intermediate stage: independent discharges in both foci with possible seizures arising from the secondary focus; disappear after excision of the primary focus;
- independent stage: seizures arise from the secondary focus and persist after excision of the primary focus.

Since this description appeared in 1967 (1), the kindling phenomenon has provided a valuable experimental model in epilepsy, allowing studies of electrophysiological and neurochemical changes arising from seizures and the testing of possible AEDs.

There is some evidence that epileptogenic foci in mesial temporal regions may arise from epileptogenic cortex surrounding distant arteriovenous malformations (2). Others believe that secondary epileptogenesis in man has not been proven (3).

References

1. Goddard GV. Development of epileptic seizures through brain stimulation at low intensity. *Nature* 1967;241:1020–21.
2. Yeh H, Privitera MD. Secondary epileptogenesis in cerebral arteriovenous malformations. *Arch Neurol* 1991;48:1121–24.
3. Morrell F. Secondary epileptogenesis in man. *Arch Neurol* 1985;42:318–35.

● ● ● ● ● ●
KLONOPIN® (CLONAZEPAM)

Tablets: 0.5 mg, 1 mg, 2 mg (see also Clonazepam).

● ● ● ● ● ●
KOJEWNIKOW'S (SYNDROME); EPILEPSIA PARTIALIS CONTINUA

Initially, Kojewnikow's syndrome referred to a condition with ongoing focal clonic activity (hemifacial, shoulder, hand, etc.) and somatomotor seizures, beginning in the same region. Subsequently, the phrase has come to connote partial focal, motor, or sensory status epilepticus.

Two types have been described (1,2):

Localized form:

* The seizure focus involves the Rolandic cortex. It is seen at any age and may be caused by circumscribed lesions of various causes (tumor, vascular, etc.). The clinical picture and prognosis depend on the underlying lesion (3).

Encephalitic form:

* It presents as a chronic partial epilepsy of childhood which is a progressive syndrome apparently due to chronic focal encephalitis (see Rasmussen's encephalitis).

References

1. Commission on Classification and Terminology of the International League Against Epilepsy. Proposal for classification of epilepsies and epileptic syndromes. *Epilepsia* 1989;30:389–99.
2. Bancaud J. Kojewnikow's syndrome (epilepsia partialis continua) in children. In: Roger J, Bureau M, Dravet C, Dreifuss FE, Perret A, Wolf P (eds.). *Epileptic syndromes in infancy, childhood and adolescence,* 2nd edition. London: John Libbey Eurotext, 1992:363–79.
3. Thomas JE, Reagan TJ, Klass DW. Epilepsia partialis continua. A review of 32 cases. *Arch Neurol* 1977;34:266–75.

• • • • • •
KUFS (DISEASE)

Kufs disease is a late form of ceroid-lipofuscinoses (see this heading)(1). Kufs disease exhibits autosomal recessive transmission with onset around 30 years of age. A typical presentation is with progressive myoclonic epilepsy without visual disturbance, but with a subsequent rapidly progressive dementia. Death usually occurs within 10 years of the onset of the disease.

Diagnosis: Dolichols are found in urinary sediments. Specific granular storage abnormalities may be confirmed histologically in endocrine glands of the skin (2).

References

1. Kufs H. Uber eine Spätform der amaurotischen idiotic und ihre heredofamiliaren Grundlagen. *Z Gesamte Neurol Psychiat* 1925;95:168–88.
2. Berkovic SF, Carpenter S, Andermann F, Andermann E, Wolfe L. Kufs disease: a critical reappraisal. *Brain* 1988;111:27–62.

LAFORA (DISEASE)

Lafora disease presents as a progressive myoclonic epilepsy. It may be distinguished from the Unverricht-Lundborg syndrome by its different clinical features (mental deterioration and more rapid progression) and the presence of Lafora bodies in particular tissue target organs (1,2). Lafora disease is a genetic condition, with autosomal recessive transmission. The onset is between 6 and 19 years of age, typically presenting in succession with tonic-clonic seizures, focal visual seizures (3) and severe myoclonic seizures, action myoclonus, and a rapidly progressive dementia. Death follows within 2–10 years of disease onset.

The EEG shows focal epileptiform discharges, frequently in the occipital region, occasionally multifocal or generalized, and activated by photic stimulation. The early EEG has normal or slow (4) background frequencies with isolated bursts of posterior spike-waves (5); polyspikes, polyspike-waves, and marked response to intermittent photic stimulation. It then progresses with background slowing, fast generalized polyspikes and polyspike waves up to 6–12 Hz, and multifocal spikes (4–6).

Diagnosis is confirmed by the presence of round or oval periodic acid Schiff-positive glycogen B particles (Lafora bodies) evident in the sweat glands on skin biopsy (7). The enzymatic abnormality is as yet unknown.

References

1. Lafora GR, Glueck B. Beitrag zur Histopathologie der myoklonischen Epilepsie. *Z Gesamte Neurol Psychiatr* 1911;6:1–14.
2. Van Heycop Ten Ham MW, De Jager H. Progressive myoclonus epilepsy with Lafora bodies: clinical-pathological features. *Epilepsia* 1963;4:95–119.
3. Tinuper P, Aguglia U, Pellissier JF, Gastaut H. Visual ictal phenomena in a case of Lafora disease proven by skin biopsy. *Epilepsia* 1983;24:214–18.
4. Yen C, Beydoun A, Drury I. Longitudinal EEG studies in a kindred with Lafora disease. *Epilepsia* 1991;32:895–99.

5. Roger J, Genton P, Bureau M. Progressive myoclonus epilepsies. In: Dam M, Gram L (eds.). *Comprehensive epileptology*. New York: Raven Press, 1990:220–21.
6. Ponsford S, Pye IF, Elliot EJ. Posterior paroxysmal discharge: an aid to early diagnosis in Lafora disease. *J Roy Soc Med* 1993;86:597–99.
7. Carpenter S, Karpati G, Sweat gland duct cells in Lafora disease: diagnosis by skin biopsy. *Neurology* 1981;31:1564–68.

• • • • • • •
LAMICTAL® (LAMOTRIGINE)

Diaminotriazine AED.

Tablets: 100 mg, 200 mg, 250 mg.

Lamotrigine (3,5-diamino-6-(2,3 dichlorophenyl)-1,2,3 triazine) is structurally unrelated to any other AED in current use.

In animal models it has shown an AED profile similar to that of phenytoin and carbamazepine. Its antiepileptic action is probably related to its inhibitory effect on glutamate release and stabilization of neuronal membrane voltage-sensitive sodium channels (1). Pharmacokinetics in normal human subjects: complete bioavailability, a very long plasma half-life (24 ± 5–7h), linear kinetics; approximately 60% protein binding (2).

Enzyme-inducing AEDs reduce its half-life; VPA increases it. In patients with intractable seizures already on other AEDs, lamotrigine reduced seizures by approximately one-third (3–6) and median seizure frequency decreased by 20-36% (6,7). The drug is well tolerated; skin rashes occur in 2–3% of patients (4,5).

Lamotrigine is approved in several countries, and has received FDA approval in the United States as adjunctive therapy for partial seizures.

References

1. Cohen AF, Land GS, Breiner DD, Yuen WC, Winton C, Peck AN. Lamotrigine, a new anticonvulsant. Pharmacokinetics in normal humans. *Clin Pharmacol Ther* 1987;42:535–41.
2. Leach MJ, Marden CM, Miller AA. Pharmacological studies on lamotrigine, a novel potential antiepileptic drug II. Neurochemical studies on the mechanism of action. *Epilepsia* 1986;27:490–97.
3. Goa KL, Ross SR, Christ P. Lamotrigine: a review of its pharmacological properties and clinical efficacy in epilepsy. *Drugs* 1993;46:152–76.
4. Richens A. Safety of lamotrigine. *Epilepsia* 1994;35(Suppl 5):S37–S40.
5. Brodie MJ. Lamotrigine. *Lancet* 1992;339:1397–1400.
6. Matsuo F, Bergen D, Faught E, Messenheimer JA, Dren AT, Rudd GD, Lineberry CG. Placebo-controlled study of the efficacy and safety of lamotrigine in patients with partial seizures. *Neurology* 1993;43:2284–91.

7. Messenheimer J, Ramsay RE, Willmore LJ, et al. Lamotrigine therapy for partial seizures: a multicenter placebo-controlled, double-blind, cross-over trial. *Epilepsia* 1994;35:113–21.

• • • • • •
LANDAU-KLEFFNER (SYNDROME)

The Landau-Kleffner syndrome (1) is characterized by the association of the following features: an acquired aphasia, epileptiform discharges on the EEG, epileptic seizures, and behavioral problems. Onset is age 3–8 years. Seizures and behavioral disturbances are common.

LANGUAGE DISTURBANCES

Progressive loss of language supervenes in previously normal children. Initial presentation is with verbal and auditory agnosia, followed by expressive problems. Resolution depends on the age of onset and early language therapy (2).

EPILEPSY

Seizures usually are infrequent. Less often, repeated seizures occur, especially at night. Clinical symptomatology is varied. Seizures may be well controlled with AEDs and usually remit by 15 years of age.

PSYCHOMOTOR DISTURBANCES

The Landau-Kleffner syndrome may present with attention deficit disorder, hyperactive behavior, personality disturbances, and affective problems.

EEG FEATURES

The EEG features of the Landau-Kleffner syndrome are nonspecific. Initially, the background rhythm is normal. Repetitive, high amplitude spikes, and spike-waves (sometimes focal) supervene (3). During slow wave sleep, continuous spike-wave discharges may be seen (4), raising a possible relation to the syndrome of epilepsy with continuous spikes and waves during slow sleep (see also this heading). High-dose steroids and, to a certain extent, benzodiazepines, ethosuximide, and valproic acid have been effective in treating seizures (5). There is a complex relationship between the aphasia, seizures, and EEG correlates (6).

References

1. Landau NM, Kleffner FR. Syndrome of acquired aphasia with convulsive disorder in children. *Neurology* 1957;7:523–30.
2. Deonna T, Peter CI, Ziegler AL. Adult follow-up of the acquired aphasia-epilepsy syndrome in childhood. Report of 7 cases. *Neuropediatrics* 1989;20:132–38.
3. Beaumanoir A. The Landau-Kleffner syndrome. In: Roger J, Bureau M, Dravet C, Dreifuss FE, Perret A, Wolf P (eds.). *Epileptic syndromes in infancy, childhood and adolescence,* 2nd edition. London: John Libbey Eurotext, 1992:231–43.
4. Hirsch E, Marescaux C, Maquet P, et al. Landau-Kleffner syndrome: a clinical and EEG study of five cases. *Epilepsia* 1990;31:756–67.
5. Marescaux C, Hirsch E, Finck S, et al. Landau-Kleffner syndrome: a pharmacological study of five cases. *Epilepsia* 1990;31:768–77.
6. Deonna T, Beaumanoir A, Gaillard F, Assal GA. Acquired aphasia in childhood with seizure disorder: a heterogeneous syndrome. *Neuropaediatrie* 1977;8:262–73.

• • • • • • •
LENNOX-GASTAUT (SYNDROME)

The Lennox-Gastaut syndrome of childhood was described in 1966 (1) and is characterized by the triad of:

- seizures: multiple seizure types, including tonic axial seizures, atonic seizures, and atypical absences;
- EEG changes with slow spike and wave discharges during wakefulness, abnormal background rhythm, and runs of rapid sharp activity during sleep;
- psychomotor retardation with personality changes.

The Lennox-Gastaut syndrome accounts for approximately 3% of childhood epilepsies (2), although higher percentages are seen in referral centers. The syndrome is more common in males, and a family history is positive in 2.5–40% of cases (3). Onset usually occurs before the age of 8 years, and the syndrome is most common at age 3–5 years. Lennox-Gastaut syndrome may appear in previously normal children (30%) or may appear secondarily in the context of a preexisting insult, such as West syndrome. Other predisposing factors include head trauma, malformations, CNS infections, tumors, cerebral dysgenesis, and vascular injuries.

SEIZURES

- The presence of *tonic seizures* is essential to making the diagnosis; they are seen during slow wave sleep or during wakefulness. These seizures involve the trunk, typically symmetrically; sometimes with lateralization. Seizures may be brief with abrupt tonic eye deviation and respiratory alteration. The EEG shows rapid bilateral rhythmic sharp activity predominantly over the vertex and anterior head regions preceded by a flattening (electrodecremental) phase, or with slow spike and waves. Postictal EEG suppression is minimal or absent;

- *Atypical absence* seizures last 5–25 seconds, with an incomplete loss of consciousness. These seizures are associated with progressive loss of tone beginning in the face or neck muscles often with eyelid flutter. The EEG shows irregular 2–2.5 Hertz bilaterally symmetric, spike and slow wave discharges. Seizures are not induced by hyperventilation or photic stimulation;
- *Atonic seizures* present as drop attacks or falls in association with a brief myoclonic movement (see also Drop attacks);
- All three seizure types may be seen in the same patient, but myoclonic seizures may predominate (3);
- Other seizure types, including generalized tonic-clonic seizures, partial complex seizures, or unilateral clonic seizures, may be seen in Lennox-Gastaut syndrome;
- Status epilepticus with obtundation may be seen with tonic seizures or more rarely with myoclonic seizures. Such an episode of status may herald the onset of the disease (2).

INTERICTAL EEG

The waking EEG shows diffuse slow spike and wave activity (2–2.5 Hertz) associated with multifocal temporal or frontal spikes, polyspikes, and slow wave discharges. Although nonspecific, the slow spike-wave EEG pattern is essential to the diagnosis of Lennox-Gastaut syndrome (4). During slow wave sleep, slow spike and slow wave discharges are seen diffusely and synchronously. Runs of 10 Hertz spikes are diagnostic.

PSYCHIATRIC DISTURBANCES

Psychiatric and behavioral disturbances are frequent and potentially severe. No specific symptomatology dominates the clinical picture, but early progressive intellectual decline with learning difficulties, aggressive behavior, and personality disturbances are common. Mental retardation is generally more severe in cases with younger age of onset of seizures.

DIFFERENTIAL DIAGNOSIS

Differential diagnosis of the Lennox-Gastaut syndrome includes myoclonic-astatic epilepsy, intermediate petit mal, ceroid-lipofuscinoses, and other symptomatic generalized epilepsies.

TREATMENT

Seizures associated with the Lennox-Gastaut syndrome are notoriously resistant to treatment, with a satisfactory response occurring in less than 20% of cases. Benzodiazepines (especially clobazam), sodium valproate, and a ketogenic diet may be useful, and carbamazepine sometimes ameliorates tonic-clonic seizures. Felbamate and lamotrigine, newer AEDs, may diminish seizure frequency, but felbamate may have serious side effects (see Felbamate (Felbatol®)) (5). Early use of corticosteroids occasionally provides surprisingly beneficial results (6). Corpus callosotomy has been used to diminish drop attacks (7).

PROGRESSION

Progressive deterioration is unfortunately the rule in Lennox-Gastaut syndrome (8). Seizures are frequent and may be interspersed with episodes of status epilepticus. There is progressive decline in intellect with psychiatric and personality problems, occasionally with psychosis. Mortality in Lennox-Gastaut syndrome is 7% (8). The clinical features may remain constant in adulthood (8) or give way to another type of epilepsy, most frequently partial. Remission is unusual (8). Poor prognostic signs include a preceding West syndrome, early onset before the age of 3 years, symptomatic etiology (3), the frequency and multiplicity of seizure types, repeated status epilepticus, and marked slowing of the background EEG frequencies.

References

1. Gastaut H, Roger J, Soulayrol R, et al. Childhood epileptic encephalopathy with diffuse slow-spike-waves (otherwise known as "petit mal variant") or Lennox-syndrome. *Epilepsia* 1966;7:139–79.
2. Beaumanoir A, Dravet C. Lennox-Gastaut syndrome. In: Roger J, Bureau M, Dravet C, Dreifuss FE, Perret A, Wolf P (eds.). *Epileptic syndromes in infancy, childhood and adolescence,* 2nd edition. London: John Libbey & Co. Ltd., 1992:115–32.
3. Chevrie JJ, Aicardi J. Childhood epileptic encephalopathy with slow spike-wave. A statistical study of 80 cases. *Epilepsia* 1972;13:259–71.
4. Gastaut H. The Lennox-Gastaut syndrome. *Electroenceph clin Neurophysiol* 1982; (Suppl 35):71–84.
5. Ritter FJ, Leppik IE, Dreifuss FE, et al. Efficacy of felbamate in chilhood epileptic encephalopathy (Lennox-Gastaut syndrome). *N Engl J Med* 1993;328:29–33.

6. Yamatogi Y, Ohtuska Y, Ishida T, Ichiba N, Ishida S, Miyake S, Oka E, Ohtahara S. Treatment of the Lennox-Gastaut syndrome with ACTH: a clinical and electroencephalographic study. *Brain Dev* 1979;1:267–76.
7. Wilson DH, Reeves AG, Gazzaniga MS. "Central" commissurotomy for intractable generalized epilepsy: series two. *Neurology* 1982;32:687–97.
8. Blume WT, David RB, Gomez MR. Generalized sharp and slow wave complexes. Associated clinical features and long term follow-up. *Brain* 1973;96:289–306.

• • • • • •
LEUKOENCEPHALITIS

Leukoencephalitis literally connotes inflammation of the white matter, but it is sometimes used less precisely to refer to certain demyelinating diseases:

- Subacute sclerosing leukoencephalitis or sclerosing panencephalitis (Van Bogaert disease) is a secondary encephalitis seen in children and adolescents following measles infection. Myoclonic, generalized, or partial seizures may herald onset and are frequent during the course of the illness. Characteristic EEG abnormalities include periodic bursts that are bilateral and generalized, synchronous with myoclonic jerks;
- Acute hemorrhagic leukoencephalopathy of Weston-Hurst is an acute, fulminating, demyelinating disorder of unclear etiology related to post-infectious encephalomyelitis;
- Progressive multifocal leukoencephalopathy is a widespread demyelinating disorder of brain and spinal cord. It has been associated with previous Papova virus infection, systemic neoplasia, or acquired immunodeficiency. Seizures are rare.

• • • • • •
LEUKOENCEPHALOPATHIES

Leukoencephalopathies are heredodegenerative disorders of the central nervous system predominantly involving white matter and due to an inborn error of metabolism. Encephalopathy is often severe and associated with seizures.

- Metachromatic leukodystrophy;
- Globoid leukodystrophy due to cerebral galactosidase deficiency (Krabbe disease);
- Pelizaeus-Merzbacher disease or sudanophilic leukodystrophy;
- Adrenoleukodystrophy (see this heading);
- Canavan disease;
- Alexander's disease.

● ● ● ● ● ●
LIDOCAINE (XYLOCAINE®)

Lidocaine is a local anesthetic occasionally used to treat status epilepticus resistant to other medications (1–4).

It has been given by slow IV infusion (1 mg/kg) with further supplementation while monitoring for blood pressure, electrocardiogram changes, and EEG changes (4).

Side effects are predominantly cardiovascular.

References

1. Lemmen LJ, Klassen M, Duiser B. Intravenous lidocaine in the treatment of convulsions. *JAMA* 1978;239:2025.
2. Morris HH. Lidocaine: a neglected anticonvulsant? *South Med J* 1979;72:1564–66.
3. Taverner D, Bain WA. Intravenous lidocaine as an anticonvulsant in status epilepticus and serial epilepsy. *Lancet* 1958;2:1145–47.
4. De Giorgio CM, Altman K, Hamilton-Byrd E, Rabinowicz A. Lidocaine in refractory status epilepticus: confirmation of efficacy with continuous EEG monitoring. *Epilepsia* 1992;33:913–16.

● ● ● ● ● ●
LIPIDOSES

Lipidoses are hereditary disorders of autosomal recessive inheritance leading to lipid deposition in neurons. Lipidoses previously were called amaurotic familial idiocies, but successive classifications have been based on analysis of abnormal storage and deposition substances, and subsequent identification of the relevant enzymatic deficiency. Lipidoses now include:

- the sphingolipidoses (see this heading);
- the ceroid-lipofuscinoses (see this heading);
- the mucolipidoses;
- disorders due to the accumulation of simple lipids, including phytanic acid (Refsum's disease), triglycerides, and cholesterol esters.

Sphingolipidoses and ceroid-lipofuscinoses may present with seizures during the course of the disease.

• • • • • •
LISSENCEPHALY
(AGYRIA-PACHYGYRIA); CORTICAL DYSPLASIA

Lissencephaly is an abnormality of cerebral cellular migration resulting in a decrease of infolding and total surface area of the cortex. Some cases are associated with a partial deletion of the short arm of chromosome 17, with or without translocation. Clinical correlates are psychomotor retardation, microcephaly, marked axial hypotonia, pyramidal signs, and typical dysmorphic facial features (1).

Ectopic cortical neurons within subcortical areas, or heterotopias, are thought to represent abnormalities of neuronal migration and differentiation. The CT head scan or MRI head scan are diagnostic (2). MRI and PET scans are helpful in identifying areas of epileptogenic potential (3,4).

Seizures are seen in 75% of cases of lissencephaly, usually infantile spasms with onset in the first year of life. The interictal EEG shows high-voltage, 6–10 Hertz paroxysmal discharges.

References

1. Dieker H, Edwards RH, Zu Rhein G, Chou SM, Hartman HA, Opitz JM. The lissencephaly syndrome. *Birth Defects* 1969;5:53–64.
2. Lee BCP, Engel M. MR of lissencephaly. *AJNR* 1988;9:804.
3. Taylor DL, Falconer MA, Bruton CJ, Corsellis JAN. Focal dysplasia of the cerebral cortex in epilepsy. *J Neurol Neurosurg Psychiatry* 1971;34:369–87.
4. Lee N, Radthe R, Gray L, Burger PC, et al. Neuronal migration disorders: positron emission tomography correlations. *Ann Neurol* 1994;35:290–97.

• • • • • •
LOADING DOSE (ORAL)

In order to avoid transient but undesirable side effects, the daily dose of AED must be gradually increased. There is a delay between the initiation of treatment and the achievement of therapeutic blood levels; up to 3 weeks for phenobarbital. To avoid this problem, a loading dose of some AEDs may be given (e.g., double the daily dose for 2 to 3 days). Although brief symptoms of toxicity may be seen, therapeutic AED levels may be reached in about 3 days. Loading doses should only be used in patients under observation. Loading doses for medications with short half-lives are not effective (see also individual AEDs, e.g., Phenytoin).

● ● ● ● ● ●
LORAZEPAM (ATIVAN®)

Lorazepam is a benzodiazepine used in the treatment of status epilepticus. It has a longer AED action than diazepam and purportedly less respiratory depression (1–4).

Lorazepam is also used in resistant neonatal seizures (5) and sublingually in repeated seizures during childhood (6).

References

1. Lacey DJ. Status epilepticus in children and adults. *J Clin Psychiat* 1988;49:33–36.
2. Treiman DM. Pharmacokinetics and clinical use of benzodiazepines in the management of status epilepticus. *Epilepsia* 1989;(Suppl 2): S4–S20.
3. Levy RJ, Krall RL. Treatment of status epilepticus with lorazepam. *Arch Neurol* 1984;41:605–11.
4. Giang DW, McBride MC. Lorazepam versus diazepam for the treatment of status epilepticus. *Pediat Neurol* 1988;4:359–61.
5. Deshmukh A, Wittert W, Shnitzler E, Mangurten HH. Lorazepam in the treatment of refractory neonatal seizures. A pilot study. *Am J Dis Child* 1986; 140:1042–44.
6. Yager JY, Seshia SS. Sublingual lorazepam in childhood serial seizures. *Am J Dis Child* 1988;142:931–32.

• • • • • •
MAGNESIUM

At the cellular level, magnesium is involved in the mechanisms of neuronal excitation by its effect in blocking calcium entry into cells. Low extracellular magnesium may increase membrane excitability. Part of the N-methyl-D-aspartic acid (NMDA) receptor-cation channel subtype of the glutamate receptor affecting neuronal excitation is regulated by Mg^{2+}, thus having theoretical antiepileptic properties, but this has not been established in animals or humans (1,2), aside from occasional case reports (3). Magnesium sulfate has been widely used by obstetricians in the United States for the empirical treatment of eclamptic seizures, although its action as an AED is questioned (4,5) (see also Eclampsia).

References

1. Krauss GL, Kaplan P, Fisher RS. Parenteral magnesium sulfate fails to control electroshock and pentylenetetrazol seizures in mice. *Epilepsy Res* 1989;4:201–206.
2. Fisher RS, Kaplan PW, Krumholtz A, Lesser RP, Rosen SA, Wolff MR. Failure of high-dose intravenous magnesium sulfate to control myoclonic status epilepticus. *Clin Neuropharmacol* 1988;11:537–44.
3. Sadeh M, Blatt I, Martonovits G, Karni A, Goldhammer Y. Treatment of porphyric convulsions with magnesium sulfate. *Epilepsia* 1991;32:712–14.
4. Kaplan PW, Lesser RP, Fisher RS, Repke JT, Hanley DF. No, magnesium sulfate should not be used in treating eclamptic seizures. Controversies in neurology. *Arch Neurol* 1988;45:1361–64.
5. Kaplan PW, Lesser RP, Fisher RS, Repke JT, Hanley DF. A continuing controversy: magnesium sulfate in the treatment of eclamptic seizures. *Arch Neurol* 1990;47:1031–32.

• • • • • •
MAGNETIC RESONANCE IMAGING (MRI)

Several studies (1–4) indicate that head MRI has advantages over head CT scanning: (a) in demonstrating small lesions, particularly in the mesial and inferior aspects of the temporal lobe where CT is limited by bone artifact;

(b) in more clearly delineating lesions revealed on CT scan. Lesions such as cavernous angiomas, with surrounding hemosiderin, cortical dysplasias (5), and hippocampal sclerosis (6), are much more readily detected with MRI than with CT or cerebral angiography. MRI spectroscopy can provide functional as well as morphologic information with regard to biochemical modifications brought about by seizures (7), although such uses are still in the realm of research. With late-onset epilepsy, MRI may reveal epileptogenic lesions not seen on CT (8).

Whereas MRI is very sensitive, interpretation of findings must be cautious. With interhemispheric asymmetry, the pathological significance may be difficult to interpret. Increased T2 signal intensity may be seen with histological lesions as well as with edema. Reversible abnormalities can occur after seizures, predominanly over the posterior head regions (7,9,10). Occasional false negative results may still occur.

References

1. Conlon P, Trimble MR, Rogers D, Callicott C. Magnetic resonance imaging in epilepsy: a controlled study. *Epilepsy Res* 1988;2:37–43.
2. Kuzniecky R, de la Sayette V, Ethier R, et al. Magnetic resonance imaging in temporal lobe epilepsy: pathological correlations. *Ann Neurol* 1987;2:341–47.
3. Latack JT, Abou-Khalil BW, Seigel GJ, Sackellares JC, Gabrielsen TO, Aisen AM. Patients with partial seizures: evaluation by MR, CT and PET imaging. *Radiology* 1986;159:159–63.
4. Kuzniecky R, Murro A, King D, Morawetz R, et al. Magnetic resonance imaging in childhood intractable partial epilepsies: pathological considerations. *Neurology* 1993;43:681–87.
5. Kuzniecky R, Garcia JH, Faught F, Morawetz RB. Cortical dysplasia in temporal lobe epilepsy: magnetic resonance imaging correlations. *Ann Neurol* 1991;29:293–98.
6. Berkovic SF, Andermann F, Olivier A, et al. Hippocampal sclerosis in temporal lobe epilepsy demonstrated by magnetic resonance imaging. *Ann Neurol* 1991;29:175–82.
7. Kramer RE, Lüders H, Lesser RP, Weinstein MR, Dinner DS, Morris HH, Wyllie E. Transient focal abnormalities of neuroimaging studies during focal status epilepticus. *Epilepsia* 1987;28:528–32.
8. Kilpatrick CJ, O'Donnell G, Rossiter S, Hopper J. Magnetic resonance imaging and late-onset epilepsy. *Epilepsia* 1991;32:358–64.
9. Yaffe K, Ferrierro D, Barkovich J, Rowley H. Reversible MRI abnormalities following seizures. *Neurology* 1995;45:104–108.
10. Henry TR, Drury I, Brunberg JA, et al. Focal cerebral magnetic resonance changes associated with partial status epilepticus. *Epilepsia* 1994;35:35–41.

●●●●●●
MAGNETOENCEPHALOGRAPHY (MEG)

Transmembrane ion movements in active neurons generate magnetic fields that may be recorded by external devices (1,2). Since the magnetic fields produced by the brain are extremely weak (10^{-12} to 10^{-15} tesla), sensitive superconducting quantum interference devices (SQUIDs) and magnetically-shielded rooms are used to record MEG. Early systems used a single probe, resulting in a long laborious testing period. More recent machines use an assembly of SQUIDs arranged radially around a central probe. Unlike electric potentials, magnetic fields are not altered by their passage through brain, bone, and surrounding tissue. Analysis of the magnetic field can provide three-dimensional localization of the generating dipole source; however, formulas to solve this problem are subject to several simplifying assumptions that may degrade accuracy of localization. Despite limitations and expense, MEG can aid in localization of interictal and ictal seizure foci (3,4).

References

1. Sato S, Smith PD. Magnetoencephalography. *J Clin Neurophysiol* 1985;2:173–92.
2. Rose DF, Smith PD, Sato S. Magnetoencephalography and epilepsy research. *Science* 1987;238:329–35.
3. Sutherling WF, Crandall PH, Cahan LD, Barth DS. The magnetic field of epileptic spikes agrees with intracranial localizations in complex partial epilepsy. *Neurology* 1988;38:778–86.
4. Stefan H, Schneider S, Abraham-Fuchs K, et al. Magnetic source localization in focal epilepsy: multichannel magnetoencephalography correlated with magnetic resonance brain imaging. *Brain* 1990;113:1347–59.

●●●●●●
MALFORMATIONS

Cerebral malformations include:

- *Malformations caused by epilepsy.* Major or minor malformations in newborns of mothers with epilepsy have been indirectly attributed to AEDs taken during pregnancy, genetic factors, and environmental factors (see Pregnancy);
- *Malformations causing epilepsy.* Epilepsy with onset in the newborn or infant presents predominantly with neonatal seizures or West syndrome (see these headings). Some effects of cerebral malformations may also appear in childhood or even in adulthood. There are a

wide variety of malformations with different pathophysiological origins, morphologies, significances, and clinical presentations. In past years, diagnosis of malformations was usually made at postmortem. With the advent of head CT and MRI head scanning, in vivo diagnosis of malformations has become easier (1).

Some malformations are associated with a characteristic clinical presentation, for example, chromosomal abnormalities, Aicardi's syndrome, or malformations with inborn errors of metabolism (2). Other malformations may present with seizures and cognitive or somatic abnormalities, including hydrancephaly, porencephaly, schizencephaly, holoprosencephaly, agenesis of the corpus callosum, or multiple malformations (2–6). Only rarely are seizures the only presenting feature. This is also the case with abnormalities of neural migration, including lissencephaly, hemimegalencephaly, macro- or micropolygyria (7–12). Previously underestimated, modern neuroimaging techniques have revealed a greater number of minor abnormalities of neuronal migration than previously thought, particularly microdysgenesis (13). These heterotopic islets of gray matter within white matter appear to be highly epileptogenic (14), but their significance (15–17) in the nonepileptic population is unknown.

References

1. Van der Knaap MS, Valk J. Classification of congenital abnormalities of the CNS. *AJNR* 1988;9:315–26.
2. Clayton PT, Thompson E. Dysmorphic syndromes with demonstrable biochemical abnormalities. *J Med Genet* 1988;25:463–72.
3. Menezes L, Aicardi J, Goutieres F. Absence of the septum pellucidum with porencephalia: a neuroradiologic syndrome with variable clinical expression. *Arch Neurol* 1988;45:542–45.
4. Miller GM, Stears JC, Guggenheim MA, et al. Schizencephaly: a clinical and CT study. *Neurology* 1984;34:997–1001.
5. Barkovich AJ, Norman D. MR imaging of schizencephaly. *AJNR* 1988; 9:297–302.
6. Serur D, Jeret JS, Wisniewski K. Agenesis of the corpus callosum: clinical, neuroradiological and cytogenetic studies. *Neuropediatrics* 1988;19:87–91.
7. Jellinger K, Gross H, Kaltenback E, Grisold W. Holoprosencephalic agenesis of the corpus callosum: frequency of associated malformations. *Acta Neuropath* (Berlin) 1981;55:1–10.
8. Gooskerns RHJM, Willemse J, Bijlsma JB, Hanlo PW. Megaencephaly: definition and classification. *Brain Dev* 1988;10:17.
9. Lee BCP, Engel M. MR of lissencephaly. *ANJR* 1988;9:804.
10. Vigevano F, Bertini E, Boldrini R, et al. Heminegalencephaly and intractable epilepsy: benefits of hemispherectomy. *Epilepsia* 1989;30:833–43.
11. Robain O, Floquet C, Heldt N, Rozenberg F. Heminegalencephaly: a clinicopathological study of four cases. *Neuropathol Appl Neurobiol* 1988;14:125–36.
12. Kuzniecky R, Andermann F, Tampieri D, Melanson D, Olivier D, Leppick I.

Bilateral central macrogyria: epilepsy, pseudobulbar palsy, and mental retardation: a recognizable neuronal migration disorder. *Ann Neurol* 1989;25:547–54.

13. Becker PS, Dixon AM, Troncoso JC. Bilateral opercular polymicrogyria. *Ann Neurol* 1989;25:90–92.

14. Smith AS, Weinstein MA, Quencer RM, et al. Association of heterotopic gray matter with seizures: MR imaging. *Radiology* 1988;168:195–98.

15. Hardiman O, Burke T, Phillips J, Murphy S, O'Moore B, Staunton H, Farrell MA. Microdysgenesis in resected temporal neocortex: incidence and clinical significance in focal epilepsy. *Neurology* 1988;38:1041–47.

16. Meencke HJ, Janz D. Neuropathological findings in primary generalized epilepsy. A study of eight cases. *Epilepsia* 1984;25:8–21 and 1985;26:368–71.

17. Lyon G, Gastaut H. Considerations on the significance attributed to unusual cerebral histological findings recently described in eight patients with primary generalized epilepsy. *Epilepsia* 1985;26:365–67.

• • • • • •
MARRIAGE

Couples contemplating marriage should be aware that:

- epilepsy is not a contraindication to marriage; in fact, marriage may provide a stabilizing influence on the course of the disease (1). Parents, however, appear not to favor marriage of their child to a patient with epilepsy (2,3). Men with early onset seizures marry less frequently and at a later age than people without epilepsy (4).
- there are genetic risks for the offspring (see Genetics); marriage between two people with epilepsy of the same type, such as idiopathic generalized epilepsy, results in a significantly increased risk of having a child with epilepsy;
- the effect of AEDs on the developing fetus with risk of malformation (see this heading), their effect on sexual activity (see Sexuality), and on the effectiveness of oral contraceptives (see this heading);
- fertility (see this heading) of the couple.

References

1. Webster A, Mawer GE. Seizures frequency and major life events in epilepsy. *Epilepsia* 1989;30:162–67.

2. Caveness WP, Gallup GH Jr. A survey of public attitudes toward epilepsy in 1979 with an indication of trends over the past thirty years. *Epilepsia* 1980;21:509–18.

3. Lai CW, Huang X, Lai YHC, Zhang Z, Liu G, Yang MZ. Survey of public awareness, understanding, and attitudes toward epilepsy in Henan province China. *Epilepsia* 1990;31:182–87.

4. Dansky LY, Andermann E, Andermann F. Marriage and fertility in epileptic patients. *Epilepsia* 1980;21:261–71.

● ● ● ● ● ●
MEMORY

Disturbances of memory are among the most common complaints of people with epilepsy. Patients typically report preservation of distant memories, but significant difficulties with acquisition, retention, and retrieval of recent memories. Verbal material is preferentially affected with left hemisphere hippocampal damage (1), presumably related to seizure foci; and visuospatial material with right hemisphere foci (2–4). Overall memory function is most impaired in people with bilateral lesions. Some of the apparent memory disturbance in people with epilepsy may be a result of their inability to register information appearing in rapid succession during standard memory tests (5).

In patients with epilepsy, memory problems may be categorized as follows:

- *Interictal:* Patients with seizure discharges affecting the temporal lobes often show evidence of memory acquisition problems in the interictal state of their disorder. Electrical stimulation of the temporal lobes affects the laying down of memory and recall (6). Frontal lobe foci occasionally produce memory disturbances (7). Possible mechanisms include: (1) underlying damage to neocortex and mesial temporal areas known to be involved in memory; (2) the possibility that frequent interictal discharges may transiently disrupt cognitive processing (8–10); (3) impairment of memory by AEDs (see Antiepileptic drugs (AEDs)).
- *Ictal:* By the definition of the International Classification of the Epilepsies (see Classification), generalized and partial complex seizures are associated with disruption of consciousness (see this heading) and, therefore, of memory. Ictal and postictal memory disturbances may be difficult to distinguish from each other. Furthermore, intermittent memory deficits may, in part, be due to subclinical seizures affecting the hippocampus and related structures (5). Seizures characterized primarily by distortion of memory are referred to as dysmnestic seizures.
- *Postictal:* During the postictal state, patients exhibit variable impairment of memory. Postictal memory disturbance may be difficult to distinguish from postictal global confusion, aphasia, or other cognitive deficits; however, some patients do appear to show a degree of anterograde or retrograde amnesia disproportionate to global cognitive disturbances in the postictal state.

References

1. Sass KJ, Spencer DD, Kim JH, Westerveld M, Novelly RA, Lencz T. Verbal memory impairment correlates with hippocampal pyramidal cell density. *Neurology* 1990;40:1694–97.
2. Milner B. Intellectual functions of the temporal lobe. *Psychol Bull* 1954;51:42–62.
3. Glowinski H. Cognitive deficits in temporal lobe epilepsy. An investigation of memory functioning. *J Nerv Ment Dis* 1973;157:129–37.
4. Delaney RC, Rosen AJ, Mattson RH, Novely RA. Memory function in focal epilepsy: a comparison of non-surgical, unilateral temporal lobe and frontal lobe samples. *Cortex* 1980;16:103–17.
5. Bridgman PA, Malamut BL, Sperling MR, Saykin AJ, O'Connor MJ. Memory during subictal hippocampal seizures. *Neurology* 1989;39:853–56.
6. Halgren E, Wilson CL, Stapleton JM. Human medical temporal-lobe stimulation disrupts both formation and retrieval of recent memories. *Brain and Cognition* 1985;4:287–95.
7. Milner B, Petrides M, Smith ML. Frontal lobes and the temporal organization of memory. *Human Neurobiol* 1985;4:137–42.
8. Halgren E, Wilson CL. Recall deficits produced by afterdischarges in the human hippocampal formation and amygdala. *Electroenceph clin Neurophysiol* 1985;61:375–80
9. Aars JHP, Binnie CD, Smit AM, Wilkins AJ. Selective cognitive impairment during focal and generalized epileptiform EEG activity. *Brain* 1984;107:293–308.
10. Shewmon DA, Erwin RJ. The effect of focal interictal spikes on perception and reaction time. I. General considerations. *Electroenceph clin Neurophysiol* 1988;69:319–37.

• • • • • •

MENINGITIS

Meningitis refers to inflammation of the coverings of the brain because of infectious, chemical, or neoplastic irritation. Seizures never result from meningitis alone; however, meningitis may progress to involve the brain (meningoencephalitis), and this, in turn, commonly results in seizures (1). Bacterial meningitis (2) is more likely to progress to seizures than is aseptic meningitis.

References

1. Annegers JF, Hauser WA, Beghi E, Nicolosi A, Kurland LT. The risk of unprovoked seizures after encephalitis and meningitis. *Neurology* 1988;38:1407–10.
2. Pomeroy SL, Holmes SI, Dodge PR, Feigen RD. Seizures and other neurologic sequelae of bacterial meningitis in children. *N Engl J Med* 1990;323:1651–57.

• • • • • •
MESIAL TEMPORAL SCLEROSIS

Bouchet and Cazauvieilh in 1825 and Sommer in 1880 described hippocampal sclerosis from autopsy specimens of patients with epilepsy. A significant percent (50–80%) of patients with cryptogenic epilepsies have a pattern of gliosis and neuronal loss in the mesial temporal area or Ammon's horn (1,2). One out of two patients with severe epilepsy who have undergone temporal lobectomy have mesial temporal sclerosis.

There has been much debate as to whether these lesions are a cause or an effect of these seizures. It is clear, however, that temporal lobe structures are highly vulnerable to anoxic insult. Scholtz believed that mesial temporal sclerosis was a result of repeated seizures. Subsequently, many authors subscribed to the belief that anoxic insult was the cause of epilepsy. Several mechanisms have been proposed (1–5):

Temporal lobe compression during birth with hippocampal herniation; cerebral edema stemming from febrile status epilepticus resulting in vascular compromise; the role of prolonged febrile convulsions.

More recently, it has been suggested that ischemic lesions may be produced by an excessive intracellular calcium or excitatory neurotransmitter—demonstrated experimentally. In man, particular aspects of neuronal death appear to be of recent origin, hence postictal.

Hippocampal sclerosis may be seen with MRI scans (6).

References

1. Falconer MA. Mesial temporal (Ammon's horn) sclerosis as a common cause of epilepsy: etiology, treatment and prevention. *Lancet* 1974;2:767–70
2. Margerison JH, Corsellis JAN. Epilepsy and the temporal lobes. *J Neurophys* 1966;89:499–529.
3. Falconer MA. Genetic and related aetiological factors in temporal lobe epilepsy. A review. *Epilepsia* 1971;12:13–31.
4. Gates JR, Cruz-Rodriguez R. Mesial temporal sclerosis: pathogenesis, diagnosis and management. *Epilepsia* 1990;31(Suppl):555–66.
5. Meldrum BS, Horton RW, Brierley JG. Epileptic brain damage in adolescent baboons following seizures indiced by allylglycine. *Brain* 1979;97:407–18.
6. Jackson GD, Berkovic SF, Tress BM, Kalnins RM, Fabingi TCA, Bladin PF. Hippocampal sclerosis can be reliably detected by magnetic resonance imaging. *Neurology* 1990;40:1869–75.

• • • • • •
METABOLIC ERRORS (INBORN)

Any inborn error of metabolism may at some time cause seizures. These are usually myoclonic and are associated with other neurological abnormalities. Some rare disorders result in severe epileptic conditions, manifesting at different ages:

- in newborns: hyperglycinemia, D-glycine-acidemia;
- in infants: phenylketonuria, pyridoxine deficiency, Tay-Sachs disease, infantile presentations of ceroid-lipofuscinoses (see under these headings);
- in children: childhood ceroid-lipofuscinoses, childhood forms of Huntington's chorea;
- in childhood and adolescence: Gaucher's disease, juvenile forms of ceroid-lipofuscinosis, Lafora body disease, cherry-red spot-myoclonus, MERRF;
- in adults: Kufs' disease.

Reference

Aicardi J. Epilepsy and inborn errors of metabolism. In: Roger J, Bureau M, Dravet C, Dreifuss FE, Perret A, Wolf P (eds.). *Epileptic syndromes in infancy, childhood and adolescence,* 2nd edition. London: John Libbey & Co. Ltd., 1992:97–102.

• • • • • •
MIGRAINE

Migraine and epilepsy are both common disorders, and causal links have been difficult to establish (1). Nevertheless, more than chance associations may appear in some circumstances.

- Seizures, particularly tonic-clonic seizures, are often associated with a vascular-type headache in the postictal phase (seizure-triggered migraine)(see also Headache).
- Complicated migraine can result in ischemic lesions that then lead to seizures (migraine-related stroke and epilepsy).
- There is controversy over whether a migraine attack can lead directly to a seizure, although numerous patients have reported this experience.
- Migraine and epilepsy are each on the differential diagnosis of episodes affecting consciousness, sensorimotor function, or behavior, and migraine may be mistaken for epilepsy.

- Several syndromes have been described that present features of both epilepsy and migraine (1), including: Bickerstaff's basilar migraine of childhood; benign epilepsy of childhood with centro-temporal spikes; benign epilepsy of childhood with occipital spike-waves; occasionally absence epilepsy of childhood; and mitochondrial encephalopathies.

Reference

Andermann F. Migraine-epilepsy relationships. *Epilepsy Res* 1987;1:213–16.

• • • • • •
MITOCHONDRIAL ENCEPHALOMYOPATHIES

A syndrome described in 1962 (1) associated with mitochondrial dysfunction in which abnormalities of the mitochondria of muscle fibers and abnormalities of the oxidation-phosphorylation coupling are implicated.

These now include: chronic progressive ophthalmoplegia, Kearns-Sayre syndrome, Leigh's and Alpers syndrome, MERRF and MELAS syndrome (see these headings).

Diagnosis is based on increased serum lactate and CSF lactate (1,2). Definitive diagnosis is made by muscle biopsy and tests of the respiratory mitochondrial chain.

The EEG is abnormal in most patients, showing focal and diffuse epileptiform discharges and focal and diffuse slowing in different patients (3).

References

1. Luft R, Ikkos D, Palmieri G. A case of severe hypometabolism of non-thyroid origin with a defect in the maintenance of mitochondrial respiratory control: a correlated clinical, biochemical and morphological study. *J Clin Invest* 1962;41:1776–1854.
2. Lombes A, Bonilla E, Dimauro S, Mitochondrial encephalomyopathies. *Rev Neurol* 1989;145:671–89.
3. Smith SJM, Harding AE. EEG and evoked potential findings in mitochondrial myopathies. *J Neurology* 1993;240:367–72.

• • • • • •
MITOCHONDRIAL MYOPATHY, ENCEPHALOPATHY, LACTIC ACIDOSIS, STROKE-LIKE EPISODES (MELAS)

MELAS syndrome results from a mitochondrial myopathy with encephalopathy that presents with episodic vomiting, growth delay, seizures, and stroke-like events. Onset is in childhood or young adult life. There may be an associated rapidly progressive dementia. Diagnosis is made on clinical grounds, in combination with elevated serum lactate and muscle biopsy demonstrating "ragged red fibers" with special staining techniques. MELAS is one of a family of disorders of the mitochondrial respiratory transport chain, including MERRF, chronic external ophthalmoplegia, Kearnes-Sayre syndrome, and Leber's optic atrophy.

Reference

Pavlakis SG, Phillips PC, Di Mauro S, De Vivo D, Rowland LP. Mitochondrial myopathy, encephalopathy, lactic acidosis, and stroke like episodes: a distinctive clinical syndrome. *Ann Neurol* 1984;16:481–88.

• • • • • •
MOGADON® (NITRAZEPAM)

Used mostly for infantile spasms; occasionally for myoclonic epilepsy and Lennox-Gastaut syndrome (1,2).

Usual daily dose 0.5–1.0 mg/kg—once or twice per day dosing.

Not available in the United States.

References

1. Baruzzi A, Michelucci R, Tassinari FA. Benzodiazepines, nitrazepam. In: Levy RH, Dreifuss FE, Mattson RH, Meldrum BS, Penry JK (eds.). *Antiepileptic drugs,* 3rd edition. New York: Raven Press: 1989:785–804.
2. Millichap JG, Ortiz WR. Nitrazepam in myoclonic epilepsies. *Am J Dis Child* 1966;112:242–48.

• • • • • •
MONOTHERAPY

Reynolds (1976) has advocated the use of a single antiepileptic medication (monotherapy) for as long as possible (1,2). Advantages of monotherapy include easier dosing, fewer drug interactions and side effects, the same or better efficacy than polypharmacy, and lower cost (1–3).

References

1. Reynolds EH, Shorvon SD. Monotherapy or polytherapy for epilepsy? *Epilepsia* 1981;22:1–10.
2. Reynolds EH, Shorvon SD, Galbraith AW, Chadwick D, Dellaportas CI, Vydelingum L. Phenytoin monotherapy for epilepsy: a long term prospective study, assisted by serum level monitoring, in previously untreated patients. *Epilepsia* 1981;22:475–88.
3. Mattson RH, Cramer JA, Collins JF, et al. Comparison of carbamazepine, phenobarbital, phenytoin and primidone in partial and secondarily generalized tonic-clonic seizures. *N Engl J Med* 1985;313:145–51.

• • • • • •

MORTALITY

An association between epilepsy and increased mortality (1–3) is elusive because sources of data, such as death certificates or insurance statistics, are difficult to compare, and epilepsy is often associated with other factors affecting mortality, e.g., trauma, stroke, brain tumor, encephalitis. Nevertheless, several studies do show that life expectancy is lower in patients with epilepsy, especially in symptomatic epilepsies (1).

- The ratio of deaths in patients with epilepsy to the total population has been found to be 1.1–2.5 per 100,000 per year (2). From 0.2 to 2% of all deaths occur in patients with epilepsy (2). The standardized mortality ratio (observed deaths over expected deaths) is 2.3–3.5 for epilepsy (1).
- The cause of death in people with epilepsy (1) may be unrelated to the epilepsy in 23–47% of cases. Causes directly related to the seizures include status epilepticus that cannot be controlled; cardiac arrhythmia during a seizure (see Arrhythmia). Causes related to the circumstances of the seizure include suffocation, aspiration, trauma received during the seizure, accidental death or drowning. Causes related more generally to epilepsy include depression leading to suicide; drug reactions. Any cause of accidental death may also incidentally affect people with epilepsy as it would the general population. Microscopic examination of tongue muscle fibers for the presence or absence of trauma may provide evidence for or against a concomitant seizure (4).
- Unexplained death represents 5–30% of deaths in patients with epilepsy (5–7). Purported causes include cardiac dysrhythmia during a seizure resulting from sympathetic stimulation or medications, cardiac ischemia, and neurogenic pulmonary edema (5–7). The commonest causes of mortality after status epilepticus are from cerebrovascular diseases and discontinuation of AEDs (8) (see also Cerebrovascular accidents and seizures).

References

1. Hauser WA, Annegers JF, Eleveback CR. Mortality in patients with epilepsy. *Epilepsia* 1980;21:399–412.
2. Massey EW, Schoenberg BS. Mortality from epilepsy. *Neuroepidemiology* 1985;4:65–70.
3. Chandra V, Bharucha NE, Schoenberg BS. Deaths related to epilepsy in the U.S. *Neuroepidemiology* 1983;2:148–55.
4. Copeland AR. Seizure disorders. The Dade county experience from 1978 to 1982. *Am J Forensic Med* 1984;211–15.
5. Jay GW, Leetsma JE. Sudden death in epilepsy. A comprehensive review of the literature and proposed mechanisms. *Acta Neurol Scand* 1981;63(Suppl 82):11–66.
6. Hirsh C, Martin D. Unexpected deaths in young epileptics. *Neurology* 1971; 21:682–90.
7. Leetsma JE, Walczak T, Hughes JR, Kalelkar MB, Teas SS. A prospective study on sudden unexpected death in epilepsy. *Ann Neurol* 1989;26:195–203.
8. Towne AR, Pellock JM, Ko D, DeLorenzo RJ. Determinants of mortality in status epilepticus. *Epilepsia* 1994;35:27–34.

• • • • • • •

MOVEMENT (SEIZURES INDUCED BY)

Certain seizures can be induced by passive or active movement of an extremity or by a startle reaction (1,2). The inciting stimulus may in some cases be proprioceptive feedback resulting from the movement. Examples of movement-sensitive epilepsy are categorized below:

- Startle-induced epilepsy: patients with lesions of the motor cortex and infantile hemiplegia may have tonic seizures involving the paralyzed side. Children with diffuse cortical lesions can exhibit tonic bilateral seizures (3,4).
- Touch-induced epilepsy: certain seizures can be induced by somesthetic stimulation without startle (5,6). Patients may thus auto-induce somatomotor seizures or sensorimotor seizures.
- Movement-induced epilepsy: unilateral or bilateral tonic seizures are seen in some patients with focal cortical lesions (7–9).
- Hyperglycemia-related epilepsy: nonketotic hyperglycemia in the elderly may predispose to partial seizures induced by active or passive movements. Seizures usually remit following normalization of hyperglycemia (10).
- Paroxysmal kinesigenic choreoathetosis and familial paroxysmal dystonic choreoathetosis are believed to be nonepileptic syndromes (11–12) that may be confused with movement-sensitive epilepsy (see also Reflex (S,E)).

References

1. Chauvel P, Louvel J, Lamarche M. Transcortical reflexes and focal motor epilepsy. *Electroenceph clin Neurophysiol* 1978;45:309–18.
2. Obeso JH, Rothwell JC, Marsden CD. The spectrum of cortical myoclonus. From focal reflex jerks to spontaneous motor epilepsy. *Brain* 1985;108:193–224.
3. Gastaut H, Tassinari CA. Triggering mechanisms in epilepsy. *Epilepsia* 1966; 7:85–138.
4. Saenz-Lope E, Herranz FJ, Masden JC. Startle-epilepsy: a clinical study. *Ann Neurol* 1984;16:78–81.
5. Beaumanoir A, Haenggeli C, Zagury S, Nahory A, Lieury C. Modalités inhabituelles de provocation de l'épilepsie sursaut. *Boll Leg It Epil* 1980;29/30:1169–73.
6. Oller-Daurella L, Dini J. Las crisis epilepticas desencadenadas por movimientos voluntarios. *Medicina Clinica* 1970;54:189–98.
7. Falconer MA, Driver MV, Serafetinides EA. Seizures induced by movement: report of a case relieved by operation. *J Neurol Neurosurg Psychiatry* 1963; 26:300–308.
8. Kennedy WA. Clinical and electroencephalographic aspects of epileptogenic lesions of the medial surface and superior border of the cerebral hemisphere. *Brain* 1959;82:147–61.
9. Perez-Borja C, Tassinari AC, Swanson AG. Paroxysmal choreo-athetosis and seizures induced by movement (reflex epilepsy). *Epilepsia* 1967;8:260–70.
10. Brick JF, Butrecht JA, Ringel RA. Reflex epilepsy and nonketotic hyperglycemia in the elderly: a specific neuroendocrine syndrome. *Neurology* 1989;39:394–99.
11. Lance JW. Familial paroxysmal dystonic choreoathetosis and its differentiation from related syndromes. *Ann Neurol* 1977;2:285–93.
12. Kertesz A. Paroxysmal kinesigenic choreo-athetosis. *Neurology* 1967;17:680–90.

• • • • • •

MULTIPLE (DISSEMINATED) SCLEROSIS

In definite multiple sclerosis, the incidence of seizures has been reported to be 1–4% (1,2). Partial seizures are usually seen and appear during the course of the illness, rarely at onset. The relationship between demyelination and seizure foci is unclear (1). The larger, non-resolving lesions seen on MRI involving cortical subcortical regions are most likely to be associated with ongoing seizures (3).

Other nonepileptic "seizures" (painful tonic spasms) responsive to carbamazepine may confuse the picture (4).

References

1. Kinnunen E, Wikstrom J. Prevalence and prognosis of epilepsy in patients with multiple sclerosis. *Epilepsia* 1986;27:729–33.
2. Ghezzi A, Montanini R, Basso PF, Zaffaroni M, Massimo E, Cazzullo CL. Epilepsy in multiple sclerosis. *Eur Neurol* 1990; 30:218–23.
3. Thompson AJ, Kermode AG, Moseley IF, MacManus DG, McDonald WI. Seizures due to multiple sclerosis: seven patients with MRI correlations. *J Neurol Neurosurg Psychiatry* 1993;56:1317–20.
4. Twomey JA, Espir MLE. Paroxysmal symptoms as the first manifestations of multiple sclerosis. *J Neurol Neurosurg Psychiatry* 1980;43:296–304.

• • • • • •
MYOCLONIC ENCEPHALOPATHY
(EARLY MYOCLONIC ENCEPHALOPATHY) (1,2)

Myoclonic encephalopathy (also called "early myoclonic encephalopathy") is a rare syndrome due to a variety of causes. The onset is in the neonatal period, with fragmentary myoclonic jerks interspersed with occasional massive myoclonus, partial seizures or infantile spasms; death usually occurs before the age of one year. Initially, the EEG shows high-voltage runs of spikes, irregular spike and slow waves separated by periods of voltage suppression. The EEG pattern may deteriorate over time to hypsarrythmia.

Myoclonic encephalopathy resembles the syndrome of "early infantile epileptic encephalopathy with suppression-burst," but the latter syndrome includes cerebral malformations, and focal myoclonus is absent.

References

1. Aicardi J. Early myoclonic encephalopathy In: Roger J, Bureau M, Dravet C, Dreifuss FE, Perret A, Wolf P (eds.). *Epileptic syndromes in infancy, childhood and adolescence,* 2nd edition. London: John Libbey & Co. Ltd., 1992:13–23.
2. Ohtahara S, Ohtahara Y, Yamatogi Y, Oka E. The early infantile epileptic encephalopathy with suppression-burst: developmental aspects. *Brain Dev* 1987;9:371–76.

• • • • • •
MYOCLONIC (EPILEPSIES)

Myoclonic epilepsies are epileptic syndromes in which myoclonus (see this heading) occurs either at onset or as a prominent feature during the course of the disease. The International Classification of the Epilepsies distinguishes between:

- idiopathic generalized epilepsies: benign myoclonic epilepsy of infancy, juvenile myoclonic epilepsy;
- cryptogenic or symptomatic generalized epilepsies: early myoclonic epilepsy with encephalopathy, infantile epileptic encephalopathy, severe myoclonic epilepsy of infancy, myoclonic absence, Lennox-Gastaut syndrome with myoclonus, myoclonic-astatic epilepsy (see these headings), progressive myoclonic epilepsies (see Myoclonic epilepsies, progressive). Myoclonic components may be seen in certain encephalopathies or partial epilepsies (Kojewnikow's syndrome).

• • • • • •
MYOCLONIC EPILEPSY IN INFANCY (BENIGN) (1)

Myoclonic epilepsy in infancy (also called "benign myoclonic epilepsy") is a rare epileptic syndrome. It begins between the fourth month and the first year of life in a previously normal infant, and in the absence of a family history of epilepsy. Myoclonic jerks are brief, mild, spontaneous, and frequent, especially during light sleep. Myoclonic epilepsy is not associated with other seizure types.

The EEG shows a normal posterior background rhythm, but generalized spike, polyspike, and slow waves occur synchronously with myoclonic jerks. Myoclonus can be induced by intermittent photic stimulation.

Myoclonic epilepsy of infancy usually responds to the early use of AEDs, for example, valproic acid. Sequelae are unusual.

Reference

Dravet C, Bureau M, Roger J. Benign myoclonic epilepsy in infants. In: Roger J, Bureau M, Dravet C, Dreifuss FE, Perret A, Wolf P (eds.). *Epileptic syndromes in infancy, childhood and adolescence,* 2nd edition. London: John Libbey & Co. Ltd., 1992:67–74.

● ● ● ● ● ●
MYOCLONIC EPILEPSY IN INFANCY AND CHILDHOOD (SEVERE) (1)

Myoclonic epilepsy of infancy and childhood was first identified in 1982 (2). This disorder begins in the first year in previously normal infants and is characterized by unilateral or generalized clonic, tonic-clonic, myoclonic, or partial seizures. Tonic seizures do not occur. Convulsions may initially be precipitated by fever and soon become frequent and prolonged. Incidence is 1/40,000 children of less than 7 years of age (3). There is no known specific etiology. Approximately 25% of patients have a history of febrile convulsions or a family history of epilepsy.

The EEG, usually normal at onset, comes to show generalized spikes, polyspikes, and slow waves, focal abnormalities, and photic sensitivity.

Myoclonic epilepsy of infancy and childhood frequently is associated with progressive ataxia, dementia, pyramidal signs, as well as worsening myoclonus. Treatment is generally ineffective.

References

1. Dravet C, Roger J, Bureau M. Severe myoclonic epilepsy in infants. In: Roger J, Bureau M, Dravet C, Dreifuss FE, Perret A, Wolf P (eds.). *Epileptic syndromes in infancy, childhood and adolescence,* 2nd edition. London: John Libbey & Co. Ltd., 1992:75–88.
2. Dravet C, Roger J, Bureau M, Dalla-Bernardina B. Myoclonic epilepsies of childhood. In: Akimoto H, Kazamatsuri H, Seino M, Ward A (eds). *Advances in Epileptology: XIIth Epilepsy International Symposium.* New York: Raven Press, 1982:135–40.
3. Hurst DL. Epidemiology of severe myoclonic epilepsy of infancy. *Epilepsia* 1990;31:397–400.

● ● ● ● ● ●
MYOCLONIC EPILEPSIES, PROGRESSIVE

Progressive myoclonic epilepsies (PME), originally delineated by Unverricht and Lundborg (1,2), are now believed to comprise a family of myoclonic syndromes. Characteristic findings in PME include massive myoclonus, focal and segmental myoclonus, tonic-clonic seizures, progressive dementia, and cerebellar or pyramidal signs.

Inheritance is usually by autosomal recessive transmission; an autosomal dominant transmission is seen when other neurological signs are present. Unverricht-Lundborg disease (see this heading) is degenerative without a known specific biochemical abnormality. Other varieties of PME have identified biochemical abnormalities: Lafora disease, ceroid-lipofuscinoses, siali-doses type I and type II, mitochondrial encephalopathies, gangliosidoses (GM1, GM2).

Clinical features of PME include (various combinations seen in different syndromes):

- a cherry-red spot in the optic fundus (lipidoses and mucolipidoses);
- early blindness (ceroid-lipofuscinoses);
- intra-cytoplasmic inclusion bodies (ceroid-lipofuscinoses);
- abnormalities of lipid metabolic enzymes in serum, leukocytes, and cutaneous fibroblasts (lipidoses);
- amyloid inclusions in skin, muscle, liver (Lafora disease).

Other forms of PME are associated with particular neurological manifestations: mitochondrial myopathies, dentato-rubro-thalamic atrophy. Ramsay Hunt syndrome (see this heading) includes a heterogeneous group of disorders.

References

1. Berkovic SF, Andermann F, Carpenter S, Wolf E. Progressive myoclonus epilepsies: specific causes and diagnosis. *N Engl J Med* 1986;315:296–305.
2. Marseille Consensus Group. Classification of progressive myoclonus epilepsies and related disorders. *Ann Neurol* 1990;28:113–16.

● ● ● ● ● ● ●

MYOCLONIC-ASTATIC (EPILEPSY) (DOOSE'S SYNDROME)

Myoclonic-astatic epilepsy is a rare epilepsy of childhood characterized in 1964 by Doose (1). Onset occurs between the ages of 7 months and 6 years, usually in children with previously normal development. The syndrome is more frequent in males (1,2). A family history of epilepsy is present in 37% of cases.

Seizure types include myoclonic-astatic seizures (see this heading); absence seizures with myoclonus tonic-clonic seizures (2). Status epilepticus is common. The EEG shows a background dominated by 4–7 Hz rhythms, with a variable array of spikes, polyspikes, and slow waves. Paroxysmal EEG patterns are increased by intermittent photic stimulation. The course of this epileptic syndrome is variable. Spontaneous remissions, as well as clinical deterioration similar to that seen in the Lennox-Gastaut syndrome, can be seen.

Doose's syndrome may overlap with the Lennox-Gastaut syndrome and early myoclonic epilepsy (see these headings).

References

1. Doose H. Das akinetische Petit Mal. *Arch Psych Nervenkr* 1964;205:637–54
2. Doose H. Myoclonic-astatic epilepsy of early childhood. In: Roger J, Bureau M, Dravet C, Dreifuss FE, Perret A, Wolf P (eds.). *Epileptic syndromes in infancy, childhood and adolescence,* 2nd edition. London: John Libbey & Co. Ltd., 1992:103–14.

• • • • • • •
MYOCLONIC-ASTATIC (SEIZURES)

The term "astatic" (loss of stasis) is gradually being replaced by "atonic" (loss of tone), but "astatic" remains in use as a modifier for certain types of seizures. Myoclonic-astatic seizures begin with symmetric myoclonus involving the upper limbs, followed by a diffuse loss of muscle tone. Injurious falls may result. Myoclonic-astatic seizures are seen in the Lennox-Gastaut syndrome (see this heading), myoclonic-astatic epilepsy of Doose (2) (see this heading), and other myoclonic epilepsies of childhood. The EEG of children with myoclonic-astatic seizures shows polyspike corresponding to the myoclonus, and slow wave discharges with the loss of tone (1,2).

References

1. Gastaut H, Broughton R. *Epileptic seizures, clinical and electrographic features, diagnosis and treatment.* Springfield: Charles C. Thomas, 1972.
2. Doose H. Myoclonic-astatic epilepsy of early childhood. In: Roger J, Bureau M, Dravet C, Dreifuss FE, Perret A, Wolf P (eds.). *Epileptic syndromes in infancy, childhood and adolescence,* 2nd edition. London: John Libbey Eurotext, 1992:103–14.

• • • • • • •
MYOCLONIC (SEIZURES)

Myoclonic seizures consist of brief and violent muscular contractions, usually bilateral, that do not affect consciousness. Myoclonic contractions may be single or multiple, lasting for seconds to hours. Contractions may be rhythmic or irregular. When the upper limbs are involved, patients may drop or throw objects. When the legs or trunk are involved, the patient may suddenly fall. Myoclonic seizures may be spontaneous or induced by flashes of light, more rarely by other triggering stimuli (see Reflex (S,E)).

The usual EEG correlate of myoclonic seizures is generalized or multifocal spikes, polyspikes, and slow waves. Scalp-recorded EEG discharges may be visible in the case of cortical myoclonus, or invisible in the case of subcortical myoclonus. Certain cortical discharges with myoclonus are detectable only with use of signal averaging techniques (1).

Myoclonic seizures are seen in idiopathic generalized epilepsies; benign myoclonic epilepsy of childhood; juvenile myoclonic epilepsy; the Lennox-Gastaut syndrome; progressive myoclonic epilepsies; and a wide variety of seizures from toxic and metabolic causes (1,2)(see also Anoxia/Hypoxia and individual headings).

References

1. Hallett M. Myoclonus: relation to epilepsy. *Epilepsia* 1985;26(Suppl 1):S67–S77.
2. Roger J, Bureau M, Dravet C, Dreifuss FE, Perret A, Wolf P (eds.). *Epileptic syndromes in infancy, childhood and adolescence,* 2nd edition. London: John Libbey Eurotext, 1992.

• • • • • •
MYOCLONUS (1–3)

Brief and involuntary contraction of one or more muscles. Myoclonus is not necessarily epileptic. Epileptic myoclonus arises from paroxysmal discharges of the central nervous system. (see Myoclonic (E), Myoclonic (S)).

References

1. Hallett M. Myoclonus: relation to epilepsy. *Epilepsia* 1985;26(Suppl 1):S67–S77.
2. Kelly JJ Jr, Sharbrough FW, Daube JR. A clinical and electrophysiological evaluation of myoclonus. *Neurology* 1981;31:581–89.
3. Obeso JA, Rothwell JC, Marsden CD. The spectrum of cortical myoclonus: from focal reflex jerks to spontaneous motor epilepsy. *Brain* 1985;108:193–224.

• • • • • •
MYOCLONUS EPILEPSY WITH
RAGGED RED FIBERS (MERRF)

This mitochondrial encephalopathy was described in 1980 (1). It is related to several other conditions involving abnormalities of mitochondrial enzymes (see Mitochondrial myopathy, encephalopathy, lactic acidosis, stroke-like episodes (MELAS)) (2). Inheritance is by maternal transmission.

The syndrome of myoclonus epilepsy with "ragged red fibers" (MERRF) is a myoclonic epilepsy with action and intention myoclonus, generalized seizures, ataxia with a variable age of onset, and rapidly progressive mental deterioration (3). MERRF and related mitochondrial disorders may be associated with deafness, optic atrophy, peripheral neuropathy, or upper motor neuron signs. The diagnosis is made by a finding of increased blood pyruvate and lactate, the presence of "ragged red fibers" on muscle biopsy, and abnormalities of the mitochondrial respiratory chain (4).

References

1. Fukuhara N, Togikuschi S, Shirakawa K, Tsubaki T. Myoclonus epilepsy associated with ragged-red fibers (mitochondrial abnormalities): disease entity or syndrome? Light and electron microscopic studies of two cases and review of literature. *J Neurol Sci* 1980;47:117–33.
2. Fukuhara N. MERRF: a clinicopathological study. Relationship between myoclonus epilepsies and mitochondrial myopathies. *Rev Neurol* 1991;147: 476–79.
3. Berkovic SF, Carpenter S, Evans A, et al. Myoclonus epilepsy and ragged-red fibers (MERRF). A clinical pathological, biochemical magnetic resonance spectrographic and positron emission tomographic study. *Brain* 1989;112:1231–60.
4. So N, Berkovic S, Andermann F, Kuznicky R, Gendron D, Quesney LF. Myoclonus epilepsy and ragged-red fibers (MERRF). Electrophysiological studies and comparison with other progressive myoclonus epilepsies. *Brain* 1989;112:1261–76.

• • • • • •
MYSOLINE® (PRIMIDONE)

Tablets of 50 mg, 250 mg; suspension 250 mg per 5 mL.

A barbiturate (see this heading) useful in treatment of generalized, partial and myoclonic seizures (see also Primidone).

NARCOLEPSY

This disorder, characterized by hypersomnolence, is presently delineated by a tetrad of symptoms: excessive wake-time somnolence, cataplexy, sleep paralysis, and hallucinations on waking and going to sleep. It has incorrectly been thought to be epileptic in nature because of its paroxysmal nature, sudden falls, and unresponsiveness. It may be distinguished from seizures by the more prolonged periods of sleep-like flaccid unresponsiveness, the absence of convulsions and postictal confusion. The EEG during such episodes shows rapid eye movement (REM) or non-rapid eye movement (non-REM) sleep. More prolonged periods of automatic behavior may occur for which the patient is amnestic, contrasting with the briefer automatisms of complex partial seizures.

Diagnosis of narcolepsy is based on its clinical features and a multiple sleep latency polygraph test showing abbreviated sleep onset into REM sleep. Treatment includes modification of sleep habit, the use of short daytime naps, and central stimulant medication.

NEONATAL (SEIZURES)

Neonatal seizures are defined as seizures occurring in the first 4 weeks of life. From 0.5% to 1.4% of all newborns will have neonatal seizures, and the number is higher in high risk newborns (1). They include the following (2):

NEONATAL SEIZURE TYPES

- *Clonic seizures,* with focal jerking in face, limbs, and axial muscles. EEG shows 1–3 per second synchronous discharges, with centrally maximal spikes and slow waves. Less often seizures will be hemiconvulsive, axial, or multifocal.

194

- *Myoclonic seizures,* with generalized or focal (particularly flexor muscles) myoclonus, associated with high-voltage EEG discharges.
- *Tonic seizures,* with focal flexion of the trunk, symmetric or asymmetric. Concurrent EEG may demonstrate a rhythmic, rapid low-voltage epileptiform discharge in the frontotemporal region ipsilateral to the flexion (3). Rarely, neonatal tonic seizures present as tonic deviation of the eyes with nystagmus in association with an occipital EEG discharge.
- *Other seizure types,* not well categorized by standard seizure classification schemes, occur in the neonatal period (3–5). The neonate may show eye opening, eyelid fluttering, oscillatory or rotatory movement of the eyes, poorly coordinated movements of the limbs, chewing, sucking, apneic episodes, and cardiac dysrhythmias. Autonomic signs can be prominent, in the form of tachycardia and increase in blood pressure. These seizures may be difficult to distinguish from normal neonatal behavior and conditions such as "fidgetiness" (6).

Any form of neonatal seizures can progress to neonatal status epilepticus (7).

ETIOLOGY OF NEONATAL SEIZURES

Seizure onset in the neonatal period mandates a search for the underlying cause or causes, which determine the ultimate prognosis. Neonatal seizures may be symptomatic (secondary) or idiopathic (cryptogenic). Several important etiologies are as follows.

- *Anoxic-ischemic encephalopathy* (see also Anoxia/Hypoxia; Hypoxia). Anoxia-ischemia is probably responsible for 50–75% of neonatal convulsions (3,7). Initially, seizures are infrequent, but subsequently become more severe 12–24 hours after birth.
- *Intracranial hemorrhages* account for about 15% of all neonatal convulsions. Intraventricular hemorrhages predominate in the premature neonate. EEGs of neonates with intraventricular hemmorhage typically show positive sharp waves with phase reversals in the Rolandic area. Prognosis in patients with intraventricular hemorrhage is guarded. Subarachnoid, subdural, or intraparenchymal hemorrhages have a better prognosis than does intraventricular hemorrhage, but outcome is still highly variable.
- *Central nervous system infections* account for about 15% of cases of neonatal convulsions (3,7). Bacterial infections predominate, but Herpes simplex encephalitis rarely may be encountered at this age.

- *Metabolic disturbances* are common causes for neonatal convulsions (8). Seizures with hypocalcemia of early onset usually respond poorly to AEDs unless the underlying problem is corrected. Late onset hypocalcemia (developing after the first week) carries a better prognosis. Hypocalcemia may be associated with hypomagnesemia.

Hypoglycemia is a potentially serious cause of neonatal seizures if it remains uncorrected. Toxic causes of seizures from alcohol or drugs are rare, but important to recognize (9). Other metabolic causes of seizures in the first month of life include hypernatremia, hyponatremia, pyridoxine deficiency (rare with modern feeding formulas), and inborn errors of metabolism (see also Metabolic errors, inborn).

- *Cerebral malformations* may lead to neonatal myoclonic seizures and an associated burst suppression pattern on the EEG.

NEONATAL SEIZURE SYNDROMES

From 10% to 25% of neonatal convulsions or neonatal status epilepticus remain idiopathic. A few of the neonatal syndromes have been highlighted by the International Classification of Epileptic Syndromes.

- *Idiopathic neonatal convulsions* (fifth day fits) (10,11) are focal or multifocal tonic seizures seen between day 3 and day 6 of life in previously normal children; the EEG changes are nonspecific. Prognosis is guarded, with the later risk of further seizures or psychomotor retardation (11). With the exception of a possible zinc deficiency (12), no etiology has been determined. Incidence of idiopathic neonatal convulsions has fallen since the 1980s (11).
- *Benign familial neonatal convulsions* (10) are clonic, apneic, or, more rarely, tonic seizures, seen in previously normal newborns at around the second to third day of life. Seizures are frequently repetitive. The EEG is normal. Diagnosis is based on a family history of a similar presentation. Inheritance is by autosomal dominant transmission with normal penetrance but variable expression. Two genetic loci (CMM6 and RMR6) on the long arm of chromosome 20 (13) have been linked to the syndrome. The risk of developing epilepsy after benign familial neonatal convulsions has been calculated at 14% (10).
- *Early myoclonic encephalopathy* (14) is a rare epileptic syndrome presenting with several seizure types: occasional myoclonic jerks which may be partial or fragmentary, massive myoclonic jerks, partial motor seizures, or tonic spasms. Seizures present in the first month of life and may be associated with major metabolic problems. The EEG shows bursts of spikes and sharply contoured spike waves, irregular and arrhythmic slow wave bursts separated by periods of relative

voltage suppression lasting 3–10 seconds. The bursts of epileptiform EEG activity are not synchronous with the myoclonic jerks. The EEG pattern deteriorates over time to hypsarrythmia or a multifocal epileptiform pattern. Neurological examination is always abnormal and prognosis is grim. (See also Myoclonic encephalopathy.)

- *Early epileptic encephalopathy with burst suppression* is a syndrome characterized by Ohtahara in 1978 (15). Clinical characteristics are similar to those of early myoclonic encephalopathy, except that neonates with Ohtahara's syndrome are less likely to show myoclonic and partial seizures. Diagnosis is made by identification of severe cerebral malformations believed to be responsible for the condition.

TREATMENT OF NEONATAL SEIZURES

Treatment of neonatal seizures consists of supportive care for the child, correction wherever possible of the underlying cause (see previous), and judicious use of AEDs—phenobarbital, phenytoin, and parenteral or rectal benzodiazepines. Chronic AED therapy may be useful, but is not necessary in all cases.

PROGNOSIS OF NEONATAL SEIZURES

The prognosis of neonatal seizures depends on the gestational age, the frequency and characteristics of the seizures, the severity of EEG abnormality, and, most importantly, on the underlying cause. Mortality ranges from 10–35% (16), mental retardation ensues in 10–25% of cases (6), infantile cerebral hemiplegia occurs in 13–25% of cases (6), and 10–25% of cases later develop epilepsy (16–18). Despite this serious prognosis, two-thirds have no sequelae (18).

References

1. Bergman I, Painter MJ, Hirsch RP, Crumrine PK, David R. Outcome of neonates with convulsive seizures treated in an intensive care unit. *Ann Neurol* 1983;14:642–47.
2. Volpe JJ. Neonatal seizures: current concepts and revised classification. *Pediatrics* 1989;84:422–28.
3. Mizrahi EM, Kellaway P. Characterization and classification of neonatal seizures. *Neurology* 1987;37:1837–44.
4. Clancy RR, Legido A, Lewis D. Occult neonatal seizures. *Epilepsia* 1988;29:256–61.
5. Connell J, Oozeer R, De Vries L, Dubowitz LMS, Dubowitz V. Continuous EEG monitoring for neonatal seizures: diagnostic and prognostic considerations. *Arch Dis Child* 1989;64:452–58.
6. Volpe JJ. Neonatal seizures. *Clin Perinatal* 1977;4:43–63.

7. Dreyfus-Brisac C, Monod N. Neonatal status epilepticus. *Electroenceph clin Neurophysiol* 1972;15:38–52.
8. Brown JK. Convulsions in the newborn period. *Dev Med Child Neurol* 1973;15:823–46.
9. Herzlinger RA, Candali SP, Vaughn HG Jr. Neonatal seizures associated with narcotic withdrawal. *J Pediatr* 1977;91:638–44.
10. Plouin P. Benign idiopathic neonatal convulsions (familial and non familial). In: Roger J, Bureau M, Dravet C, Dreifuss FE, Perret A, Wolf P (eds.). *Epileptic syndromes in infancy, childhood and adolescence,* 2nd edition. London, John Libbey Eurotext, 1992:3–11.
11. North KN, Storey GNB, Henderson-Smart DJ. Fifth day fits in the newborn. *Austr Paediatr J* 1989;25:284–87.
12. Goldberg HJ, Sheely EM. Fifth day fits: an acute zinc deficiency syndrome? *Arch Dis Child* 1982 57:633–35.
13. Leppert M, Anderson VE, Quattelbaum T, et al. Benign familial neonatal convulsions linked to genetic markers on chromosome 20. *Nature* 1989;337:647–48.
14. Aicardi J. Early myoclonic encephalopathy. In: Roger J, Bureau M, Dravet C, Dreifuss FE, Perret A, Wolf P (eds.). *Epileptic syndromes in infancy, childhood and adolescence,* 2nd edition. London: John Libbey & Co. Ltd., 1992:13–23.
15. Ohtahara S. Clinical electrical delineation of epileptic encephalopathies in childhood. *Asian Med J* 1978;21:7–17.
16. Holden KR, Mellits ED, Freeman JM. Neonatal seizures I. Correlation of prenatal and perinatal events with the outcome. *Pediatrics* 1982;70:165–76.
17. Rose AL, Lombroso CT. Neonatal seizures states: a study of clinical, pathological and electro-encephalographic features in 137 full-term babies with a long term follow-up. *Pediatrics* 1970;45:405–25.
18. Lombroso CT. Prognosis in neonatal seizures. *Adv Neurol* 1983;34:101–13.

● ● ● ● ● ●
NEUROPATHIES (AND AEDS)

Peripheral neuropathy is a potential side effect of chronic use of AEDs. Electrophysiological abnormalities (slowed conduction times) may be detected in a majority of patients on long-term therapy. Clinical signs, including paresthesias or decreased reflexes, occur in up to 38% of some populations. Phenytoin has been primarily implicated, although phenobarbital, carbamazepine (1,2), or phenytoin and phenobarbital (3) can also induce neuropathy. Histologic examination reveals axonopathy with secondary demyelinization (4). The role of folate deficiency has been debated.

References

1. Geraldini C, Faedda MT, Sideri G. Anticonvulsant therapy and its possible consequence on peripheral nervous system: a neurographic study. *Epilepsia* 1984;25:502–505.

2. Taylor JW, Murphy MJ, Rivey MP. Clinical and electrophysiologic evaluation of peripheral nerve function in chronic phenytoin therapy. *Epilepsia* 1985;26:416–20.
3. Shorvon SD, Reynolds EH. Anticonvulsant peripheral neuropathies: a clinical and electrophysiological study of patients on single drug treatment with phenytoin, carbamazepine or barbiturates. *J Neurol Neurosurg Psychiatry* 1982;45:620–26.
4. Ramirez JA, Mendell JR, Warmolts JR, Griggs RC. Phenytoin neuropathy: structural changes in the sural nerve. *Ann Neurol* 1986;19:162–67.

• • • • • •
NIEMANN-PICK (DISEASE)

Niemann-Pick disease is a sphingolipidosis described in 1914 (1), characterized by accumulation of sphingomyelin in the reticulo-endothelial system. Inheritance is by autosomal recessive transmission, with Ashkenazy Jews at relatively high risk. Four clinical forms of Niemann-Pick disease have been described. Group A, the most common, has an onset in the first year of life. Patients have hepatosplenomegaly, severe and rapidly progressive cognitive decline, cherry-red spots in the optic fundi (25%), myoclonic seizures, and a variety of other neurological abnormalities. Death is usual by age 5 years. The other groups of Niemann-Pick disease show less marked hepatosplenomegaly, onset later in life, and a more gradual progression (2). Diagnosis of Niemann-Pick disease in any of its forms depends on the clinical picture and biopsy (e.g., rectal or splenic) for determination of a deficit in sphingomyelinase activity.

References

1. Niemann A. Ein unbekanntes Krankheitsbild. *Jahrb Kinderheilk* 1914;79:1–10.
2. Crocker AC, Farbers PC. Niemann-Pick disease: a review of 18 patients. *Medicine* 1958;37:10–95.

• • • • • •
NIGHT TERRORS

Night terrors are a nonepileptic, intermittent, paroxysmal phenomenon occurring in the early hours of sleep in children between 18 months and 5 years of age. Children characteristically arouse their parents with an alarming scream, but recall nothing unusual when they are themselves awakened. Occurrence usually is in slow wave sleep. The interictal EEG is normal; information is not available on EEGs during night terrors. Night terrors are best considered age-dependent normal sleep behaviors, to be distinguished from nocturnal seizures of childhood, panic attacks, and nightmares.

Reference

Gastaut H, Broughton R. *Epileptic seizures, clinical and electrographic features, diagnosis and treatment.* Springfield: Charles C. Thomas, 1972.

• • • • • •
NITRAZEPAM (MOGADON®)

Nitrazepam is a sedative and hypnotic with AED properties of the benzodiazepine family (see Benzodiazepines) used in symptomatic generalized epilepsies, West syndrome, atypical absences, and complex partial seizures. The drug is not presently approved for use in the United States.

Reference

Levy RH, Mattson R, Meldrum B, Penry JK, Dreifuss FE (eds.). *Antiepileptic drugs,* 3rd edition. New York: Raven Press, 1989.

• • • • • •
NYSTAGMUS (EPILEPTIC)

A synonym for "oculoclonic epileptic seizure" (1). During seizures, there may be tonic deviation of the eyes to a position of extreme lateral gaze; a clonic component may rhythmically interrupt this excursion with rapid jerky movements toward the midline, producing nystagmus (2).

Nystagmus during a seizure may include horizontal, vertical or unilateral, disconjugate, or seesaw movements. Conjugate horizontal eye movements are most common. Nystagmus rarely is the sole symptom of a seizure (3). The mechanism of epileptic nystagmus is presumed to be activation of eye movement centers controlling saccades and pursuit movements by the seizures. In obtunded patients, the localizing value of epileptic nystagmus is limited. Video-EEG correlative studies have identified epileptic foci in the hemisphere contralateral to the fast-phase of the nystagmus, predominantly in parieto-temporal regions, but also in ipsilateral and contralateral frontal and occipital regions (3–7). In awake patients, epileptic nystagmus usually localizes to the contralateral junctional zone. When presenting as a simple partial seizure, the epileptic discharge frequency is usually above 10 Hz (7).

References

1. Gastaut H. *Dictionary of epilepy. Part 1: Definitions.* Geneva: World Health Organization, 1973.
2. Gastaut H, Broughton R. *Epileptic seizures, clinical and electrographic features, diagnosis and treatment.* Springfield: Charles C. Thomas, 1972:114–16.
3. Beun AM, Beintema DJ, Binnie CD, Debets RMC, Overweg J, van Heycop Ten Ham MW. Epileptic nystagmus. *Epilepsia* 1984;25:609–14.
4. Furman JMR, Crumrine PK, Reinmuth OM. Epileptic nystagmus. *Ann Neurol* 1990;27:686–88.
5. Tusa RJ, Kaplan PW, Hain TC, Naidu S. Ipsiversive eye deviation and epileptic nystagmus. *Neurology* 1990;40:662–65.
6. Kaplan PW, Lesser RP. Vertical and horizontal epileptic gaze deviation and nystagmus. *Neurology* 1989;39:1391–93.
7. Kaplan PW, Tusa RJ. Neurophysiologic and clinical correlations of epileptic nystagmus. *Neurology* 1993;43:2508–14.

OCCASIONAL (SEIZURES)

"Occasional seizures" is a phrase used primarily in Europe to connote isolated or symptomatic seizures associated with environmental factors, such as sleep deprivation, acute illness, stress, etc.

OCCIPITAL (EPILEPSY)
(PARTIAL EPILEPSY WITH OCCIPITAL PAROXYSMS)

Partial epilepsy with occipital paroxysms is a rare epileptic syndrome of childhood described in 1982 (1,2). The condition was previously confused with basilar migraine (3). There is a family history of epilepsy in 36%, and of migraine in 16% of cases (1). The usual age of onset is 15 months to 17 years, with a mean of 7 years.

Clinical characteristics of the seizures depend on whether they occur during wakefulness or sleep (1). Nocturnal seizures are predominantly partial motor seizures with eye opening, tonic deviation of the eyes and head. Daytime seizures present with elementary visual phenomena (amaurosis, scotomas, phosphenes) or elaborate phenomena (hallucinations, illusions). Hemiclonic, adversive, or generalized tonic-clonic seizures may be seen. One-third of the cases suffer diffuse headache with nausea and vomiting suggesting migraine.

The EEG in cases of partial epilepsy with occipital paroxysms shows normal background frequencies and interictal high-voltage spike and slow wave discharges occurring in runs at 1–3 Hertz. These paroxysms are maximal in the occipital regions and are always decreased by eye opening and increased during slow wave sleep (2). Generalized spike and slow wave discharges and Rolandic spikes are less common EEG patterns.

A similar clinical and EEG picture may be seen with other widespread occipital lesions (5) or occipital calcification (6). Occipital spike-waves do not necessarily indicate a benign epilepsy or even an epilepsy (7). In partial epilepsy with occipital paroxysms, seizures may be resistant to treatment, but usually remit after 3–9 years (4).

References

1. Gastaut H. L'épilepsie bénigne de l'enfant à pointe-ondes occipitales. *Rev EEG Neurophysiol Clin* 1982;12:179–201.
2. Beaumanoir A. Infantile epilepsy with occipital focus and good prognosis. *Eur Neurol* 1983;22:43–52.
3. Camfield PR, Metrakos K, Andermann F. Basilar migraine, seizures and severe epileptiform EEG abnormalities. *Neurology* 1978:28:584–88.
4. Panayiotopoulos CP. Benign childhood epilepsy with occipital paroxysms: a 15 years prospective study. *Ann Neurol* 1989;26:51–56.
5. Newton R, Aicardi J. Clinical findings in children with occipital spike-wave complexes suppressed by eyes opening. *Neurology* 1983;33:1526–29.
6. Gobbi G, Sorrenti G, Santucci M, Rosi PG, Ambrosetto P, Michelucci R, Tassinari CA. Epilepsy with bilateral occipital calcifications: a benign onset with progressive severity. *Neurology* 1988;38:1100–1106.
7. Fois A, Malandrini F, Tomaccini D. Clinical findings in children with occipital paroxysmal discharges. *Epilepsia* 1988;29:620–23.

• • • • • •
OCCIPITAL (SEIZURES)

Occipital seizures are characterized by simple partial seizures, sometimes with secondary generalization. Seizures consist of predominantly visual symptoms (see Visual (S)). Seizure discharges in primary visual cortex produce simple visual symptoms, whereas discharges in the temporo-parieto-occipital association cortex result in complex hallucinations, illusions, or epileptic nystagmus (see Nystagmus (epileptic))(1). Occipital seizures may also start with contralateral tonic or clonic deviation of the eyes of the head (see Versive (S)). Seizure activity may spread forward to the temporal lobe, resulting in a complex partial seizure. When the focus is in the supracalcarine area, the spread may involve the supra-Sylvian convexity, resulting in frontal or parietal symptoms. Spread to the contralateral occipital lobe may be rapid (2). Occipital epilepsy may be difficult to distinguish from migraine (see this heading), and overlap syndromes do exist.

Occipital seizures belong to several syndromes (3):

• *Benign epilepsy of childhood with occipital spike waves;* (see Benign epilepsies).

- *Bilateral occipital calcifications with epilepsy.* In this syndrome, seizures begin in early childhood. Visual or somatomotor symptoms predominate, but complex partial seizures may develop. Children have normal or diminished intelligence, and dyslexia is common. Many children continue to suffer seizures and psychomotor retardation, although a few cases remit (4).
- *Sturge-Weber syndrome.*
- *Occipital seizures with posterior cerebral artery infarction* (5). Posterior cerebral artery infarction from thromboembolic vascular disease, trauma, or migraine can result in partial seizures, together with hemianopsia and sometimes hemiparesis. Head CT or MRI may show occipital porencephaly.
- *Mitochondrial encephalomyopathies* (see this heading).
- Other symptomatic or cryptogenic focal epilepsies.

References

1. Kaplan PW, Tusa RJ. Neurophysiologic and clinical correlations of epileptic nystagmus. *Neurology* 1993;43:2508–14.
2. Commission on Classification and Terminology of the International League Against Epilepsy. Proposal for classification of epilepsies and epileptic syndromes. *Epilepsia* 1989;30:389–99.
3. Huott AD, Madison DS, Niedermeyer E. Occipital lobe epilepsy: a clinical and electroencephalographic study. *Eur Neurol* 1974;11:325–39.
4. Gobbi G, Sorrenti G, Santucci M, Rossi PG, Ambrosetto P, Michelucci R, Tassinari CA. Epilepsy with bilateral occipital calcifications: a benign onset with progressive severity. *Neurology* 1988;38:913–20.
5. Remillard GR, Ethier R, Andermann FA. Temporal lobe epilepsy and perinatal occlusion of the posterior cerebral artery. A syndrome analogous to infantile hemiplegia and a demonstrable etiology in some patients with temporal lobe epilepsy. *Neurology* 1974;24:1100–1109.

• • • • • •

OLFACTORY (SEIZURES)

Seizures with olfactory manifestations may present as an illusion of an increase in the sense of smell, or a hallucination, with distorted smells. Olfactory hallucinations are usually of a disagreeable nature: the smell of organic decomposition, chemical smells, burning rubber, or other unidentifiable unpleasant smells.

These seizures are also referred to as "uncinate" seizures because of their frequent involvement of the uncus, orbitofrontal cortex, and mesial temporal cortex. Uncinate seizures should raise the suspicion of a symptomatic partial epilepsy and may warrant evaluation for underlying frontal or temporal lesions. Nevertheless, many such cases are benign.

Reference

Bancaud J. Sémiologie clinique des crises épileptiques d'origine temporale. *Rev Neurol* 1987:143:392–400.

• • • • • •
OROPHARYNGEAL (SEIZURES)

Oropharyngeal seizures present as increased salivation, speech arrest, gustatory hallucinations, lip-smacking or chewing, occasionally epigastric discomfort, fear, autonomic signs, or hemifacial spasms. Opercular or supra-insular epileptic discharges have been identified. Seizures are seen with symptomatic or cryptogenic partial epilepsies.

The term "oropharyngeal seizure" is also used for the common benign epilepsy of childhood with centro-temporal spikes. Seizures in this setting include increased salivation, difficulty speaking, swallowing or gargling, chewing movements or clonic movements of the jaw, inability to move the tongue, forced contraction of the tongue, inability to open the mouth, swallowing of saliva, pharyngeal constriction, gum or tongue tingling.

• • • • • •
OXCARBAZEPINE (TRILEPTAL®)

Oxcarbazepine is a keto analog of carbamazepine (CBZ). It is in use in several countries and is in phase II clinical trials in the United States. It is believed to have similar efficacy, but fewer adverse events than CBZ, possibly because it is not metabolized to the 10–11 epoxide (1,2). Hyponatremia, however, can be a problem.

References

1. Dam M, Ekberg R. Löyning Y, et al. A double-blind study comparing oxcarbazepine and carbamazepine in patients with newly diagnosed previously untreated epilepsy. *Epilepsy Res* 1989;3:70–76.
2. Friis ML, Kristensen O, Boas J, et al. Therapeutic experiences with 947 epileptic outpatients in oxcarbazepine treatment. *Acta Neurol Scand* 1993;87:224–27.

P-300

Numerous studies using scalp and depth electrodes provide evidence of widespread long-latency positive and negative waves generated above the brain stem. The P-300 is a symmetric midline positive potential with a latency of approximately 250–600 msec produced by a number of modalities, including the presentation of unpredictable, infrequent stimuli. A hippocampal origin has been postulated (1). The absence of P-300 is reported to be a predictor of structural or functional abnormalities of the hippocampus in patients with epilepsy originating in the temporal lobe (2).

References

1. Halgren E, Squires N, Wilson C, Rohrbaugh, Babb T, Crandall P. Endogenous potentials generated in the human hippocampal formation and amygdala by infrequent events. *Science* 1980;210:803–805.
2. Puce A, Kalnins RM, Berkovic SF, Donnan GA, Bladin PF. Limbic P3 potentials, seizure localization, and surgical pathology in temporal lobe epilepsy. *Ann Neurol* 1989;26:377–85.

PARALDEHYDE

Paraldehyde is a hypnotic and AED used in the treatment of status epilepticus or repeated seizures associated with alcohol withdrawal. Although it can be effective, it is irritating when given parenterally, may cause pulmonary complications, and is difficult to administer since it dissolves plastic tubing. Paraldehyde is little used in Europe; it is no longer available in the United States.

Reference

Ramsay RE. Pharmacokinetics and clinical use of parenteral phenytoin, phenobarbital and paraldehyde. *Epilepsia* 1989;30(Suppl 2): S1–S3.

• • • • • •
PARASITOSES

Parasites are relatively unusual causes for seizures in developed nations; however, they are the most common cause of seizures in certain regions of the world. Malaria due to plasmodium falciparum is the main cause of childhood seizures in Africa. Cysticercosis (taenia solium) is the primary cause of recurrent seizures in Central America, South America, and sub-Saharan Africa. Parasitic seizures are usually seen in the child or young adult (50% of cases) (1–3), and may cause adult-onset epilepsy in almost 30% of a rural population (3).

Parasite-induced seizures may be associated with acute, subacute, or chronic encephalopathies secondary to migration of parasite eggs, larvae, or adults to the cerebral parenchyma. Migrating organisms include cysticercosis, filariasis (brancroftii), distomatoses, bilharziasis, loaiasis, and numerous other parasites. Alternatively, seizures can result from an allergic reaction or antigenic response following therapy (sudden death of a parasite) in cases of distomatosis, cysticercosis, and loaiases. Toxoplasmosis, amebiasis due to acanthamoeba can produce an acute meningitis with seizures. Seizures can result from focal cerebral parasitic disease with abscess (amebiasis histolitica), cysts (hydatidosis, paragominiasis, cysticercosis), or calcifications (toxoplasmosis, cysticercosis, paragominiasis).

The clinical characteristics of parasitic seizures are not specific. About half of parasitic seizures are partial. Seizure incidence varies with the degree of infestation, number of cysts, localization, size, and evolution. Seizures are the presenting manifestation of parasitic disease in 30% of cases. Status epilepticus is infrequent. Residual calcifications, recurrent seizures, and multiple cysts before albendazole therapy carry the highest relapse rate in neurocysticercosis after AED withdrawal (4).

Diagnosis of parasite-related seizures is made by head CT scan or MRI showing multiple, disseminated cysts of different ages with variable degrees of calcification.

Treatment is advocated by some for the parasitosis and the resulting seizure disorder but there is controversy regarding effectiveness (5–7).

In the case of malaria, antimalarial drugs may themselves cause seizures (8).

References

1. MacCormick G, Zee CS, Heinden J. Cysticercosis cerebri. Review of 127 cases. *Arch Neurol* 1982;39:534–39.
2. Sotelo J, Guerrero V, Rubio F. Neurocysticercosis: a new classification based on active and inactive forms. A study of 753 cases. *Arch Int Med* 1985;145:442–45.
3. Garcia JJ, Gilman R, Martinez M, et al. Cysticercosis as a major cause of epilepsy in Peru. *Lancet* 1993;341:197–200.

4. Del Brutto OH. Prognostic factors for seizure recurrence after withdrawal of anti-epileptic drugs in patients with neurocysticerosis. *Neurology* 1994;44:1706–1709.
5. Kramer LD. Medical treatment of cysticercosis—ineffective. *Arch Neurol* 1995; 52:101–102.
6. Del Brutto OH. Medical treatment of cysticercosis—effective. *Arch Neurol* 1995; 52:102–104.
7. Hachinski V. Medical treatment of cysticercosis—neither effective nor ineffective. *Arch Neurol* 1995;52:104.
8. Commission on tropical diseases of the International League Against Epilepsy. Relationship between epilepsy and tropical diseases. *Epilepsia* 1994;35:89–93.

● ● ● ● ● ● ●

PARIETAL (EPILEPSIES)

Parietal lobe seizure foci are less common than are foci in the temporal or frontal lobes, but they are not rare [about 6% (1)]. Parietal seizures may present as simple partial seizures or secondary generalized seizures. Somatosensory seizures (see this heading) may induce symptoms in any body part, but face, tongue, or hand symptoms are most frequent in accordance with the large representation of these regions in the somatosensory homunculus (2). Paracentral lobule epileptic activity may cause focal sensory symptoms in the genital area, and sometimes postural rotatory features (possibly from anterior spread of seizure activity). Infero-lateral parietal foci may cause vertigo (see Vertiginous (S)), spatial disorientation, a falling sensation, or nausea (2). Visual symptoms of posterior parietal seizure discharges include bright lights, metamorphopsia, or hallucinations (1–3). These symptoms may be difficult to distinguish from migraine (see this heading). Nondominant parietal foci can cause an illusion of partial body displacement (asomatognosia). Dominant hemisphere disturbances affect language.

In diagnosing parietal lobe epilepsy, scalp EEG is frequently negative or may be misleading (1), and intracranial EEG may be unhelpful (3). Functional mapping can enable safe resection of epileptogenic lesions with excellent surgical results (3).

References

1. Sveinbjornsdottir S, Duncan JS. Parietal and occipital lobe epilepsy: a review. *Epilepsia* 1993;34:493–521.
2. Commission on Classification and Terminology of the International League Against Epilepsy. Proposal for classification of epilepsies and epileptic syndromes. *Epilepsia* 1989;30:389–99.
3. Williamson, PD, Boon PA, Thadani VM, et al. Parietal lobe epilepsy: diagnostic considerations and results of surgery. *Ann Neurol* 1992;31:193–201.

• • • • • •
PAROXYSMAL EEG BURSTS

Paroxysmal EEG bursts are commonly seen with epilepsy, but many paroxysmal EEG events are normal (e.g., runs of vertex waves) or normal variants (e.g., 14–&-6 per second positive pikes). EEG paroxyms may be single, rhythmic, or periodic over time. Spatial distribution is similarly variable, ranging from focal to bilateral, multifocal, or diffuse. In epilepsy, the interictal EEG may reveal paroxysmal (epileptiform) discharges occurring as single events or in bursts (1). They may be divided into several categories:

- *Spike*: A high frequency biphasic phenomenon lasting 70 msec or less, measured at its half-height. Spike morphologies can also be mono- or triphasic. Spikes are predominantly surface-negative potentials with amplitudes varying from about 20 microvolts to several millivolts. Some electroencephalographers also include an aftergoing single slow wave in the definition of an EEG spike.
- *Sharp wave:* Similar to a spike, but with duration of 70–200 msec.
- *Polyspike:* A sequence of several successive spikes.
- *Spike-waves:* A rhythmical pattern of spikes alternating with slow waves.
- *Polyspike-wave:* A rhythmical pattern of several spikes followed by slow waves.
- *Slow spike and wave:* Spike-slow wave rhythms at frequencies less than 3 per second. Slow spike-waves (sometimes called atypical spike-waves) are commonly seen in the Lennox-Gastaut syndrome.

References

1. Shorvon SD. The routine EEG. In: Dam M, Gram L (eds.). *Comprehensive epileptology.* New York: Raven Press, 1991.
2. International Federation of Societies for Electroencephalography and Clinical Neurophysiology. Glossary of terms most commonly used by clinical electroencephalographers. *Electroenceph clin Neurophysiol* 1974;37:538–48.

• • • • • •
PAROXYSMAL NOCTURNAL DYSTONIA

This syndrome was delineated in 1981 (1)

- *Clinical picture:* seizures may appear at any age in previously normal patients; dystonic or ballistic movements occur repeatedly for 15–50 seconds after awakening from slow wave sleep. They occur frequently: 2–20 times per night; the interictal and ictal EEG recording are normal, and seizures remit with carbamazepine.

- *Pathogenesis:* like kinesigenic paroxysmal choreoathetosis, the pathogenesis is unclear and the phenomenon may be nonepileptic in nature (2). Nonetheless, ablation of cerebral cortex in the region of Brodmann's areas 6 and 8 (the localization of ictal discharges seen on stereotactic EEG) has eradicated seizures (3).

References

1. Lugaresi E, Cirignotta F. Hypnogenic paroxysmal dystonia: epileptic seizures or a new syndrome? *Sleep* 1981;4:121–38.
2. Lance JW. Familial paroxysmal dystonic choreoathetosis and its differentiation from related syndromes. *Ann Neurol* 1977;2:285–93.
3. Colicchio G. Unclassified nocturnal seizures: case reports. 17th Epilepsy International Congress. September 1987 (abstract).

● ● ● ● ● ●

PARTIAL (SEIZURES)
(SEIZURES WITH FOCAL ONSET)

Partial seizures result from anatomical or functional neuronal activation restricted to part of one hemisphere (1). The signs and symptoms depend on the origin and spread of the seizure discharge. They may remain localized, spread in one or more directions, remain limited to within one hemisphere, spread to the contralateral hemisphere, or involve both hemispheres with subsequent secondary generalization. The first clinical sign in the course of the seizure may have localizing value. If the epileptic focus is in a clinically silent area, spread to an area that induces a recognizable clinical correlation may result in false localization.

Partial seizures are divided into three groups:

- simple partial seizures with no alteration in consciousness (see Consciousness);
- partial complex seizures involving alteration in the level of consciousness, but insufficient to induce a generalized tonic-clonic seizure;
- simple or complex partial seizures may secondarily generalize.

Partial seizures may evolve in a number of ways:

- simple partial seizures may remain simple partial;
- simple partial seizures may progress to complex partial;
- complex partial seizures may remain complex partial;
- simple partial seizures may secondarily generalize;
- complex partial seizures may secondarily generalize;

- simple partial seizures may become complex partial that subsequently secondarily generalize.

The EEG during simple partial seizures may show rhythmic spike or sharp wave discharges, with or without slow waves, maximal in the region of the seizure focus. A generalized EEG voltage depression (electrodecremental pattern) may occur at the seizure focus at the start of an ictal event. Extremely localized seizures or deeply situated cortical seizures may have no scalp EEG correlate. The interictal EEG in cases of simple partial seizures may show spikes, sharp waves, spike and slow waves, sharp waves, rhythmic slow waves, focal slowing, or no changes. Focal EEG abnormalities are most common over temporal regions, next most often over frontal regions.

There are numerous etiologies for partial seizures (see Etiology). Partial seizures may be mistaken for absence seizures or psychogenic seizures (2).

Two types of complex partial seizures have been described: type 1 with simple partial onset leading to impairment of consciousness, with or without automatisms; type 2 with impairment of consciousness at the onset, with or without stereotyped automatisms. With type 1 complex partial seizures, typified by a motionless stare, the EEG ictal discharge remains in the temporal region. Type 2 seizures have a much more diffuse scalp representation. Some authors believe that anterior temporal lobectomy produces better results with type 1 seizures (3,4). These results remain to be confirmed in other patient populations.

References

1. Commission on Classification and Terminology of the International League Against Epilepsy. Proposal for revised clinical and electroencephalographic classification of epileptic seizures. *Epilepsia* 1981;22:489–501.
2. Theodore WH, Porter RJ, Penry JK. Complex partial seizures: clinical characteristics and differential diagnosis. *Neurology* 1983;33:1115–21.
3. Delgado-Escueta AV, Walsh GO. Type 1 complex partial seizures of hippocampal origin: excellent results of anterior temporal lobectomy. *Neurology* 1985; 35:143–54.
4. Walsh GO, Delgado-Escueta AV. Type II complex partial seizures: poor results of anterior temporal lobectomy. *Neurology* 1984;34:1–13.

● ● ● ● ● ●
PETIT MAL

Petit mal is a term initially suggested by Esquirol in 1815 (1) and promoted by Calmeil in 1824 (2). The discovery of the EEG hallmark of 3/second bilateral spike and wave discharges by Gibbs, Davis, and Lennox in 1943

(3) led to the delineation of an electroclinical syndrome and subsequent description of the petit mal triad by Lennox: absence; myoclonic seizures; akinetic seizures. This categorization has led to confusion in studies of the prognosis of petit mal epilepsy since children with simple absence seizures have a more benign outcome than do children with the full triad. The term "petit mal" also suffers from common usage to depict any "little" or "minor" seizure. In adults, this usually indicates complex partial or simple partial seizures. The modern term for "petit mal" is "absence" (4) (see also Absence (S,E)).

References

1. Esquirol J. De l'Epilepsie. In: Traité des Maladies Mentales. Tome 1. Paris: Baillère, 1838:274–75.
2. Calmeil LF. De l'Epilepsie Etudiée sous le rapport de son siège et de son influence sur la production de l'aliénation mentale. Thèse, Paris 1824.
3. Gibbs FA, Davis H, Lennox WG. The EEG in epilepsy and in conditions of impaired consciousness. *Arch Neurol Psychiatry* 1935;34:1134–48.
4. Commission of Classification and Terminology of the International League Against Epilepsy. Proposal for Revised Classification of Epilepsies and Epileptic Syndromes. *Epilepsia* 1989;30:389–99.

• • • • • •
PETIT MAL (INTERMEDIATE)

Intermediate petit mal is a concept proposed by Pazzaglia and Lugaresi in the 1970s (1) to represent a clinical condition intermediate between petit mal and petit mal variant. Clinically, the absences are those of typical absence type with normal background EEG recording. The spike and slow wave discharges, however, resemble those of the generalized symptomatic epilepsies, with 1.5–2.5 per second or asymmetric discharges. Absences appear early in childhood with intermediate petit mal: 50% of the children have brain damage. Generalized tonic-clonic seizures are seen in two-thirds of cases, tonic seizures in one-fourth, and myoclonic seizures, partial seizures, absence status epilepticus in occasional cases. Prognosis is poor in three-fourths of the cases because of mental retardation and persistence of seizures.

The concept of intermediate petit mal has been revised more recently to include a continuum of seizure types between absence, typical absence, and atypical absence without a clear demarcation of intermediate forms (2,3).

References

1. Lugaresi E, Pazzaglia P, Franck L, Roger J, Bureau-Paillas M, Ambrosetto G, Tassinari CA. Evolution and prognosis of primary generalized epilepsies of the

Petit Mal absence type. In: Lugaresi E, Pazzaglia P, Tassinari CA (eds.). *Evolution and prognosis of epilepsies.* Bologna: Aulo-Gaggi, 1973:1–22.

2. Berkovic SF, Andermann F, Andermann E. Gloor P. Concepts of absence epilepsies: discrete syndromes or biological continuum? *Neurology* 1987;37:993–1000.
3. Holmes GL, McKeever M, Adamson M. Absence seizures in children: clinical and electroencephalographic features. *Ann Neurol* 1987;21:268–73.

• • • • • •
PHENOBARBITAL

With the exception of bromides (see this heading), phenobarbital was the first major anticonvulsant, introduced in 1912 (1). Proprietary names for medications containing phenobarbital include: Luminal ®, Aparoxal®, Epanal®, Gardenal®, Kaneuron®, Ortenal®(2). Phenobarbital is the most prescribed AED in the world because of its low cost and long record of safe use. Sedative properties do limit its use when other AEDs are available. It is effective in all forms of epilepsy with the exception of typical absence.

Tablets of 15, 30, 60, and 100 mg; elixir 20 mg/5mL, 30 mg/7.5mL. Ampules IV containing 65 mg/mL or 130 mg/mL.

GENERAL PROPERTIES

Phenobarbital is a weak acid with pKa = 7.3. Drug ionization and diffusion depend on the internal pH.

PHARMACOKINETICS

Pharmacokinetics are linear. Oral bioavailability is excellent, with 80–90% absorption, except in the newborn. The speed of absorption after oral intake depends on the formulation of the tablet, gastric acidity, stomach contents, and gastric emptying. Peak plasma levels are seen 1–18 hours after ingestion. Volume of distribution is 0.54–0.75 l/kg in adults and 0.41–1.31 in young children. Phenobarbital is bound to serum proteins with a binding fraction of 45–54% for adults, 49–67% for children, and 36–43% for newborns. Salivary levels (reflecting unbound drug) of phenobarbital are about 35% of serum levels, but salivary measurements may be unreliable since they depend on salivary pH. The serum half-life of phenobarbital is 46–136 hours in adults, 21–78 hours in 5–10-year-old children, and 59–182 hours in newborns. Steady state serum levels are achieved 15–21 days after starting the medication without a loading dose. Phenobarbital induces hepatic enzymes, resulting in accelerated biotransformation of other drugs and endogenous and exogenous steroids. Elimination of phenobarbital is decreased by a number of enzyme inhibitors. Valproic acid produces a consistent increase of barbiturate levels. Optimal plasma concentrations of phenobarbital are 15–30 mg/l, or 64–130 micromol/l.

SIDE EFFECTS

Benign side effects of phenobarbital are frequent; severe side effects are rare.

- CNS: sedation in 69% of patients (3). There is often a paradoxical excitation in children, the elderly, or those with cognitive deficits, even with small doses. Phenobarbital commonly inteferes with learning in children. Irritability, aggressiveness, and depression are relatively common. Abrupt stopping of medication may lead to withdrawal symptoms. Dyskinesias are rare (4).
- Barbiturate-related connective tissue disorders: barbiturate-induced rheumatism, Dupuytren's contractures, plantar fibromas, Ledderhosen syndrome, Peyronie's disease, thickening of the facies (5).
- Enzyme induction: increase in hepatic enzymes, lowering of calcium, phosphate, 25-hydroxycalciferol, folate levels, macrocytosis, decrease in effectiveness of oral contraceptives.
- Peripheral neuropathies rare, subclinical.
- Hemorraghic diathesis in the newborn of mothers taking phenobarbital.
- Passage of PB into maternal milk may lead to sedation of the child.
- Idiosyncratic reactions: rashes (less that 3% of cases), rare hypersensitivity syndrome (6).

References

1. Feely M, O'Callagan M, Duggan B, Callaghan N. Phenobarbitone in previously untreated epilepsy. *J Neurol Neurosurg Psychiatry* 1980;43:365–68.
2. Levy RH, Mattson R, Meldrum B, Penry JK, Dreifuss FE (eds.). *Antiepileptic drugs,* 3rd edition. New York: Raven Press, 1989.
3. Smith DB, Mattson RH, Cramer JA, Collins JF, Novelly RA, Craft B, and the Administration Cooperative Epilepsy Cooperative Study Group. Results of a nationwide Veterans Administration Cooperative Study comparing the efficacy and toxicity of carbamazepine, phenobarbital, phenytoin and primidone. *Epilepsia* 1987:28(Suppl 3):S50–S58.
4. Wisnitzer M, Younkin D. Phenobarbital-induced dyskinesia in a neurologically-impaired child. *Neurology* 1984;34:1600–1601.
5. Mattson RH, Cramer JA, McCutchen CB, and the Veterans Administration Epilepsy Cooperative Study Group. Barbiturate-related connective tissue disorders. *Arch Intern Med* 1989;149:911–14.
6. Shapiro PA, Antonioli DA, Peppercorn MA. Barbiturate-induced submassive hepatic necrosis. *Am J Gastroenterol* 1980;74:270–73.

• • • • • •
PHENYTOIN
(PHT, DIPHENYLHYDANTOIN, DILANTIN®) (1)

Phenytoin (PHT, diphenylhydantoin, Dilantin®) is a drug of choice for partial and tonic-clonic seizures. It is of less (or no) efficacy in absence and myoclonic seizures. PHT is probably the most widely used AED drug in the United States.

PHARMACOKINETICS

For a certain dosage range, phenytoin possesses linear kinetics, meaning that serum levels and rate of excretion are proportional to administered dose. At higher dosages, however, PHT saturates the hepatic excretion capacity, and drug is excreted at a constant rate independent of dose (zero order kinetics). The practical consequence of this is that PHT serum levels may rise precipitously after a small increase in dose. PHT is well absorbed orally, with bioavailability in the 20–90% range. Peak plasma levels after oral intake are dose-dependent, peaking in 3–12 hours. Protein binding is significant, with 87–93% of PHT bound to albumin. Phenytoin free levels, which are correlated with biologic activity, may therefore change with alterations in serum proteins or other drugs that bind to serum proteins. The usual "therapeutic range" for PHT is 10–20 mg/L (40–80 micromol/L), but higher levels may be needed to control seizures without causing toxicity. Free serum levels may be measured by special techniques, and therapeutic free levels are 1–2 mg/L. Salivary levels reflect the free fraction and are approximately 10% of serum total levels. Serum half-life of phenytoin ranges from 8–60 (usually 24) hours for adults, and from 12–22 (usually 16) hours for children. Steady state serum levels are achieved without a loading dose in approximately 5–10 days. The volume of distribution for PHT is 0.5–0.8/L/kg. Enzyme induction (see Phenobarbital; Antiepileptic drugs/(AEDs)) occurs to a significant extent with PHT. Metabolism of PHT is inhibited by isoniazid, disulfiram, cimetidine, and many other agents. Free serum fraction of PHT is increased by acetylsalicylic acid, phenylbutazone, certain sulfa drugs, heparin, and valproic acid.

SIDE EFFECTS

Side effects of PHT occur typically with serum levels in excess of 20 mg/L, but some individuals cannot tolerate even much lower levels. As with all AEDs, ideal serum ranges are specified under an assumption of monotherapy. Typical PHT side effects include anorexia, nausea, dysarthria, dizziness, diplopia, nystagmus, ataxia, confusion, and obtundation.

- Sedation with change in cognitive function and psychomotor retardation is usually insidious and moderate (2,3), but may be no more than is seen on carbamazepine (4). There may occasionally be progressive mental deterioration, sometimes called phenytoin encephalopathy.
- Gingival hyperplasia occurs in 30–60% of patients, believed to relate to a salivary deficit of IgA.
- Cerebellar syndrome occurs more often in patients with preexisting cerebellar lesions.
- Chronic peripheral neuropathy, usually subclinical.
- Enzyme induction may lead to abnormalities in phosphorus and calcium metabolism (osteomalacia) and decreased effectiveness of oral contraceptives.
- Endocrine and metabolic changes.
- Respiratory insufficiency, rarely described (5,6).
- Abnormalities in immunologic function, occasionally causing lymphomas (not to be confused with the lymphadenopathies of hypersensitivity syndromes).
- Dyskinesias, rare asterixis, myoclonias, oro-facial dyskinesias, or dystonias that may be confused with seizures (7).

References

1. Levy RH, Mattson R, Meldrum B, Penry JK, Dreifuss FE (eds.). *Antiepileptic drugs,* 3rd edition. New York: Raven Press, 1989.
2. Dodrill CB, Troupin AS. Psychotropic effects of carbamazepine in epilepsy: a double-blind comparison with phenytoin. *Neurology* 1977;27:1023–28.
3. Dodrill CB, Temkin NR. Motor speed is a contaminating factor in evaluating the cognitive effects of phenytoin. *Epilepsia* 1989;30:453–57.
4. Dodrill CB, Troupin AS. Neuropsychological effects of carbamazepine and phenytoin: a reanalysis. *Neurology* 1991;41:141–43.
5. Hazlett DR, Ward GW, Madison DS. Pulmonary function loss in diphenylhydantoin therapy. *Chest* 1974;66:660–64.
6. Smith RJ, Man GCW, McLean DR. Diphenylhydantoin and pulmonary function. *J Canad Sc Neurol* 1979;6:21–25.
7. Osorio I, Burnstine TH, Remler B, Manon-Espaillat R, Reed RC. Phenytoin-induced seizures: a paradoxical effect at toxic concentrations in epileptic patients. *Epilepsia* 1989;30:230–34.

• • • • • • •
PHONATORY (SEIZURES)

Phonatory seizures present with speech arrest (aphemic, anarthric seizures) or difficulty with enunciation (dysarthric seizures). Internal language is intact. Speech arrest commonly is found with foci at the foot of the third frontal convolution, associated with salivation, hemifacial or oropharyngeal movements, or in the supplementary motor area. Foci in the dominant inferior frontal cortex and the anterior portion of the medial frontal gyrus may also lead to phonatory seizures.

Phonatory seizures may also comprise positive symptoms, with uncontrolled vocalization, palilalia, grunts, whines, or cries.

• • • • • • •
PHOSPHATE-CALCIUM METABOLISM

Since 1968 it has been known that chronic ingestion of AEDs induces abnormalities in calcium and phosphate metabolism. AEDs induce hepatic microsomal enzymes with a resultant increase in hydroxylation of vitamin D3 to 25-hydroxycalciferol. Other mechanisms are also likely (1). The clinical impact of this problem has not been fully established, but metabolic consequences include hypocalcemia, hypophosphatemia, increase in serum alkaline phosphatase, and decrease in serum 25-hydroxycalciferol levels. X-rays may show demineralization of bone, and in extreme cases the clinical picture is consistent with osteomalacia and rickets. Although changes in phosphatase and 25-hydroxycalciferol levels are frequent (2), there is rarely an effect on bone density (3). Vitamin D3 supplements may only occasionally be helpful (4), particularly for sedentary patients with poor sun exposure or patients on renal dialysis (5).

References

1. Offermann G. Chronic antiepileptic drug treatment and disorders of mineral metabolism. In: Oxley J, et al. (eds.). *Antiepileptic therapy: chronic toxicity of antiepileptic drugs.* New York: Raven Press, 1983:175–84.
2. Ala-Houhala M, Korpela R, Kivikko M, Koskinen T, Koskinen M, Koivula T. Long-term anticonvulsant therapy and vitamin D metabolism in ambulatory pubertal children. *Neuropediatrics* 1986;17:212–16.
3. Zanzi I, Roginsky MS, Rosen A, Cohn SH. Skeletal mass in patients receiving chronic anticonvulsant therapy. *Mineral Electrolyte Metab* 1981;5:240–48.
4. Christiansen C, Rodbro P, Tjellessen L. Pathophysiology behind anticonvulsant osteomalacia. *Acta Neurol Scand* 1983;(Suppl 94):21–28.
5. Pierides AM, Ellis HA, Ward M, et al. Barbiturate and anticonvulsant treatment in relation to osteomalacia with hemodialysis and renal transplantation. *Br Med J* 1976;1:190–93.

• • • • • •
PHOTOCONVULSIVE (SEIZURES) (INDUCED SEIZURES)

Intermittent light stimulation, whether by the interruption of a steady light source or the appearance of light, intermittently, may trigger seizures. Photoconvulsive seizures are not to be confused with a photomyoclonic EEG response (see this heading). Photoconvulsive stimuli in the environment include changing light sources, for example, moving from relative darkness to a brightly lit region, when traveling down tree-lined avenues on a sunny day, when watching a revolving wheel, helicopter blades, or stroboscopic lights in a discotheque or EEG laboratory.

Photoconvulsive seizures are usually generalized tonic-clonic or myoclonic, but they may also take the form of absence or partial motor.

Children, adolescents, and young adults are most susceptible to photoconvulsive seizures. Photosensitivity usually disappears by the third decade of life (1). Alcohol withdrawal is also a risk factor for photoconvulsive or photomyoclonic responses.

Television epilepsy is a type of reflex epilepsy in response to watching certain TV images. These seizures usually develop in late childhood and are generalized or rarely partial. Factors responsible include flickering images, screen brightness, geometric figures, and rarely actual content of the picture (2). EEG photosensitivity is common but not invariable with TV epilepsy.

In some patients, visual patterns rather than simple light may induce seizures (3–5). Visual scanning of pictures or objects with geometric and contrasting contours, for example, vertical bands on wallpaper, Venetian blinds, or radiators, may induce seizures. The EEG often demonstrates bilateral synchronous spike and slow waves in pattern-sensitive epilepsy.

References

1. Jeavons PM, Bishop A, Harding GFA. The prognosis of photosensitivity. *Epilepsia* 1986;27:569–73.
2. Darby AJ. Television epilepsy. The role of patterns. *Electroenceph clin Neurophysiol* 1979;47:163–71.
3. Kogeorgos J, Henson RA, Scott DF. Pattern sensitive epilepsy: a case report. *J Neurol Neurosurg Psychiatry* 1979;42:635–39.
4. Chatrian GE, Lettich E, Miller LH, Green JR. Pattern-sensitive epilepsy. Part 1: An electrographic study of its mechanisms. *Epilepsia* 1970;11:125–49.
5. Chatrian GE, Lettich E, Miller LH, Green JR, Kupfer C. Pattern-sensitive epilepsy. Part 2: Clinical changes, tests of responsiveness and motor output, alterations of evoked potentials and therapeutic measures. *Epilepsia* 1970;11:151–62.

• • • • • •
PHOTOSENSITIVITY

Photosensitivity refers to the triggering of seizures or bursts of spike and slow wave activity on the EEG by light. Photosensitivity is not a synonym for epilepsy.

PHOTOSENSITIVE EPILEPSIES

Photosensitivity is frequently familial. The condition is more frequent in women, generally appears at puberty, and disappears in the third decade of life (1). There is no single photosensitive epilepsy; rather, there are photosensitivity components in a number of epileptic syndromes. As per Jeavons (2):

- pure photosensitive epilepsy: Seizures supervene only under certain circumstances of daily living (see Induced (S); Reflex (E));
- palpebral myoclonias with absence (see Absence (S,E));
- auto-induced epilepsy (see Reflex (E));
- pattern-sensitive epilepsy (seizures provoked by light);
- epilepsies with photosensitivity causing spontaneous or provoked seizures; spontaneous seizures with spike and slow waves or polyspike and slow waves; with or without myoclonus during intermittent photic stimulation. Frequent forms include juvenile myoclonic epilepsy, epilepsy with tonic-clonic seizures on wakening, absence epilepsy of childhood (3), i.e., the idiopathic generalized epilepsies. Photosensitivity may also be seen in symptomatic generalized epilepsies and partial epilepsies (3);
- seizures brought on only by intermittent photic stimulation, but without spontaneous seizures during normal activity. In such cases, individuals cannot be considered as having epilepsy.

PHOTOSENSITIVITY WITHOUT EPILEPSY

Bickford and associates (4) distinguished two types of abnormal EEG response to intermittent photic stimulation: photomyoclonic reactions involving only the anterior scalp regions corresponding to muscle artifact and with no link to seizures; a photoconvulsive response consisting of spike and slow wave or polyspike and slow wave generalized bilateral synchronous symmetric discharges. The paroxysmal response to intermittent photic stimulation is frequently seen in patients with epilepsy but may also be recorded following head trauma in children or adolescents, or during alcohol and sedative drug withdrawal.

References

1. Jeavons PM, Bishop A, Harding GFA. The prognosis of photosensitivity. *Epilepsia* 1986;27:569–73.
2. Binnie CD, Jeavons PM. Photosensitive epilepsies. In: Roger J, Bureau M, Dravet C, Dreifuss FE, Perret A, Wolf P (eds.). *Epileptic syndromes in infancy, childhood and adolescence,* 2nd edition. London, John Libbey Eurotext, 1992: 299–305.
3. Wolf P, Gooses R. Relation of photosensitivity to epileptic syndromes. *J Neurol Neurosurg Psychiatry* 1986;49:1386–91.
4. Bickford RG, Daly D, Keith HM. Convulsive effects of light stimulation in children. *Am J Dis Child* 1953;86:170–83.

● ● ● ● ● ●
POLYPHARMACY

Until recently, two or three AEDs were frequently prescribed simultaneously with the intention of potentiating the effect of each medication and in the hope that smaller doses might minimize undesirable side effects. When seizures persisted despite treatment, other AEDs were added with a reluctance to remove the initial AED.

More recent studies show that the interactions between the different AEDs are rarely beneficial and that their toxicity is frequently additive. Since 1977, the advantages of decreasing polypharmacy have been emphasized: a decrease in side effects and even a decrease in seizure frequency (1,2). However, reduction of polypharmacy to monotherapy is not always possible (3). A small number of patients (approximately 10%) may benefit from therapy using two AEDs (4,5). Additionally, the withdrawal course of an AED may be stormy; patients should be warned, and the long-term therapeutic goal explained.

References

1. Milano Collaborative Group for Studies on Epilepsy. Long term intensive monitoring in the difficult patient. Preliminary results of 16 months of observations. Usefulness and limitations. In: Gardner-Thorpe G, et al. (eds.). *Antiepileptic drug monitoring.* Kent, U.K.: Pitman Med Publ., 1977:197–213.
2. Shorvon SD, Reynolds EH. Unnecessary polypharmacy for epilepsy. *Br Med J* 1977;1:1635–37.
3. Albright P, Bruni J. Reduction of polypharmacy in epileptic patients. *Arch Neurol* 1985;42:797–99.
4. Bourgeois B. Combination of valproate and ethosuximide: antiepileptic and neurotoxic interaction. *J Pharmacol Exp Ther* 1988;247:1128–32.
5. Lorenzo NY, Bromfield EB, Theodore WH. Phenytoin and carbamazepine: combination versus single-drug therapy for intractable partial seizures. *Ann Neurol* 1988;24:136.

• • • • • •
PORENCEPHALY

Porencephaly is a condition in which a brain cavity allows communication between the ventricular and subarachnoid spaces. This may be caused (1) by a malformation, (2) as a result of cerebral infarction in the neonatal period (see Occipital (S)). Seizures are a frequent consequence of porencephaly.

• • • • • •
PORPHYRIA

Seizures occur in 10–30% (1–3) of cases of acute intermittent porphyria and can also be seen in porphyria cutanea tarda (4), mixed porphyrias, and hereditary coproporphyria. Most AEDs are problematic because of their porphyrogenic potential, demonstrated in vitro and in vivo (5,6). Diazepam, clonazepam, clorazepate, bromides (see also this heading), valproate, and magnesium sulfate have all been advocated as being safer than most AEDs (2,4–9).

References

1. Waldenström J. Studien uber porphyrie. *Acta Med Scand* 1937;82(Suppl):1–254.
2. Kaplan PW, Lewis DV. Juvenile acute intermittent porphyria with hypercholesterolemia and epilepsy. *J Child Neurol* 1986;1:38–45.
3. Goldberg GA. Acute intermittent porphyria. *Quart J Med* 1959;28:183–208.
4. D'Alessandro R, Rocchi E, Cristina E, et al. Safety of valproate in porphyria cutanea tarda. *Epilepsia* 1988;29:159–62.
5. Tschudy DP, Valsamis M, Magnussen CR. Acute intermittent porphyria: clinical and selected research aspects. *Ann Intern Med* 1974;83:851–64.
6. Magnussen CR, Doherty JM, Hess RA, et al. Grand mal seizures and acute intermittent porphyria. *Neurology* 1975;25:1121–25.
7. Reynolds, NC Jr, Miska RM. Safety of anticonvulsants in hepatic porphyrias. *Neurology* 1981;31:480–84.
8. Shedlofsky SI, Bonkowsky HL. Seizure management in hepatic porphyrias: results from a cell-culture model of porphyria. *Neurology* 1984;34:399.
9. Sadeh M, Blatt I, Martonovits G, Karni A, Goldhammer Y. Treatment of porphyric convulsions with magnesium sulfate. *Epilepsia* 1991;32:712–14.

• • • • • •
POSITRON EMISSION TOMOGRAPHY
SCANNING (PET)

Positron emission tomography scanning (PET) is a new technique useful in imaging neurochemical processes and blood flow in the brain. Like EEG, but unlike CT and MRI, PET illustrates functional (rather than morphological) features of the brain. PET scanning has proven useful in localization of seizure foci and in exploration of the underlying neurochemical mechanisms of epilepsy (1).

The principle of PET is as follows: (1) a radioactive isotope that "homes" to a particular part of brain is prepared in a cyclotron; (2) the isotope is injected intravenously into a patient; (3) the isotope localizes to a certain region of brain, or set of cells, or of neuroreceptors according to the binding affinity of the receptor, cerebral blood flow, and several other factors; (4) the isotope releases a positron, which travels a short distance and decays to paired gamma rays traveling in opposite directions; (5) scintillation counters detect the gamma rays; (6) computerized tomographic techniques generate an image of the isotope localization in brain; (7) interpretation of images is performed in accordance with various models of tracer distribution, binding, decay and with an understanding of the underlying biology.

The most commonly employed radioisotope for PET is ^{18}F-fluorodeoxyglucose (FDG). FDG is transported into neurons in proportion to glucose consumption of neurons, and is trapped there (2). PET with FDG, therefore, images a representation of cerebral energy metabolism. The other energy substrate for brain is oxygen, and ^{15}O-O_2 PET images can also portray energy metabolism in brain (3). Ligands have been produced to mark location of neuroreceptors for opiates, dopamine, acetylcholine, norepinephrine, serotonin, and benzodiazepines (1).

FDG PET studies have demonstrated that brain regions near partial seizure foci are hypometabolic during the interictal period and hypermetabolic during seizures (4–6). The region of hypometabolism may extend beyond the actual zone of the electroencephalographic focus (4,5,7) and may fluctuate with time; nevertheless, it provides a useful regional marker for the epileptogenic process. Interictal hypometabolism with PET can be used in the decision process for selecting patients for surgery (5).

PET studies with ^{15}O-O2 are useful in delineating brain regions involved in ongoing cognitive processes, because the oxygen isotope has a half-life of 2 minutes and so can be adminstered before and during performance of a cognitive function (8). PET studies with neurotransmitter receptor markers give clues to neurochemical mechanisms of epilepsy. Opiate receptors, for example, increase in the region of a seizure focus, possibly as an inhibitory control mechanism (9). Benzodiazepine receptors in contrast are said to decrease in the region of a seizure focus (10). Volumetric MRI shows a correlation between decreased FDG-PET and hippocampal/temporal lobe volumes (11).

PET studies do suffer from some limitations. They are expensive and require highly specialized equipment and personnel. PET studies average metabolic activity over minutes, so rapid events cannot be discriminated. Spatial resolution is in theory about 0.5 cm under ideal conditions, but actual resolution may be less. Registration and comparison of PET images with MRI and CAT requires meticulous superimposition of images. The tracer kinetic models upon which interpretations depend are not always simple. Changes in cerebral blood flow and in concentration of endogenous compounds that may compete with the radioactive label may greatly affect the results. Finally, PET, as one slice in time, gives little information on cause and effect: are changes causative, reactive, or essentially coincidental? Despite these limitations, PET remains a useful tool for localizing seizure foci and a promising approach to understanding the neurochemistry of the brain.

References

1. Fisher RS, Frost JJ. Epilepsy. *J Nucl Med* 1991;32:651–59.
2. Sokoloff L. Mapping of local cerebral functional activity by measurement of local cerebral glucose utilization with 14C deoxyglucose. *Brain* 1979;102: 653–58.
3. Franck G, Salmon E, Sadzot B, Maquet P. Epilepsy—the use of oxygen-15-labeled gases. *Sem Neurol* 1989;9:307–16.
4. Abou-Khalil BW, Siegel GJ, Sackellares JC, Gilman S, Hichwa R, Marchall R. Positron emission tomography studies of cerebral glucose metabolism in chronic partial epilepsy. *Ann Neurol* 1987;22:480–86.
5. Engel J Jr, Kuhl DE, Phelps ME, Mazziotta JC. Interictal cerebral glucose metabolism in partial epilepsy and its relation to EEG changes. *Ann Neurol* 1982;12:510–17.
6. Kuhl DE, Engel J Jr, Phelps ME, Selin C. Epileptic pattern of local cerebral metabolism and perfusion in humans, determined by emission computed tomography of 18 FDG and 13NH3. *Ann Neurol* 1980;3:348–60.
7. Holmes MD, Kelly K, Theodore WH. Complex partial seizures. Correlations of clinical and metabolic features. *Arch Neurol* 1988;45:1191–93.
8. Petersen SE, Fox PT, Posner MI, Mintun M, Raichle ME. Positron emission tomographic studies of the cortical anatomy of single-word processing. *Nature* 1988;331:585–89.
9. Frost J, Mayberg HS, Fisher RS, et al. Mu-opiate receptors measured by positron emission tomography are increased in temporal lobe epilepsy. *Ann Neurol* 1988;23:231–37.
10. Savic I, Persson A, Roland P, Pauli S, Sedvall G, Widen L. In vivo demonstration of reduced benzodiazepine receptor binding in human epileptic foci. *Lancet* 1988;2:863–66.
11. Gaillard WD, Bhatia S, Bookheimer SY, et al. FDG-PET and volumetric MRI in the evaluation of patients with partial epilepsy. *Neurology* 1995;45:123–26.

• • • • • •
POSTOPERATIVE (SEIZURES)

Seizures occuring within a few weeks of craniotomy occur in approximately 5% of cases (1), although the incidence varies widely by type of preoperative lesion and the population studied. It is difficult to distinguish seizures due to surgery from those due to the underlying brain disorder that necessitated surgery. Among postoperative seizures, 45% occur in the first week (particularly in the first 48 hours), 65% occur during the first month (2). Late seizures may herald relapse.

Risk factors for postoperative seizures include arteriovenous malformations, aneurysm, meningiomata, trauma, lesions situated in the centroparietal region, and preoperative seizures. The risk of epilepsy after ventricular shunting procedures has been estimated at 9.4% (15.2% in children under 1 year of age to 6.9% above 50 years of age). The site of shunt placement is an important determinant of postoperative seizure frequency, with frontal 55% and parietal 7% (3). In cases at high risk for postoperative seizures, treatment with a medication such as phenytoin before surgery and for a limited time thereafter may have a prophylactic role (2).

References

1. Lee ST, Lui TN, Chang CN, Cheng WC, Wang DJ, Heimburger RF, Lin CG. Prophylactic anticonvulsants for prevention of immediate and early post-craniotomy seizures. *Surg Neurol* 1989;31:361–64.
2. North JB, Penhall RK, Hanieth A, Frewin DB, Taylor WB. Phenytoin and post-operative epilepsy. *J Neurosurg* 1983;15:672–77.
3. Dan NG, Wade MJ. The incidence of epilepsy after ventricular shunting procedures. *J Neurosurg* 1986;65:19–21.

• • • • • •
POST-TRAUMATIC (EPILEPSY)

Post-traumatic epilepsy is defined as an epilepsy (spontaneous recurrent seizures) due to head trauma and appearing after a certain "incubation" period (1). Early (situation-related) seizures occurring within the first 8 days usually do not recur, but are a risk factor for epilepsy. Late seizures (recurrent) occurring after the first week correspond to true post-traumatic epilepsy.

The incidence of post-traumatic epilepsy is difficult to determine. Head trauma during war produces an incidence of post-traumatic epilepsy varying between 25% and 50% (2–4). Head trauma sustained in civilian life produces a lower incidence of epilepsy, estimated to be 0.5–5% (1,5).

RISK FACTORS

Several risk factors predict development of post-traumatic epilepsy after injury. These factors, listed below, may be incorporated into a predicitive mathematical formula (4,7).

The Severity of Head Trauma.
- Head injuries: Seizure incidence depends on the extent of injury (limited to one lobe or multiple lobes); the site of injury (centroparietal > temporal > occipital > frontal) (4,7); the level of consciousness at the time of head trauma, (awake: 33%, coma: 58%); the presence of a foreign body (49%); intracranial hematoma or neurological deficit (hemiparesis, aphasia, visual field cut) (7–9).
- Closed head injury: Injuries must be severe to significantly increase the incidence of epilepsy (10). Risks for epilepsy after closed head injury are high with an intracranial hematoma or hemorrhagic contusion, a focal neurological deficit, depressed skull fracture, or posttraumatic amnesia exceeding 24 hours (5). Almost every patient with epilepsy relates a history of some minor head trauma, for example, a fall from a swing, a hard blow from a soccer ball, or a tumble from the crib. Presuming that this injury failed to result in penetrating head injury, focal neurological deficit, several hours of coma, or amnesia, then it is unlikely to be the cause of the epilepsy. This is especially true if the injury occurred many years before.
- Between 5% and 36% of patients with early seizures in the first week after injury will have late seizures (11). Early seizures are a risk factor for later seizures, although this risk may be different for children and adults (5).

The Electroencephalogram.
Several studies have revealed that only early presence of spikes evolving to a focus of slow waves increases a subsequent risk of late onset epilepsy (11–13).

Genetic factors have an indirect effect (11).

LATENCY

The incubation period of post-traumatic epilepsy is variable: 55% of seizures appear in the first year (14); 80% of patients will have had their seizure by the second year (15). The incubation period is shortened with early seizures, prolonged post-traumatic amnesia, large cerebral lesions, and Rolandic injury (15). Latency is longer in children. Very late-onset epilepsy is unusual. If no seizures are seen during the first 3 years, the risk of late-onset epilepsy is low (4).

CLINICAL CHARACTERISTICS

Post-traumatic seizures are generalized in approximately half the cases (14), partial motor in one-third of cases (15). Other seizure types are rarer. Status epilepticus occurs in 4% of cases (15). The EEG is normal at time of seizure onset in approximately 20% of cases, shows focal slow waves in approximately 30%, and demonstrates bursts of spikes and slow waves in 20–40% of cases (17). Generalized sharp waves may appear late, particularly with frontal lesions. Head CT scan or MRI is effective in localizing older lesions from head trauma, such as cerebral contusions or chronic subdural hematoma.

PROGNOSIS

In cases of post-traumatic epilepsy, 50% of patients remit within 5 years (8). In those who do not, seizures tend to become less severe and frequent over time. Frequency of seizures early in the course is important (4). Patients with post-traumatic epilepsy could have a shortened life expectancy, but this may not be due directly to the epilepsy (13).

TREATMENT

Prophylaxis has been proposed empirically (15,18,20), and on theoretical grounds (21), but trials with phenobarbital and phenytoin (4,10,20) as prophylaxis have not been shown to be effective. Prophylactic therapy might be useful in high risk groups, but definitive studies remain to be performed (22).

References

1. Jennett B. *Epilepsy after non-missile injuries.* London: Heinemann, 1975.
2. Hughes JR. Post-traumatic epilepsy in the military. *Military Medicine* 1986; 151:416–19.
3. Caveness WF, Liss HR. Incidence of post-traumatic epilepsy. *Epilepsia* 1961; 2:123–29.
4. Weiss GH, Salazar AM, Vance SC, Grafman JA, Jabbari S. Predicting post-traumatic epilepsy in penetrating head injury. *Arch Neurol* 1986;43:771–73.
5. Annegers JF, Grabow JD, Grower RV, Laws ER, Eleveback LR, Kurland LT. Seizures after head trauma. A population study. *Neurology* 1980;30:638–789.
6. Feeney DM, Walker AE. The prediction of post-traumatic epilepsy: a mathematical approach. *Arch Neurol* 1979;36:8–12.
7. Weiss GH, Feeney DM, Caveness WF, Dillon JD, Kistler JP, Mohr JP, Rish BL. Prognostic factors for the occurrence of post-traumatic epilepsy. *Arch Neurol* 1983;40:7–10.

8. Caveness WF, Meirowski AM, Rish BL, Mohr JP, Kistler JP, Dillon JD, Weiss GH. The nature of post-traumatic epilepsy. *J Neurosurg* 1979;50:545–53.

9. Salazar AM, Jabbari B, Vance SC, Grafman JA, Amin D, Dillon JD. Epilepsy after penetrating head injury. I. Clinical correlates: a report of the Vietnam Head Injury Study. *Neurology* 1985;35:1406–14.

10. Jennett B. Assessment of the severity of head injury. *J Neurol Neurosurg Psychiatry* 1976;39:647–55.

11. Evans JH. The significance of early post-traumatic epilepsy. *Neurology* 1963;13:207–12.

12. Hahn YS, Fuchs S, Flannery AM, Barthel MJ, McLone DG. Factors influencing post-traumatic seizures in children. *Neurology* 1988;22:864–67.

13. Courjon J. A longitudinal electro-clinical study of 80 cases of post-traumatic epilepsy observed from the time of the original trauma. *Epilepsia* 1971;11:29–36.

14. Walker EA, Blumer D. The fate of World War II veterans with post-traumatic seizures. *Arch Neurol* 1989;46:23–26.

15. Caveness WF. Epilepsy, a product of trauma in our time. *Epilepsia* 1976;17:207–15.

16. Masquin A, Courjon J. Prognostic factors in post-traumatic epilepsy. *Epilepsia* 1963;4:285–97.

17. Jennett B, Van de Sande J. EEG prediction of post-traumatic epilepsy. *Epilepsia* 1975;16:251–56.

18. Rapport RL, Penry JK. A survey of attitudes toward the pharmacological prophylaxis of post-traumatic epilepsy. *J Neurosurg* 1973;38:159–66.

19. McQueen JK, Blackwood DHR, Kalbag RM, Johnson AL. Low risk of late post-traumatic seizures following severe head injuries: implications for clinical trials of prophylaxis. *J Neurol Neurosurg Psychiatry* 1983;46:899–904.

20. Young B, Rapp RP, Norton JA, Haack D, Tibbs PA, Bean JR. Failure of prophylactically administered phenytoin to prevent late post-traumatic seizures. *J Neurosurg* 1983;58:236–41.

21. McNamara JO. Development of new pharmacological agents for epilepsy: lessons from the kindling model. *Epilepsia* 1989;30(Suppl 1):S13–S18.

22. Deymeer F, Leviton A. Post-traumatic seizures: an assessment of the epidemiologic literature. *Central Nervous System Trauma* 1985;2:33–42.

• • • • • •
POSTURAL (SEIZURES)

Postural seizures are characterized by the assumption of an unusual posture. Seizures may affect any part of the body including the trunk, thorax, abdomen, or one or more limbs. The cortical seizure localization is variable.

• • • • • •
PREGNANCY

Studies investigating the interactions between epilepsy and pregnancy have led to numerous and contradictory conclusions (1,2). Several aspects of the problem have been considered (3):

THE EFFECT OF PREGNANCY ON EPILEPSY

- New onset epilepsy may appear in pregnancy due to simple coincidence (4), because of the rare appearance of a benign tumor (e.g., meningioma), or as the manifestation of an arteriovenous malformation (5). It is also plausible (but difficult to prove) that hormonal changes during pregnancy can bring out a seizure tendency in predisposed women.
- Among pregnant women with a history of epilepsy, seizure frequency remains constant in 50% (15–93%); increases in 25% (2–75%); and decreases in 25% (0–53%) (2,6–8).
- Alterations in seizure frequency may be explained in part by changes in AED metabolism during pregnancy (9). Factors include decreased intestinal absorption, increase in the volume of distribution, decrease in protein binding, increased hepatic metabolism, increase in renal clearance, drug interaction with other medications, and variable compliance because of the fear of potential teratogenic effect of AEDs.

THE EFFECT OF EPILEPSY ON PREGNANCY

Spontaneous abortions are no more frequent (13%) in women with epilepsy than in the general population (10). During pregnancy, tonic-clonic seizures may produce a transient cardiac acceleration (11) and fetal hypoxia, but only status epilepticus has been associated with clear fetal morbidity (1). Folate deficiency-induced megaloblastic anemias are more frequent during pregnancy. Hemorrhages seen during labor and delivery may be due to hepatic metabolic changes that decrease vitamin K-dependent coagulation factors.

ANTIEPILEPTIC DRUGS AND TERATOGENESIS (12)

Accurate evaluation of the relative risks of particular AEDs with congenital malformations is difficult given the different study methodologies used, the low percentage of pregnant women with epilepsy (4%), and variability in prescription and therapy practices. Additionally, proper comparison (control) groups cannot be studied since it would be unethical to withhold AED from pregnant women with epilepsy. Within the framework of these severe methodological limitations, studies (2,13–16) suggest the following risk for birth defects:

- Normal population: 1.8–3.0% (13);
- Women with epilepsy not on AEDs: 2.0–4.8% (13);
- Women with epilepsy on AEDs: 4.0–8.0% (13,14). Risk is increased by polypharmacy: 6.5% with monotherapy versus 15.6% with polytherapy (15). The increased risk may, however, be because of factors requiring polytherapy, rather than simply polytherapy itself.
- Risk for teratogenesis has a multifactorial origin, with contributions from metabolic and genetic factors (16–18), folate deficiency (19), and abnormal immune response. The period of risk for birth defects is maximal in the first two months of pregnancy (6), and is not exclusively dependent on exposure to any one specific AED (15,16).

TYPES OF MALFORMATIONS

Major malformations include cardiac and skeletal malformations, genito-urinary, cleft lip and palate (17,18,20). Minor malformations include cranio-facial and digital dysmorphia. All AEDs have been implicated: phenobarbital (20), phenytoin (12, 21), carbamazepine (22), sodium valproate (23), trimethadione (15,24), and benzodiazepines (25). Risks are particularly high with trimethadione and paramethadione. Valproic acid and, to a lesser extent, carbamazepine are associated with spina bifida. Presence of dysraphic complications often may be detected by the 20th week of gestation with real-time ultrasound and measurement of alpha fetoprotein in maternal serum or amniotic fluid.

PRACTICAL CONSIDERATIONS (3)

The physician should discuss with the patient the relative risks of seizures during pregnancy versus the teratogenic risks of medications. Both mother and fetus are at risk from tonic-clonic seizures or partial seizures with falls. Milder forms of seizures are not clearly associated with increased fetal risk, and a decision may be made not to treat these seizures during pregnancy.

Teratogenic risk increases with polytherapy. The goal is to use the fewest medications required to control potentially injurious seizures. AED serum levels (see Anticonvulsant/antiepileptic drug levels) fluctuate during pregnancy and should be evaluated frequently. Many AEDs, for example, phenytoin and sodium valproate, are highly protein-bound; therefore, measurement of free drug levels may be useful, as total plasma levels may be misleading (26).

Vitamin supplements, including vitamin D and folate (19,27), are recommended. Vitamin K (Mephyton®) in the last few weeks of pregnancy can decrease the risk of hemorrhagic disease of the newborn, secondary to depletion of coagulation factors by AEDs (28).

References

1. Janz D, Fuchs H. Sind antiepileptische Medikaments nahrend der Schwangerschaft schädlich? *Dtsch Med Wschr* 1964;89:241–43.
2. Janz D, Bossi L, Dam M, Helge H, Richens A, Schmidt D. *Epilepsy, pregnancy and the child.* New York: Raven Press, 1982.
3. Commission on Genetics, Pregnancy and the Child. International League Against Epilepsy. Guidelines for the care of epileptic women of childbearing age. *Epilepsia* 1989;30:409–10.
4. Knight AH, Rhind EG. Epilepsy and pregnancy: a study of 153 pregnancies in 59 patients. *Epilepsia* 1975;16:99–110.
5. Haas JF, Janish W, Staneczek W. Newly diagnosed primary intracranial neoplasms in pregnant women: a population based assessment. *J Neurol Neurosurg Psychiatry* 1986;49:874–88.
6. Schmidt D, Canger R, Avanzini G, et al. Changes of seizure frequency in pregnant epileptic women. *J Neurol Neurosurg Psychiatry* 1983;46:751–55.
7. Bardy AH. Incidence of seizures during pregnancy, labor and puerperium in epileptic women. *Acta Neurol Scand* 1987;75:356–60.
8. Gjerde IO, Strandjord RE, Ulstein M. The course of epilepsy during pregnancy. A study of 78 cases. *Acta Neurol Scand* 1988;78:198–205.
9. Hopkins A. Epilepsy and anticonvulsant drugs. *Br Med J* 1987;294:497–501.
10. Annegers JF, Baumgartner KB, Hauser WA, Kurland LT. Epilepsy, antiepileptic drugs and the risk of spontaneous abortion. *Epilepsia* 1988;29:451–58.
11. Teramo K, Hiilesma V, Bardy A, Saarikoski S. Fetal heart rate during a maternal grand mal epileptic seizure. *J Perinatal Med* 1979;7:3–6.
12. Meadow SR. Anticonvulsant drugs and congenital abnormalities. *Lancet* 1962;2:1296.
13. Bossi L. Fetal effects of anticonvulsants. In: Morselli PL, Pippenger CE, Penry JK (eds.). *Antiepileptic drug therapy in pediatrics.* New York: Raven Press, 1983.
14. Janz D. The teratogenic risk of antiepileptic drugs. *Epilepsia* 1975;16:159–69.
15. Kaneko S, Otani K, Fujushima Y, Ogawa Y, Nomura Y, Ono T, Nakane Y, Teranishi T. Goto M. Teratogenicity of antiepileptic drugs: analysis of possible risk factors. *Epilepsia* 1988;29:459–67.
16. Kelly TE, Edwards P, Rein M, Miller JQ, Dreifuss FE. Teratogenicity of anticonvulsant drugs. II: A prospective study. *Am J Med Genet* 1984;19:435–44.
17. Friis ML, Hauge M. Congenital heart defects in live-born children of epileptic parents. *Arch Neurol* 1985;42:374–76.
18. Friis ML. Epilepsy among parents of children with facial clefts. *Epilepsia* 1979;20:60–76.
19. Dansky LV, Andermann E, Rosenblatt D, Sherwin AL, Andermann F. Anticonvulsants, folates levels and pregnancy outcome: a prospective study. *Ann Neurol* 1987;21:176–82.

20. Seip M. Growth retardation, dysmorphic facies and minor malformations following massive exposure to phenobarbitone in utero. *Acta Paed Scand* 1976; 65:617–21.
21. Hanson JW, Smith DW. The fetal hydantoin syndrome. *J Pediatr* 1975; 87:285–90.
22. Jones KL, Lacro RV, Johnson KA, Adams J. Pattern of malformations in the children of women treated with carbamazepine during pregnancy. *N Engl J Med* 1989;320:1661–66.
23. Diliberti JH, Farndon PA, Dennis MR, Curry CJR. The fetal valproate syndrome. *Am J Med Genet* 1984;19:473–81.
24. Zachai EH, Mellman WJ, Neiderer B, Hanson JW. The fetal trimethadione syndrome. *J Pediatr* 1975;87:280–84.
25. Laegreid L. Teratogenic effects of benzodiazepine use during pregnancy. *J Pediatr* 1989;31:114–26.
26. Tomson T, Lindbom U, Ekguist B, Sundquist A. Epilepsy and pregnancy: a prospective study of seizure control in relation to free and total plasma concentrations of carbamazepine and phenytoin. *Epilepsia* 1994;35:122–30.
27. Yerby MS. Risks of pregnancy for women with epilepsy. *Epilepsia* 1992;33:523–27.
28. Yerby MS. Problems and management of the pregnant woman with epilepsy. *Epilepsia* 1987;28(Suppl 3):S29–S36.

• • • • • •
PREVALENCE

In a study of epilepsy, prevalence represents the number of patients with epilepsy in a given population at a given time, over the population number at the same time. Studies in different countries give prevalence figures for epilepsy ranging from 1.5 to 49 cases per 1,000 inhabitants. These variations may be ascribed to the different methodologies used in the study, collection, and case ascertainment of epilepsy, as well as true prevalence differences due to local factors, such as parasitoses.

• • • • • •
PRIMARY (GENERALIZED EPILEPSIES)

The term "primary generalized epilepsies" was used to refer to generalized epilepsies not due to cerebral lesions, but linked to an epileptic predisposition, frequently hereditary. No longer used, the term has been replaced by the Commission on Classification of the International League Against Epilepsy by the term "idiopathic generalized epilepsies" (see Idiopathic (E)).

• • • • • •
PRIMIDONE (PRM, MYSOLINE®) (1)

Primidone is used for the treatment of patients whose seizures do not respond to the first-line AEDs. It may be a useful adjunct in treatment of partial, generalized tonic-clonic, and myoclonic seizures. Primidone is metabolized to phenylethylmalonamide and phenobarbital, each of which have antiepileptic activity. The major action of PRM may be via phenobarbital. PRM itself has a 3–12 hour half-life and thus must be taken three or four times daily. Sedation can be extreme with PRM, especially in the early stages after initiation of therapy. The V.A. cooperative study of partial seizures (2) found no advantage of PRM over phenobarbital, carbamazepine, or phenytoin, and several patients discontinued therapy early because of sedation.

References

1. Levy RH, Mattson R, Meldrum B, Penry JK, Dreifuss FE (eds.). *Antiepileptic drugs,* 3rd edition. New York: Raven Press, 1989.
2. Mattson RH, Cramer JA, Collins JF, et al. Comparison of carbamazepine, phenobarbital, phenytoin, and primidone in partial and secondarily generalized tonic-clonic seizures. *N Engl J Med* 1985;313:145–51.

• • • • • •
PROGABIDE (GABRENE®)

Progabide (PGB) is a synthetic molecule produced with the aim of increasing cerebral GABA concentrations. Its principal metabolite (PGA) also has antiepileptic properties. PGB has been studied in Europe, but is not available in the United States. The drug has some documented efficacy, but there is a high incidence of hepatotoxicity, limiting its utility.

Reference

Levy RH, Mattson R, Meldrum B, Penry JK, Dreifuss FE (eds.). *Antiepileptic drugs,* 3rd edition. New York: Raven Press, 1989.

• • • • • •
PROGNOSIS

Many studies have investigated the prognosis of epilepsy. Comparison of prevalence and incidence ratios have suggested that the mean duration of epilepsy is approximately 12–13 years (1), although this theoretical value does not take into consideration either the age of onset of epilepsy, the clinical type, or the response to treatment. Remission rates for epilepsy with treatment vary between 10% and 82% (2), according to when the study was done, retrospective versus prospective methodology, and the length of follow-up. One study in 1968 with follow-up of 1–10 years showed a remission rate of 10–38% (3). A study in 1979 with 20 year follow-up showed that 42% of patients were in remission at 5 years, 65% at 10 years, 76% at 20 years (4). Generally accepted values would indicate that 50–82% of patients are in remission after 2–5 years (5,6).

After being free from seizures for several years, from 17% (7) to 49% (8,2) of patients will relapse after tapering AEDs. Relapses occur predominantly in the first year, particularly in the first six months (9).

Predictive prognostic factors include age of onset (see Age of onset), severity of epilepsy, numbers of seizures before treatment, the numbers of types of seizures, history of status epilepticus, the numbers of medications required to control the disease, and the length of time before seizure control was obtained (10). Complex partial seizures, especially with secondary generalization, are relatively likely to recur after cessation of medication (11).

Epilepsy that has not been controlled after two years of treatment represents a significant risk for chronic epilepsy (12). Some authorities believe that the long-term risk may be decreased by early treatment of seizures (7,12,13); however, this concept remains controversial. An abnormal EEG when treatment is stopped increases the chance of relapse (10). A normal EEG does not exclude a relapse. The presence of neurologic or psychiatric deficits worsens the prognosis.

Mortality with epilepsy is discussed under this heading.

References

1. Hauser WA, Kurland LT. The epidemiology of epilepsy in Rochester, Minnesota, 1935 through 1967. *Epilepsia* 1975;16:1–66.
2. Shorvon SD. The temporal aspects and prognosis in epilepsy. *J Neurol Neurosurg Psychiatry* 1984;4:1157–65.
3. Rodin EA. *The prognosis of patients with epilepsy.* Springfield: Charles C. Thomas, 1968:455.
4. Annegers JG, Hauser WA, Elveback LR. Remission of seizures and relapse in patients with epilepsy. *Epilepsia* 1979;20:729–37.
5. Goodridge DMG, Shorvon SD. Epileptic seizures in a population of 6000. *Br Med J* 1983;287:641–47.
6. Delgado-Escueta AV, Treiman DM, Wahs GO. The treatable epilepsies (second of two parts). *N Engl J Med* 1983;308:1576–84.
7. Oller-Daurella L, Oller FV L. Suppression of antiepileptic treatment. *Eur Neurol* 1987;27:106–13.
8. Overweg J, Binnie CD, Oosting J, Rowan AJ. Clinical and EEG prediction of seizure recurrence following antiepileptic drug withdrawal. *Epilepsy Res* 1987;1:272–83.

9. Callaghan N, Garrett A, Goggin T. Withdrawal of anticonvulsant drugs in patients free of seizures for 2 years. *N Engl J Med* 1988;318:942–46.
10. Schmidt D. Prognosis of chronic epilepsy with complex partial seizures. *J Neurol Neurosurg Psychiatry* 1984;47:1274–78.
11. Reynolds EH, Elwes RCD, Shorvon SD. Why does epilepsy become intractable? Prevention of chronic epilepsy. *Lancet* 1983; ii:952–54.
12. Elwes RDC, Johnson AJ, Shorvon SD, Reynolds EH. The prognosis for seizure control in newly diagnosed epilepsy. *N Engl J Med* 1984;311:944–47.

● ● ● ● ● ● ●

PROLACTIN

Prolactin is a lactogenic hormone secreted by the pituitary, under influence of dopaminergic systems in the hypothalamus. Serum prolactin levels rise briefly after approximately 80–90% of generalized tonic-clonic seizures, 50–80% of complex partial seizures, and 15% of partial seizures (1–4). Prolactin does not rise after nonconvulsive or convulsive status epilepticus or with absence seizures (5,6), but will rise after repetitive seizures (7). Prolactin rises are more frequent after temporal lobe complex partial seizures than those involving the frontal lobe (8). Interictal spike and slow wave discharges have a variable effect (9,10). Measurement of serum prolactin may help to distinguish psychogenic from epileptic seizures (11). Unfortunately, a long list of conditions can lead to false positive studies, including sleep, exercise, stress, general anesthesia, surgery, breast stimulation, recent sexual activity, estrogens, endometriosis, hypothyroidism, phenothiazines, opiates, L-dopa, bromocriptine, ergots, metoclopramide, several AEDs, and pituitary adenomas (12). The effects of syncope, cardiac arrhythmia, migraine, transient cerebral ischemia, and hypoglycemia on serum prolactin levels are not yet established.

Specificity of the prolactin test for epilepsy can be improved by showing a two- or three-fold rise from a time 5–20 minutes after a possible seizure compared to baseline. This baseline should ideally be taken at the same time on another (seizure-free) day, but a sample obtained an hour after an episode is probably a reasonable approximation. It is logistically difficult to obtain venous blood immediately after most possible seizures, since the patient is rarely in a medical setting. A recent study (13) demonstrates that capillary blood prolactin may be assayed accurately after application to filter paper, raising the possibility of obtaining prolactin samples in the home setting.

References

1. Yerby MS, Vanbelle G, Friel PN, Wilensky AJ. Serum prolactin in the diagnosis of epilepsy: sensibility, specificity, and predictive value. *Neurology* 1987; 37:1224–26.
2. Sperling MR, Pritchard PB, Engel J, Daniel C, Sagel J. Prolactin in partial epilepsy: an indication of limbic seizures. *Ann Neurol* 1986;20:716–22.

3. Wroe SJ, Henley R, John R, Richens H. The clinical value of serum prolactin measurement in the differential diagnosis of complex partial seizures. *Epilepsy Res* 1989;3:248–52.

4. Wyllie E, Lüders H, MacMillan JP, Gupta M. Serum prolactin levels after epileptic seizures. *Neurology* 1984;34:1601–1604.

5. Bilo L, Meo R, Striano S. Serum prolactin evaluation after 'minor' generalized seizures monitored by EEG. *J Neurol Neurosurg Psychiatry* 1988;51:308–309.

6. Tomson T, Lindbom U, Nilsson BY, Svanborg E, Anderson DEH. Serum prolactin during status epilepticus. *J Neurol Neurosurg Psychiatry* 1989;52:1435–37.

7. Bauer J, Kaufmann P, Klingmuller D, Elger CE. Serum prolactin response to repetitive seizures. *J Neurol* 1994;241:242–45.

8. Meierkord J, Shorvon S, Lightman S, Trimble M. Comparison of the effects of frontal and temporal lobe partial seizures on prolactin levels. *Arch Neurol* 1992;49:225–30.

9. Molaie M, Cruz A, Culebras A. The effect of epileptiform discharges on neurohormonal release in epileptic patients with complex partial seizures. *Neurology* 1988;38:759–62.

10. Aminoff MJ, The effect on plasma prolactin levels of interictal epileptiform EEG activity. *J Neurol Neurosurg Psychiatry* 1986;49:702–705.

11. Trimble MR. Serum prolactin in epilepsy and hysteria. *Br Med J* 1978;2:1682.

12. Frantz AG. Prolactin. *N Engl J Med* 1978;298:201–207.

13. Fisher RS, Chan DW, Bare M, Lesser RP. Finger-stick prolactin measurement for diagnosis of seizures. *Ann Neurol* 1991;29:187–92.

• • • • • •
PROPHYLAXIS

Seizure prophylaxis involves the institution of AED therapy in patients at risk for seizures following damage to the brain, such as with head injury, CNS neurosurgical interventions, intracranial hemorrhage (1), encephalitis, etc. The prevention of postoperative epilepsy in patients who have undergone intracranial surgery is controversial (2,3). As there is some potential toxicity from AED therapy, the decision to treat prophylactically involves an evaluation of the risk/benefit ratio. With subarachnoid hemorrhage, prophylaxis is frequently advised. Following intracranial hemorrhage or head trauma without depressed skull fracture, prophylaxis may not be warranted. The EEG may be useful in determining the need for drug therapy.

References

1. North JB, Penhall RK, Havieh R, Hahn CS, Challen RG, Frewin DB. Postoperative epilepsy: a double-blind trial of phenytoin after craniotomy. *Lancet* 1980;i:384–86.

2. Richardson AE, Uttley D. Prevention of postoperative epilepsy. *Lancet* 1980;i:650.

• • • • • •
PSEUDOPERIODIC (OR PERIODIC) LATERALIZED EPILEPTIFORM DISCHARGES (PLEDS)

A term coined by Chatrian (1), PLEDs refers to sharp waves, spikes (alone or in association with slow waves), or more complex wave forms occuring at quasi-regular intervals (0.3 to 12 seconds) over one hemisphere. Independent contralateral PLEDs, or more rarely synchronous ones, may occur. PLEDs are usually a transient phenomenon lasting from 1 day to several weeks. PLEDs appear in acute cerebral pathologies. Stroke is the most frequent; other causes include tumors, encephalitis (e.g., herpes simplex), cerebral abscesses, toxic/metabolic/anoxic encephalopathies, or head trauma (2). No cause can be found in 20–30% of cases (3).

Most patients with PLEDs have focal seizures with or without generalization, as well as a propensity for further seizures (3,4).

A poor outcome may be seen when associated with structural lesions (4).

References

1. Chatrian GE, Shaw CM, Leffman H. The significance of periodic lateralized epileptiform discharges in EEG: an electrographic, clinical and pathological study. *Electroenceph clin Neurophysiol* 1964;17:177–93.
2. Snodgrass SM, Tsuburaya K, Ajmone-Marsan C. Clinical significance of periodic lateralized epileptiform discharges: relationship with status epilepticus. *J Clin Neurophysiol* 1989;6:159–72.
3. Schraeder PL, Singh N. Seizure disorders following periodic lateralized epileptiform discharges. *Epilepsia* 1980;21:647–53.
4. Walsh JM, Brenner RP. Periodic lateralized epileptiform discharges—long-term outcome in adults. *Epilepsia* 1987;28:533–36.

• • • • • •
PSYCHOGENIC (SEIZURES)

Psychogenic seizure is a term used to refer to a nonepileptic seizure. The term is potentially misleading since it connotes an epileptic seizure triggered by psychological factors, which is not its meaning. Psychogenic seizures may simulate generalized tonic-clonic convulsions (2), complex partial seizures (3), or other seizure types. They may coexist with epileptic seizures (4). Diagnosis may be suspected with a history of responsiveness during the generalized episodes, suggestibility of onset or offset of the seizure, side-to-side head turning, or alternate left and right limb thrashing (2). Precipitation nearly exclusively in stressful situations is almost diagnostic. Video-EEG recording may be needed to differentiate them from real seizures (5).

Treatment of psychogenic seizures includes education of patient and family as to the nature of the process, followed by psychotherapy. With therapy, many patients may recover from the psychogenic seizures, but prognosis is dependent upon the severity of the underlying psychosocial problems.

References

1. Hopkins A. Pseudoseizures. *Quart J Med* 1989;71:473–75.
2. Gates JR, Ramani V, Whalem S, Loewenson R. Ictal characteristics of pseudo seizures. *Arch Neurol* 1985;42:1183–87.
3. Desai BT, Porter RJ, Penry JK. Psychogenic seizures: a study of 42 attacks in six patients, with intensive monitoring. *Arch Neurol* 1982;39:202–209.
4. Sackellares JC, Giordani B, Berent B, Seinberg M, Dreifuss FE, Vanderzant CW, Boll TJP. Patients with pseudo-seizures: intellectual and cognitive performance. *Neurology* 1985;35:116–19.
5. King DW, Gallagher BB, Murvin AJ, Smith DB, Marcus DJ, Hartlage LC, Ward LC. Pseudoseizures: diagnostic evaluation. *Neurology* 1982;32:18–23.

• • • • • •
PSYCHOMOTOR (SEIZURES, EPILEPSY)

The term "psychomotor" seizure is an old synonym for "complex partial" (the current official term), "temporal lobe," or "limbic" seizure. Since not all complex partial seizures have psychologic or motor activity, the term has fallen into disfavor. However, it is still in widespread common use in the United States.

Reference

Gastaut H. *Dictionary of epilepsy. Part 1: Definitions.* Geneva: World Health Organization, 1973.

• • • • • •
PSYCHOSES

Several hundreds of studies have been published relating epilepsy and psychosis. The nature of the relationship is of both practical and theoretical interest. The incidence of psychosis among people with epilepsy is approximately 7%, clearly higher than in the nonepileptic population. Marked variation in published values may be due to methodological factors such as collection bias. For example, no cases of psychosis were reported in 245 patients with epilepsy seen in a general practice (1), but 16% of patients with epilepsy being evaluated for seizure surgery showed evidence of psychosis (2).

Psychosis associated with epilepsy may be ictal, postictal, interictal, or a combination (3).

- *Ictal:* Status epilepticus or intense seizures resulting in a confusional state with psychotic elements. Examination generally reveals delirium, as well as more cardinal symptoms of psychosis.
- *Postictal:* Complex partial or tonic-clonic seizures may lead to paranoid states with confusion lasting hours to weeks (4). Affective psychoses may also occur after complex partial seizures (5). In a practical sense, it is often difficult to distinguish ictal from postictal psychoses, especially since subtle complex partial seizures may occur during sleep.
- *Interictal:* Slater and Beard (6) promulgated the concept that some patients with temporal seizure foci tend to develop a schizophreniform psychosis after 10–15 years of recurrent seizures. Risk is higher for patients with left temporal foci (6–11). Certain features differentiating this from essential schizophrenia have been noted, including the relative preservation of affect with epilepsy-associated schizophreniform psychosis (6,7). A complex relationship exists between interictal psychosis and seizure frequency, in that some patients deteriorate after a flurry of seizures, and some deteriorate after a long seizure-free interval. The latter phenomenon may relate to the value of seizures (electroshock therapy) in treatment of some psychoses. In 1958 Landolt (12) described "forced normalization" of the EEG by an unknown process, with improvement of the seizure disorder, but appearance of a psychosis. Psychosis may be precipitated by improvement in seizures from medications (13–15) or surgery (15). Many patients remit after a schizophreniform episode, but in approximately 50% the evolution is chronic with acute exacerbations.

Mechanisms of psychosis in epilepsy are poorly understood. Psychodynamic factors, such as frightening experiences during the seizure, diminished emotional adaptability and lability, recurrent disorientation of time sense and memory, and intrusive ictal hallucinations may play a role. Organic factors associated with temporal and extratemporal lesions are also potentially important.

Neurotransmitter changes may relate epilepsy and psychosis. Defects in dopamine systems may underlie epilepsy and psychosis (16). Engel and colleagues (17) have postulated the importance of the endogenous opiate system in epileptiform psychosis, and opiate receptors are increased in the region of clinical complex partial seizure foci. In an animal model, intermittent subclinical discharges in the temporal lobe may produce kindling (see this heading) of the mesolimbic system (18) with consequent psychosis.

Patients with epilepsy-associated psychosis require treatment or careful observation, even for brief postictal psychosis, since psychosis is distressing and potentially dangerous. Joint management by a neurologist and psychiatrist is useful. Psychotropic medications (see this heading), including phenothiazines, butyrophenones, and tricyclics, can lower seizure threshold; however, this is not an absolute contraindication to their use. Epilepsy-associated psychosis may respond best to a combination of AED and neuroleptic medication. Duration of neuroleptic therapy may vary from hours to years, depending on individual circumstances.

References

1. Pond DA, Bidwell BH. A survey of epilepsy in fourteen general practices. II: Social and psychological aspects. *Epilepsia* 1959;1:285–99.
2. Falconer M. Reversibility by temporal lobe resection of the behavioral abnormalities of temporal lobe epilepsy. *N Engl J Med* 1973;289:451–55.
3. Bruens JH. Psychoses in epilepsy. *Psychiatr Neurol Neurochir* 1971;74:175–92.
4. Savard G, Andermann F, Remillard GH, Olivier A. Postictal psychosis following partial complex seizures is analogous to Todd's paralysis. In: Wolf P, Dam M, Janz D, Dreifuss FE (eds.). *Advances in epileptology,* Vol 16. New York: Raven Press, 1987.
5. Lyketsos CG, Stoline AM, Longstreet P, Ranen NG, Lesser R, Fisher R, Folstein M. Mania in temporal lobe epilepsy. *Neuropsychol Behav Neurol* 1993;6:19–25.
6. Slater E, Beard AW. The schizophrenia-like psychoses of epilepsy. *Br J Psychiatry* 1963;109:95–150.
7. Perez MM, Trimble MR. Epileptic psychosis. Diagnostic comparison with process schizophrenia. *Br J Psychiatry* 1980;137:245–49.
8. Glaser GH. The problem of psychosis in psychomotor temporal lobe epilepsies. *Epilepsia* 1964;5:272–78.
9. Flor-Henry P. Psychosis and temporal lobe epilepsy. A controlled investigation. *Epilepsia* 1969;10:363–95.
10. Sherwin I. Psychosis associated with epilepsy: significance of the laterality of the epileptogenic lesion. *J Neurol Neurosurg Psychiatry* 1981;44:83–85.
11. Conlon P, Trimble MR, Rogers D. A study of epileptic psychosis using magnetic resonance imaging. *Br J Psychiatry* 1990;156:231–35.
12. Landolt H. Some clinical and electroencephalographic correlations in epileptic psychoses. *Electroenceph clin Neurophysiol* 1953;5:121.
13. Fischer M, Korskjaer G, Pedersen E. Psychotic episodes in Zarondan treatment. *Epilepsia* 1965;6:325–34.
14. Pakalnis A, Drake ME, John K, Kellum JB. Forced normalization. Acute psychosis after seizure control in seven patients. *Arch Neurol* 1987;44:289–92.
15. Trimble MR. The relationship between epilepsy and schizophrenia: a biochemical hypothesis. *Biol Psychiatr* 1977;12:299–304.
16. Engel J Jr, Caldecott-Hazard S, Bandler R. Neurobiology of behavior: anatomic and physiologic implications related to epilepsy. *Epilepsia* 1986;27(Suppl 2): S3–S13.

17. Frost JJ, Mayberg HS, Fisher RS, et al. Mu-opiate receptors measured by positron emission tomography are increased in temporal lobe epilepsy. *Ann Neurol* 1988;23:231–37.
18. Stevens JR, Livermore A. Kindling of the mesolimbic dopamine system: animal model of psychosis. *Neurology* 1978;28:36–46.

● ● ● ● ● ●
PSYCHOSOCIAL (PROBLEMS)
(SEE ALSO BEHAVIOR; EMPLOYMENT)

Since 1981 more than 5,000 articles have appeared addressing social, emotional, or psychiatric problems associated with epilepsy (1). Psychosocial difficulties impinge on aspects of daily living in obvious ways, but characterization for study can be difficult. Measurement tools have included the MMPI (Minnesota Multiphasic Personality Inventory) and WPSI (Washington Psychosocial Seizure Inventory) (2).

People with epilepsy find it more difficult to drive, work, marry, and obtain education. Contributors to these difficulties include seizures, medication side effects, underlying neurological conditions, and, perhaps most important, ongoing social stigma attached to epilepsy. In the United States, the Disabilities Act of 1990 makes discrimination against people with epilepsy illegal. Psychosocial difficulties are usually more marked in patients seeking specialized consultation for frequent seizures (3). Most people with epilepsy may lead full lives with minimal restrictions on activities.

References

1. Levin R, Banks S, Berg B. Psychosocial dimensions of epilepsy: a review of the literature. *Epilepsia* 1988;29:805–16.
2. Dodrill CB, Breyer DN, Diamond MB, Dubinsky BL, Geary BB. Psychosocial problems among adults with epilepsy. *Epilepsia* 1984;25:168–75.
3. Trostle JA, Hauser WA, Sharbrough FN. Psychologic and social adjustment to epilepsy in Rochester, Minnesota. *Neurology* 1989;39:633–37.

● ● ● ● ● ●
PSYCHOTROPIC MEDICATIONS

Psychotropic medications are among the most commonly prescribed medications. Concern arises because phenothiazines, butyrophenones, tricyclic antidepressants, and lithium, as well as newer agents such as maprotiline and fluoxitine, may occasionally precipitate seizures in predisposed individuals (1,2). In toxic doses, psychotropic medications can precipitate seizures in normal individuals (3). Most psychotropic medications have a convulsant effect in animals, and the package insert usually states that they are contraindicated in epilepsy. However, psychotropic medications are often beneficial for psychiatric conditions in people with epilepsy (4), and properly monitored use is generally safe. One study (5) of patients receiving psychotropic or antidepressant agents, including chlorpromazine, thioridazine, thiothixene, haloperidol, lithium, protriptyline, desipramine, doxepine, trazodone, and amoxapine, showed improvement in psychiatric status in 86% of the patients. Seizures were improved in 64% and worsened in only 10%. Some AEDs, such as carbamazepine and valproic acid, may directly benefit psychiatric symptoms (6).

References

1. Trimble M. Non-monoamine oxidase inhibitor antidepressant and epilepsy: a review. *Epilepsia* 1978;19:241–50.
2. Luchins DJ, Olivier AP, Wyatt RJ. Seizures with antidepressants: an in vitro technic to assess relative risk. *Epilepsia* 1984;25:25–32.
3. Crone P, Newman B. The problem of tricyclic antidepressant poisoning. *Postgrad Med J* 1979;55:528–32.
4. Robertson MM, Trimble MR, Townsend HRA. Phenomenology of depression in epilepsy. *Epilepsia* 1987;28:364–72.
5. Ojemann LM, Baugh Bookman C, Dudley DL. Effect of psychotropic medications on seizure control in patients with epilepsy. *Neurology* 1987;37:1525–27.
6. Post RM, Altshuler LL, Ketter TA, Denicoff K, Weiss SR. Antiepileptic drugs in affective illness. Clinical and theoretical implications. *Adv Neurol* 1991; 55:239–277.

• • • • • •
PYKNOLEPSY

"Pyknoepilepsy" is a term introduced by Sauer in 1916, and subsequently used by German authors to describe the condition now known as "absence epilepsy" or "petit mal" (see this heading).

Reference

Sauer H. Uber gehaufte kleine Anfalle bei Kindern (pycnolepsie). *Mschr Psychiatr Neurol* 1916;40:276–300.

• • • • • •
PYRIDOXINE

Pyridoxine deficiency cause seizures in neonates and infants (1,2) because of its role as a cofactor in the synthesis of GABA, the major inhibitory neurotransmitter in the brain. It is the single biochemical abnormality giving rise to a chronic seizure disorder in humans (3). Pyridoxine dependency may result in seizures during intrauterine life and infancy (4–6). Seizures and the EEG (showing high-voltage, generalized spike discharges) respond rapidly to treatment with pyridoxine.

References

1. Reilly RH, Killam KF, Jenney EH, Marshal WH, Tausig T, Apter NS, Pfeiffer C. Convulsant effects of isoniazid. *JAMA* 1953;152:1317–21.
2. Coursin DB. Convulsive seizures in infants with pyridoxine deficient diet. *JAMA* 1954;154:406–408.
3. Swaiman KF, Millstein TM. Pyridoxine-dependency and penicillin. *Neurology* 1970;20:78–81.
4. Hunt AD Jr, Stokes J Jr, McCrory WW, Stroud J. Pyridoxine dependency: report of a case of intractable convulsions in an infant controlled by pyridoxine. *Pediatrics* 1954;13:140–45.
5. Bejsovec M, Kulenda Z, Ponca E. Familial intrauterine convulsions in pyridoxine dependency. *Arch Dis Child* 1967;42:201–207.
6. Waldinger C, Berg RB. Signs of pyridoxine dependency manifest at birth in siblings. *Pediatrics* 1968;32:161–68.

RACE

A racial predisposition to epilepsy has yet to be demonstrated. The incidence of epilepsy is higher in developing countries than in the industrialized nations (1). This may be due to several acquired conditions, among them poor perinatal care, malnutrition of child and mother, infectious diseases (especially brain parasites), and head trauma.

In studies of multiracial societies (2), a higher incidence of epilepsy is noted in black adults (3), more than in children (4) or adolescents (5).

References

1. Shorvon SD, Farmer PJ. Epilepsy in developing countries: a review of epidemiological socio-cultural and treatment aspects. *Epilepsia* 1988;29(Suppl 1):S36–S54.
2. Davenport CB. The ecology of epilepsy: racial and geographic distribution of epilepsy. *Arch Neurol Psy* 1923;9:554–66.
3. Haerer AF, Anderson DN, Schoenberg BS. Prevalence and clinical features of epilepsy in a biracial United States population. *Epilepsia* 1986;27:66–75.
4. Shamansky SL, Glaser GH. Socio-economic characteristics of childhood seizures disorders in the New Haven area: an epidemiological study. *Epilepsia* 1979;20:457–74.
5. Cowan LD, Bodensteiner JB, Leviton A, Doherty L. Prevalence of the epilepsies in children and adolescents. *Epilepsia* 1989;30:94–106.

RAMSAY HUNT (SYNDROME)
(DYSSYNERGIA CEREBELLARIS MYOCLONICA)

The Ramsay Hunt syndrome was described in 1921 (1). In this heterogeneous syndrome (2), two groups have been identified (3,4): Ramsay Hunt syndrome with epilepsy, and Ramsay Hunt syndrome with ataxia and progressive myoclonus. Seizures and cognitive abnormalities are infrequent and mild in the latter variety. Phenotypically, patients resemble those with Baltic myoclonic epilepsy (see Baltic myoclonus), Mediterranean myoclonic epilepsy (3), or one of the other myoclonic epilepsies seen around the world. Storage abnormalities and mitochondrial dysfunction are lacking in the Ramsay Hunt syndrome.

Seizures in Ramsay Hunt syndrome may be myoclonic, tonic-clonic, or multifocal partial. As suggested by its alternate title, "dyssynergia cerebellaris myoclonica," cerebellar findings may be prominent (see also Ataxia; Cerebellum). The typical EEG shows bursts of spike and slow wave activity overlying an otherwise normal background with marked photosensitivity. Progression of the clinical picture is usually slow.

References

1. Hunt JR. Dyssnergia cerebellaris myoclonica-primary atrophy of dentate system. A contribution to the pathology and symptomatology of the cerebellum. *Brain* 1921;44:490–538.
2. Marseille Consensus Group. Classification of progressive myoclonus epilepsies and related disorders. *Ann Neurol* 1990;28:113–15.
3. Genton P, Michelucci R, Tassinari CA, Roger J. The Ramsay Hunt revisited: Mediterranean myoclonus versus mitochondrial encephalomyopathy with ragged-red fibres and baltic myoclonus. *Acta Neurol Scand* 1990;81:8–15.
4. Marsden CD, Harding AE, Obeso JA, Lu CS. Progressive myoclonic ataxia (the Ramsay Hunt syndrome). *Arch Neurol* 1990;47:1121–25.

● ● ● ● ● ●
RASMUSSEN'S (SYNDROME)

Rasmussen described this syndrome in 1958 based on his extensive surgical experience with epilepsy (1,2). Previously normal children develop partial motor seizures with increasing frequency and resistance to treatment. There is progressive intellectual decline and neurological deficit. A hallmark is progressive unilateral paresis. Head MRI and CT show unilateral focal lesions. Selective cortical resection and hemispherectomy has variable results in arresting the process. Pathological examination of operative resected brain tissue shows inflammatory lesions, especially around brain venules. The reason for the unilateral progressive disease is unknown. A viral etiology has been hypothesized, but no virus has been identified. An immune complex disease and vasculitis have also been postulated (3).

Hemispherectomy has shown promising results for treatment of seizures in this condition, with acceptable post-surgical neurologic deficits (4). Rasmussen's encephalitis may be associated with an antibody to the GluR$_3$ subtype of the glutamate receptor and may respond to plasmapheresis (S) (see also Hemispherectomy).

References

1. Piatt JH, Hwang PA, Armstrong DC, Becker LE, Hoffman HJ. Chronic focal encephalitis (Rasmussen syndrome): six cases. *Epilepsia* 1988;29:268–79.
2. Rasmussen T, Andermann F. Update on the syndrome of chronic encephalitis and epilepsy. *Cleve Clin J Med* 1989;56:S181–S184.
3. Andrews JM, Thompson JA, Pysher TJ, Walker ML, Hammond ME. Chronic encephalitis, epilepsy, and cerebrovascular immune complex deposits. *Ann Neurol* 1990;28:88–90.
4. Vining EPG, Freeman JM, Brandt J, Carson BS, Uematsu S. Progressive unilateral encephalopathy of childhood (Rasmussen's syndrome): a reappraisal. *Epilepsia* 1993;34:639–50.
5. Rogers SW, Andrews PI, Gahring LC, et al. Autoantibodies to glutamate receptor GluR$_3$ in Rasmussen's encephalitis. *Science* 1994;265:648–51.

∙ ∙ ∙ ∙ ∙ ∙ ∙
RECURRENCE (RATE)

- Recurrence rate after a first isolated seizure (see First seizure).
- Recurrence rate after stopping treatment (see Cure; Prognosis; Relapse).

∙ ∙ ∙ ∙ ∙ ∙ ∙
REFLEX EPILEPSY/
SEIZURES AND TRIGGERED SEIZURES

Seizures may be triggered (provoked, induced) by a specific stimulus. The situation in which the seizure occurs is usually referred to as the trigger. However, this situation does not imply that a unique mechanism is responsible in all patients (1). The terms "reflex seizures" or "reflex epilepsy" are misleading, since simple reflex loops are not usually involved in triggered epilepsy. Seizures may be triggered by:

- light causing generalized or partial seizures;
- eye closure or eye blinking (2). Interruption of visual input and appropriate receptive input has been implicated causing myoclonic seizures, absence seizures, and palpebral myoclonus with absences (see Absence (S,E));
- auditory stimuli: partial seizures;
- reading: partial or generalized seizures;
- speech, spontaneous or during reading (3,4): partial seizures;
- movement: partial seizures;
- eating: partial or generalized seizures
- gastric distention or abdominal pain (5): partial or atonic seizures (9);

- sensory stimuli, cutaneous (6);
- immersion in hot water (7,8): partial seizures;
- dressing (10): tonic seizures;
- physical exercise (11,12);
- cognitive activity: thinking (13), decision making (14), card playing, checkers, chess, and others (15), mental arithmetic. Whatever the stimulus, it always involves situations that place the patient in a decision-making mode with its particular emotional or psychological context. Seizures are almost always myoclonic, absence, or generalized tonic-clonic.

Seizures may be classified under two headings:

- generalized seizures with a simple trigger (light) or a complex trigger (intellectual activity);
- partial seizures. Triggering afferent stimuli reach a pathological cortical zone. Multifocal lesions may explain why a particular patient may have seizures triggered by light, movement, and hot water (16).

References

1. Gastaut H, Tassinari CA. Triggering mechanisms in epilepsy. The electro-clinical point of view. *Epilepsia* 1966;7:85–138.
2. Terzano MG, Parrino L, Manzoni GG, Manci D. Seizures triggered by blinking when beginning to speak. *Arch Neurol* 1983;40:103–106.
3. Geschwind N, Sherwin I. Language-induced epilepsy. *Arch Neurol* 1967; 16:25–31.
4. Lee SL, Sutherling WW, Persing JA, Butler AB. Language-induced seizure. A case of cortical origin. *Arch Neurol* 1980;37:433–36.
5. Gastaut H, Poirier F. Experimental, or reflex, induction of seizures. Report of a case of abdominal (enteric) epilepsy. *Epilepsia* 1964;5:256–70.
6. Scollo-Lavizzari G, Hess R. Sensory precipitation of epileptic seizures. Report of two unusual cases. *Epilepsia* 1967;8:157–61.
7. Roos RAC, Van Dijk JG. Reflex-epilepsy induced by immersion in hot water—case report and review of the litterature. *Eur Neurol* 1988;28:6–10.
8. Satishchandra P, Shivaramakrishana A, Kaliperumal VG, Schoenberg BS. Hot-water epilepsy: a variant of reflex epilepsy in Southern India. *Epilepsia* 1988; 29:52–56.
9. Lenoir P, Ramet J, De Meinleir L, D'Allest AM, Desprachine B, Loob H. Bathing-induced seizures. *Pediat Neurol* 1989;5:124–25.
10. Cirignotta F, Montagna P, Lugaresi E, Gervasig L. Seizures provoked by dressing. *Arch Neurol* 1982;39:785–86.
11. Simpson RK, Grossman RG. Seizures after jogging. *N Engl J Med* 1989;321:835.
12. Ogunyemi AO, Gomez MR, Klass DW. Seizures induced by exercise. *Neurology* 1988;38:634–36.
13. Wilkins AJ, Zifkin B, Andermann F, McGovern E. Seizures induced by thinking. *Ann Neurol* 1982;11:608–12.

14. Mutani R, Ganga A, Agnetti V. Reflex epilepsy evoked by decision making: report of case. *Schweiz Arch Neurol Neurochir Psychiat* 1980;127:61–67.
15. Senanayake N. Epileptic seizures evoked by card games, draught, and similar games. *Epilepsia* 1987;28:356–61.
16. Moritomo T, Hayakawa T, Sugie H, Awaya Y, Fukuyama Y. Epileptic seizures precipitated by constant light, movement in daily life, and hot water immersion. *Epilepsia* 1985;26:237–42.

ARITHMETIC (SEIZURES INDUCED BY CALCULATION)

In very rare patients with idiopathic generalized epilepsy, performing mathematical calculations may bring about a seizure (1,2). Seizures may be myoclonic, tonic-clonic, or absence. Seizures may also be caused by the decision-making process.

References

1. Senanayake N. Epilepsia arithmetices revisited. *Epilepsy Res* 1989;3:167–73.
2. Yamamoto J, Egawa I, Yamamoto S, Shimizu A. Reflex epilepsy induced by calculation using a Soroban, a Japanese traditional calculator. *Epilepsia* 1991;32:39–43.

AUDITORY STIMULI-INDUCED SEIZURES

Seizures produced by sounds may have different precipitating mechanisms:

- A sudden unexpected sound may cause a startle or jump, "startle epilepsy" (see Movement, seizures produced by).
- Rhythmic or monotonous sounds without the element of surprise (e.g., the sound of a running motor) may produce seizures.
- Music-induced seizures. Partial seizures with a spike-wave correlate on the EEG in the temporal region may be caused in some patients by specific melodies, certain types of music, or repetition of the same music (1). In some cases, the sound frequency appears to be important (2), but in most cases it appears that the affective significance of the music is of greater importance.
- Voice-induced seizures. Partial seizures may be induced by a particular voice (3).

References

1. Newman P, Saunders M. A unique case of musicogenic epilepsy. *Arch Neurol* 1980;37:244–45.

2. Poskanzer DG, Brown AE, Miller H. Musicogenic epilepsy caused by a discrete frequency band of church bells. *Brain* 1962;85:77–79.
3. Ramani V. Audiogenic epilepsy induced by a specific television performer. *N Engl J Med* 1991;325:134–35.

AUTO-INDUCED SEIZURES

Voluntarily-induced seizures:

• A patient may bring about an interrupted exposure to light (usually of direct sunlight or other intense light sources) by rapidly moving his fingers or hands between himself and the light source, by shaking his head while facing the sun, by looking through venetian blinds, or by rapid eye blinking (1–5). Television screens are sometimes used (6). Absence seizures are most frequently seen; occasionally myoclonic seizures or generalized tonic-clonic seizures follow absence seizures. These are classified in the group of photosensitive idiopathic generalized epilepsies. Although half the patients may be mentally subnormal, patients with normal intelligence may also bring on their seizures. Self-induced photosensitive epilepsy is usually seen at the age of five and is often discovered accidentally. For reasons not clearly understood, they may continue to be induced during childhood and adolescence. Auto-induced epilepsies are not very rare.
• Less frequently, seizures may be brought on by hyperventilation (7,8), leading to absence seizures and generalized tonic-clonic seizures.

References

1. Ames FR, Saffer D. The sunflower syndrome. A new look at self-induced photosensitive epilepsy. *J Neurol Sci* 1983;59:1–11.
2. Andermann K, Berman S, Cooke PM, Dickson J, Gastaut H, Kennedy A, Margerison J, Pond A, Tizard JM, Walsh JPM. Self-induced epilepsy. A collection of self-induced epilepsy cases composed with some other photoconvulsive cases. *Epilepsia* 1967;8:162–70.
3. Darby CE, deKorte RA, Binnie CD, Wilkins AJ. The self-induction of epileptic seizures by eye closure. *Epilepsia* 1980;21:31–42.
4. Kogeorgos J. Henson RA, Scott DF, Pattern sensitive epilepsy: a case report. *J Neurol Neurosurg Psychiatry* 1979;42:635–39.
5. Terzano MG, Parrino L, Manzoni GC, Mancia D. Seizures triggered by blinking when beginning to speak. *Arch Neurol* 1983;40:103–106.
6. Andermann F. Self-induced television epilepsy. *Epilepsia* 1971; 12:269–75.
7. Fabisch W, Darbyshire K. Report of an unusual case of self-induced epilepsy with comments on some psychological and therapeutic aspects. *Epilepsia* 1965; 6:335–40.
8. Green JB. Self-induced seizures. *Arch Neurol* 1966;11:579–86.

READING (SEIZURES INDUCED BY)

Reading epilepsy is a form of reflex epilepsy (see this heading). Bickford distinguished two types (1):

- *Primary reading epilepsy:* This form of reflex epilepsy is usually triggered by reading out loud. After a variable period of reading time, jerking of the jaw occurs, followed by generalized tonic-clonic seizures. Seizures arise only during reading, and patients are otherwise normal. The interictal EEG is unremarkable, but the ictal EEG shows bilateral or focal spikes. Etiology is multifactorial, with an apparent influence of proprioceptive stimulation arising from oculomotor, pharyngeal, and laryngeal musculature. There is also a possible triggering role of mental effort (2,3);

- *Secondary reading epilepsy* (4): In secondary reading epilepsy, cortical lesions are apparent. Partial seizures may be associated with temporo-parieto-occipital epileptiform discharges induced by reading; they sometimes occur spontaneously.

References

1. Bickford RG, Whelan JL, Klass DW, Corbin KB. Reading epilepsy. *Trans Amer Neurol Assoc* 1956;81:100–102.
2. Kartsounis LD. Comprehension as the effective trigger in a case of primary reading epilepsy. *J Neurol Neurosurg Psychiatry* 1988;51:128–30.
3. Christie S, Guberman A, Tansley BW, Courure M. Primary reading epilepsy: investigation of critical seizure-provoking stimuli. *Epilepsia* 1988;29:288–93.
4. Critchley M, Cobb W, Sears TA. On reading epilepsy. *Epilepsia* 1959;1:403–17.

• • • • • •
REFRACTORY (EPILEPSIES)

Refractory epilepsies are those in which seizures do not respond satisfactorily to AEDs. Synonyms include intractable, difficult to treat, unstable, or chronic epilepsies.

Intractable epilepsies occur in a heterogeneous group of patients (1,2):

- *Pseudo-resistance:* In this group, seizures are refractory not because of the nature of the seizures, but because of inadequate therapy. There may be diagnostic error with one of the imitators of epilepsy, such as syncope, psychogenic seizures, complicated migraine, etc. Seizures may be classified into an incorrect category, resulting in a suboptimal choice of AED. An underlying remediable neoplastic or metabolic condition may be left untreated. AEDs may be used in a suboptimal fashion. Compliance may be poor (see this heading).

* *True refractory seizures:* When refractory seizures persist despite adequate treatment. Approximately 20–25% of patients with new onset epilepsy will have refractory seizures (3). Some patients who are initially believed to have refractory seizures will respond to different or more aggressive antiepileptic therapy. Other putatively refractory patients improve with reduction in polypharmacy (4–7). Patients who are truly refractory to conventional AED therapy, by reason of continued seizures or unacceptable medication side effects, may be candidates either for protocol AED therapy or epilepsy surgery (see Surgery in epilepsy).

References

1. Aicardi J. Clinical approach to the management of intractable epilepsy. *Dev Med Child Neurol* 1988;30:429–40.
2. Janz D. Neurological morbidity of severe epilepsy. *Epilepsia* 1988;29(Suppl 2):S1–S8.
3. Reynolds EH, Elwes RD, Shorvon SD. Why does epilepsy become intractable? Prevention of chronic epilepsy. *Lancet* 1983;ii:952–54.
4. Porter RJ, Penry JK, Lacy JR. Diagnostic and therapeutic reevaluation of patients with intractable epilepsy. *Neurology* 1977;27:1006–11.
5. Sutula TP, Sackellares JC, Miller JQ, Dreifuss FE. Intensive monitoring in refractory epilepsy. *Neurology* 1981;31:243–47.
6. Theodore WH, Porter RJ. Removal of sedative hypnotic antiepileptic drugs from the regimen of patients with intractable epilepsy. *Ann Neurol* 1983; 13:320–24.
7. Theodore WH, Schulman EA, Porter RJ. Intractable seizures: long-term follow-up after prolonged inpatient treatment in an epilepsy unit. *Epilepsia* 1983; 24:336–43.
8. Elwes RDC, Shorvon SD, Reynolds EH. Epileptics refractory to anticonvulsants. *Neurology* 1984;34:263.

• • • • • •
RELAPSE (1)

Relapse represents the appearance of a seizure in a patient with previously controlled epilepsy (see Cure; Prognosis). Relapse may occur during a period of remission that variably extends from years to tens of years. The risk of relapse should be weighed in the decision to stop treatment.

After several years of freedom from seizures while on AEDs, the risk of relapse after medication taper is approximately 30% (2). Most relapses occur in the first 6–12 months, but a certain percentage do relapse years after stopping treatment.

Factors predisposing to relapse include decrease or discontinuation of AEDs, intercurrent disease, sleep deprivation, stress, alcohol, drug withdrawal (2–4). The reason for relapse is often not clear. In cases of recurring seizures, the decision to resume AED therapy, like that to initiate it in the first place, must be individualized.

References

1. Shorvon SD. The temporal aspects and prognosis in epilepsy. *J Neurol Neurosurg Psychiatry* 1984;4:1157–65.
2. Callaghan N, Garrett A, Goggin T. Withdrawal of anticonvulsant drugs in patients free of seizures for 2 years. *N Engl J Med* 1988;318:942–46.
3. Oller-Daurella L, Oller FVL. Suppression of antiepileptic treatment. *Eur Neurol* 1987;27:106–13.
4. Overweg J, Binnie CD, Oosting J, Rowan AJ. Clinical and EEG prediction of seizure recurrence following antiepileptic drug withdrawal. *Epilepsy Res* 1987;1:272–83.

• • • • • •
REMISSION

Remission is a period during which seizures disappear spontaneously or in response to therapy. Remission rate is usually expressed as a ratio of those patients in remission to the total number in a particular population of patients with epilepsy.

• • • • • •
RETT (SYNDROME) (1)

Rett syndrome (or Rett's syndrome) is a progressive encephalopathy of unknown etiology occurring only in young females. The syndrome presents a stereotyped evolution, with normal development up to 7–18 months, then developmental arrest followed by progressive mental deterioration and loss of the use of the hands with onset between the age of 9 months and 3 years, gait apraxia, axial ataxia, autism, dementia, respiratory problems, and seizures. After the age of 10 years, there is usually a progressive mental and physical deterioration with cachexia (2–4).

Seizures appear in 75% of cases, usually relatively late in the course, and include a variety of seizure types with variable response to treatment. EEG shows a marked change during the sleep-wake cycle. Waking

The diagnosis is based on the clinical and EEG characteristics, since the characteristics of the seizures alone are not specific; centro-temporal spikes may be seen in other disorders or even in normal children. Electrical status epilepticus of sleep (ESES) (epilepsy with continuous spikes and waves during slow sleep/ESES (electrical status epilepticus during slow sleep) may be confused with benign Rolandic epilepsy (11).

References

1. Blom S, Heijbel J, Bergfors PG. Benign epilepsy with centro-temporal foci. Prevalence and follow-up study of 40 patients. *Epilepsia* 1972;13:609–19.
2. Cavazzuti GB. Epidemiology of different types of epilepsy in school age children of Modena, Italy. *Epilepsia* 1980;21:57–62.
3. Heijbel J, Blom S, Rasmuson M. Benign epilepsy of childhood with centrotemporal EEG foci: a genetic study. *Epilepsia* 1975;16:285–93.
4. Lerman P. Benign partial epilepsy with centrotemporal spikes. In: Roger J, Bureau M, Dravet C, Dreifuss FE, Perret A, Wolf P (eds.). *Epileptic syndromes in infancy, childhood and adolescence,* 2nd edition. London: John Libbey Eurotext, 1992:189–200.
5. Santanelli P, Bureau M, Magaudda A, Gobbi G, Roger J. Benign partial epilepsy with centrotemporal (or rolandic) spikes and brain lesion. *Epilepsia* 1989;30:182–88.
6. Loiseau P, Duché B. Benign childhood epilepsy with centrotemporal spikes. *Cleve Clin J Med* 1989;56(Suppl 1):S17–S22.
7. Loiseau P, Beaussart M. The seizures of benign childhood epilepsy with rolandic paroxysmal discharges. *Epilepsia* 1973;14:381–89.
8. Lombroso CT. Sylvian seizures and mid-temporal spike foci in children. *Arch Neurol* 1967;17:52–59.
9. Loiseau P, Duché B, Cordova S, Dartigues JF, Cohadon S. Prognosis of benign childhood epilepsy with centrotemporal spikes: a follow-up study of 168 patients. *Epilepsia* 1988;29:229–35.
10. Doose M, Baier WK. Benign partial epilepsy and related conditions: multifactorial pathogenesis with hereditary impairment of brain maturation. *Eur J Pediatr* 1989;149:152–58.
11. Beaumanoir A, Ballis T, Varfis G, Ansari K. Benign epilepsy of childhood with rolandic spikes. *Epilepsia* 1974;15:301–15.
12. Ambrosetto G, Tassinari GA. Antiepileptic drug treatment of benign childhood epilepsy with rolandic spikes: is it necessary? *Epilepsia* 1990;31:802–805.
13. Fejerman N, Di Blasi AM. Status epilepticus of benign partial epilepsies in children report of two cases. *Epilepsia* 1987;28:351–55.

S

•••••••
SABRIL® (SEE VIGABATRIN)

A new AED not yet available in the United States. A new drug application (NDA) has been filed and approval is pending.

•••••••
SANTAVUORI-HALTIA (DISEASE) (1,2)

Santavuori-Haltia disease is an early infantile form of the ceroid-lipofuscinoses, rarely seen outside Finland. The incidence is 1 per 13,000 inhabitants, and the disease is transmitted by an autosomal recessive mode.

Onset occurs between the ages of 8 and 18 months, with progressive mental retardation, myoclonus, generalized seizures, blindness, and bilateral pyramidal signs. Death ensues by approximately 10–13 years of age.

EEGs at the beginning of the illness show generalized slowing, and later reveal generalized voltage suppression without ictal activity. The histological diagnosis is discussed under the heading of ceroid-lipofuscinoses.

References

1. Santavuori P. Infantile type of so-called neuronal ceroid-lipofuscinosis. Part 1: a clinical study of 15 patients. *J Neurol Scand* 1973;18:257–67.
2. Haltia M. Infantile type of so-called neuronal ceroid-lipofuscinosis. *J Neurol Sci* 1973;18:269–85.

•••••••
SCANS (CT; MRI)

INDICATIONS

- Neuroimaging, including computerized tomography (CT) and magnetic resonance imaging (MRI)(see also Magnetic resonance imaging (MRI)), is an essential investigation in all seizures of unknown cause.
- Imaging is also used in the pre-surgical work-up for seizure surgery.

- CT or MRI are usually not helpful in established, nonprogressive neurological disorders; however, scanning or repeat scanning is often important with a deterioration in a previously stable clinical condition.

LIMITS

- Head CT and MRI provide morphological information representing cerebral anatomy. They do not directly reflect function. An epileptogenic lesion or focus may not necessarily correspond to an anatomical or CT scan abnormality (1–3).
- Head CT provides poor visualization of the temporal regions: approximately one-third of epilepsies involving the temporal lobe have normal CT scans, but abnormal MRI images (see MRI).
- There is the danger of attributing seizures to abnormal CT scan signals that have no pathological significance, e.g., diffuse cortical atrophy, ventricular dilatation in elderly patients (2).
- Certain areas of decreased attenuation on CT scans may be produced transiently following seizures and may resemble astrocytomas with vasogenic edema (4–7).

References

1. Gloor P. Contributions of electroencephalography and electrocorticography to the neurosurgical treatment of the epilepsies. *Adv Neurol* 1975;8:59–106.
2. Janati A, Nowack WJ, Shah H, Lucy DD. A correlative study of electroencephalography and computed tomography in partial complex seizures in adults. *J Epilepsy* 1989;2:175–79.
3. Spencer SS, Spencer DD, Williamson PD, Mattson RH. The localizing value of depth electroencephalography in 32 patients with refractory epilepsy. *Ann Neurol* 1982;12:248–53.
4. Goulatia RK, Verma A, Mishra NK, Ahuja GK. Disappearing CT lesions in epilepsy. *Epilepsia* 1987;28:523–27.
5. Kramer RE, Luders H, Lesser RP, Weinstein MR, Dinner DS, Morris HH, Wyllie E. Transient focal abnormalities of neuroimaging studies during focal status epilepticus. *Epilepsia* 1987;28:528–32.
6. Yaffe K, Ferrierro D, Barkovich J, Rowley H. Reversible MRI abnormalities following seizures. *Neurology* 1995;45:104–108.
7. Henry TR, Drury I, Brunberg JA, et al. Focal cerebral magnetic resonance changes associated with partial status epilepticus. *Epilepsia* 1994;35:35–41.

● ● ● ● ● ●
SCHOLASTIC ACTIVITIES

Many school children with epilepsy experience scholastic difficulties: 21–69% (1–4). Reasons include absenteeism because of seizures, medication toxicity, problematic relationships with teachers and schoolmates, and parental fear. Each of the preceding factors contribute to behavioral problems, inattention (5), and selective cognitive deficits (3). Some scholastic problems may be due to focal cortical deficits or subclinical seizure activity (6).

Parents as well as medical and educational personnel should encourage as normal a life-style as possible, with active participation in sports (see Sports for discussion of limits) and peer group activities. Accommodations should be made for children with special learning problems within the system. If this is not feasible, special schools are available.

References

1. Rodin EP, Lennick P, Dendrill Y, Lin Y. Vocational and education problems of epileptic patients. *Epilepsia* 1972;13:149–60.
2. Jennekens-Schinkel A, Linschooten-Duikersloot EMEM, Bouma PAD, Peters ACB, Stisnen TH. Spelling errors made by children with mild epilepsy: writing-to-dictation. *Epilepsia* 1987;28:555–63.
3. Seidenberg M, Beck N, Geisser M, et al. Neuropsychological correlates of academic achievement of children with epilepsy. *J Epilepsy* 1988;1:23–29.
4. Trimble MR, Corbett J. Behavioural and cognitive disturbances in epileptic children. *Ir Med J* 1978;73(Suppl 1):21–28.
5. Stores G. School-children with epilepsy at risk for learning and behaviour problems. *Dev Med Child Neurol* 1978;20:502–508.
6. Kasteleijn-Nolst T, Bakker DJ, Binnie CD, Buerman A, Van Raajj M. Psychological effects of subclinical epileptiform EEG discharges. I: Scholastic skills. *Epilepsy Res* 1988;2:111–16.

* * * * * *

SCOTOSENSITIVE (SEIZURES)

Scotosensitive seizures are triggered by darkness. Typically, they include palpebral myoclonic movements with absence seizures caused by suppression of central vision (see also Photoconvulsive (S); Induced (S); Reflex (S,E)).

Reference

Panayiotopoulos CP. Fixation-off sensitive epilepsy in eyelid myoclonia with absence seizures. *Ann Neurol* 1987;22:87–89.

* * * * * *

SECONDARY GENERALIZED (SEIZURES)

In contrast to primary generalized epilepsies, the phrase "secondary generalized epilepsies" is used to refer to a number of epilepsy syndromes, including West and Lennox-Gastaut syndromes, presumed to be secondary

to either fixed or progressive diffuse cerebral damage. Secondary generalized epilepsies are distinguished from "secondarily" generalized epilepsies,
which begin focally. At present, the phrase "secondary generalized epilepsies" is little used; the Commission for Classification of the International
League Against Epilesy groups these disorders under the group of cryptogenic or symptomatic generalized epilepsies.

• • • • • •
SELF-MEDICATION

A patient may change the AED therapy from that prescribed, e.g., stopping treatment in the belief that therapy is ineffective or causing side effects;
or the patient may modify the amount and timing of AED doses (usually
a diminution) (see also Compliance).

The patient may take other drugs in addition to AEDs, e.g., those prescribed to another family member or by another doctor who is unaware
of ongoing AED therapy. Undesirable drug interactions may arise, which
may either increase or decrease AED levels. Some drugs may decrease
seizure threshold (theophylline, antihistamines, stimulants, tricyclic antidepressants, phenothiazines, certain antibiotics, e.g., metronidiazole).

• • • • • •
SENSORY (SEIZURES)

These are partial seizures with auditory, gustatory, olfactory, or visual symptomatology (see these headings).

• • • • • •
SEQUELAE
(TRAUMATIC CONSEQUENCES OF SEIZURES)

Seizures frequently cause injury.

- *Head trauma*
  Minor head trauma is frequent; severe trauma is rare. In one series
  of over 12,000 patients, only three had serious brain or intracranial
  injury (1). The concept of a "dementia pugilistica" with progressive
  cognitive decline following repeated head injuries has not been sub-
  stantiated in patients with epilepsy.

- *Fractures*
  These may occur from falls or intense muscle contraction during tonic-clonic seizures (c.f. fractures during electroconvulsive therapy) in patients with osteoporosis. Hip fractures, Colles' fractures, and spinal fractures are the most common (2,3). Bilateral upper humeral fractures may also be seen (4).

References

1. Russell-Jones DL, Shorvon SD. The frequency and consequences of head injury in epileptic seizures. *J Neurol Neurosurg Psychiatry* 1989;52:659–62.
2. Annegers JF, Melton III LJ, Sun CA, Hauser WA. Risk of age-related fractures in patients with unprovoked seizures. *Epilepsia* 1989;30:348–55.
3. Lindgren L, Walloe A. Incidence of fracture in epileptics. *Acta Orthop Scand* 1977;48:356–61.
4. Finelli PF, Cardi JK. Seizure as a cause of fracture. *Neurology* 1989;39:858–60.

* * * * * *

SEX/GENDER

With few exceptions (1,2), epidemiological studies show that there is a higher prevalence and incidence of epilepsy in males, with a male to female ratio of 1.2 to 1 (3). Unequal rates may be due to recruitment bias (in certain countries where women receive less attention), head injury (which is commoner in men), and genetic factors (absence epilepsy of childhood—frequently seen in girls, epilepsy with centro-temporal spikes—more frequently seen in boys).

References

1. Pond D, Bidwell B, Stein L. A survey of 14 general practices. Part 1: Medical and demographic data. *Psychiat Neurol Neurochirurg* 1960;63:217–36.
2. Gomez JG, Arcinegas E, Torres J. Prevalence of epilepsy in Bogota, Colombia. *Neurology* 1978;28:90–95.
3. Sander JWA, Shorvon SD. Incidence and prevalence studies in epilepsy and their methodological problems. A review. *J Neurol Neurosurg Psychiatry* 1987;50:829–39.

* * * * * *

SEXUALITY

During the interictal period, patients with epilepsy may have impaired sexuality. Evaluation of sexual problems is subjective and further complicated by the reluctance of patients to talk about this subject. Therefore, quantification of the frequency of sexual problems is difficult (1,2). Hypersexuality or sexual deviation appear to be rare, whereas hyposexuality (decreased libido, impotence, or frigidity) is relatively common (3). Sexual disturbances in epilepsy depend on several factors:

- Location of the seizure focus: Seizures arising from the temporal lobe have been implicated to a greater degree than those from other regions.
- Early age of onset of seizures predisposes to sexual dysfunction.
- AEDs often affect endocrine function, causing, for example, a decrease in free testosterone levels (1,4) (see Hormones). The various AEDs—sedative or not, enzyme-inducers or not— may have different effects on sexuality (5).
- Mood and behavioral problems seen in certain patients with epilepsy may introduce secondary problems with sexual relations.

Partial seizures with foci in temporal, anterior cingulate, peri-Sylvian, or parietal areas rarely may engender genital sensations or sexual reactions during the seizures (6,7). Nonspecific sexual disinhibition may occur during ictal automatisms or the postictal period (8).

References

1. Brodie MJ. Anticonvulsants and sexual function. In: Chadwick D (ed.). Fourth International Symposium on sodium valproate and epilepsy. Royal Society of Medicine Services International Congress and Symposium. Series no 152, published by Royal Society of Medicine Services Ltd., 1989;228–35.
2. Jensen P, Jensen JB, Sorensen PS, et al. Sexual dysfunction in male and female patients with epilepsy: a study of 86 outpatients. *Arch Sex Behav* 1990;19:1–14.
3. Saunders M, Rawson M. Sexuality in male epileptics. *J Neurol Sci* 1970;10: 577–83.
4. Toone BK, Wheeler M, Nanjee M, Fenwick P, Grant R. Sex hormones, sexual activity and plasma convulsant levels in male epileptics. *J Neurol Neurosurg Psychiatry* 1983;46:824–26.
5. Mattson RH, Cramer JA, Collins JF, et al. Comparison of carbamazepine, phenobarbital, phenytoin, and primidone in partial and secondarily generalized tonic-clonic seizures. *N Engl J Med* 1985;313:145–51.
6. Remillard GN, Andermann F, Testa GF, et al. Sexual ictal manifestations predominant in women with temporal lobe epilepsy: a finding suggesting sexual dimorphism in the human brain. *Neurology* 1983;33:323–30.
7. Calleja J, Carpizo R, Berciano J. Orgasmic epilepsy. *Epilepsia* 1988;29:635–39.
8. Spencer SS, Spencer DD, Williamson PD, Mattson RH. Sexual automatisms in partial complex seizures. *Neurology* 1983;33:527–33.

• • • • • • •
SIALIDOSES

The sialidoses are a group of disorders of lysosomes due to alpha-N-acetyl neuraminidase abnormalities (1). In certain phenotypes, a deficit in beta-galactosidase has been reported. Transmission is autosomal recessive. Features include a progressive myclonic epilepsy, bilateral cherry-red spots seen on fundoscopic examination, and enzymatic abnormalities in leukocytes and fibroblast cultures (2).

Two phenotypes have been described:

- *Type I (cherry-red spot myoclonus)* (3): Onset occurs during adolescence with myoclonus, progressive blindness with cerebellar signs, tonic-clonic seizures, and peripheral neuropathy. In this form, dementia typically does not occur.
- *Type II (beta-galactosidase deficiency)* (4): This type is predominantly seen in Japan. Onset occurs in the second to third decade. Clinical presentation is similar to that of Type I sialidosis, but Type II may be associated with facial dysmorphism and deafness.

References

1. Lowden JA, O'Brien JS. Sialidosis: a review of human neuraminidase deficiency. *Am J Hum Genet* 1979;31:1–18.
2. Tsiji S, Yamada T, Tsutsumi A, Miyatake T. Neuraminidase deficiency and accumulation of sialic acid in lymphocytes in adult type sialidosis with partial B-galactosidase deficiency. *Ann Neurol* 1982;11:541–43.
3. Rapin I, Goldticher S, Katzman R, Engel J Jr, O'Brien JS. The cherry-red spot myoclonus syndrome. *Ann Neurol* 1978;3:234–42.
4. Sakuraba H, Suzuki Y, Akagi M, Sakai M, Amano N. B-galactosidase-neuraminidase deficiency, clinical, pathological and enzymatic studies in postmortem cases. *Ann Neurol* 1983;13:497–503.

• • • • • •
SINGLE PHOTON EMISSION COMPUTED TOMOGRAPHY (SPECT)

Single photon emission computerized tomography (SPECT) is a cerebral imaging technique using a systemically injected or inhaled radiolabelled tracer to measure regional cerebral blood flow (1). Commonly employed tracers include Xenon[133] (2–5), iodine markers (6), hexamethyl-propylene amine oxime (HMPAO) with ^{99}Tc-technetium (7–10). SPECT is in some ways similar to PET (see Positron emission tomography scanning (PET)); however, SPECT is less expensive and does not require an on-site cyclotron.

PET in turn provides higher theoretical spatial resolution and ability to image brain metabolism and neuroreceptors more directly.

Cerebral blood flow is often decreased interictally, in the region of a seizure focus, and increased markedly during partial or tonic-clonic seizures (4,6,8,10,11). Localization of a seizure focus can be accomplished in 50–75% of cases with injection of radiolabelled tracer immediately after a seizure, followed by imaging. The sensitivity and selectivity of SPECT in epilepsy remain under study.

References

1. Holman BL, Hill TC, Polak JF, Lee RGL, Royal HD, O'Leary DH. Cerebral perfusion imaging with I-123 labeled amines. *Arch Neurol* 1984;41:1060–63.
2. Hougaard K, Ojkaw T, Sviensdottir E, Skonhog E, Ingvar DH, Lassen A. Regional cerebral blood flow in focal cortical epilepsy. *Arch Neurol* 1976;33:527–35.
3. Valmier J, Touchon J, Daures P, Zanca M, Baldy-Moulinier M. Correlations between cerebral blood flow variations and clinical parameters in temporal lobe epilepsy: an interictal study. *J Neurol Neurosurg Psychiatry* 1987;50:1306–11.
4. Duncan R, Patterson J. Regional cerebral blood flow in epilepsy studied with xenon enhanced CT. *J Neurol Neurosurg Psychiatry* 1988;51:1366–67.
5. Fish DR, Lewis TT, Brooks DJ, Zikha E, Wise RJS, Kendall BE. Regional cerebral blood flow of patients with focal epilepsy studied using xenon enhanced CT brain scanning. *J Neurol Neurosurg Psychiatry* 1987;50:1584–88.
6. Lee BI, Markand ON, Welman HN, et al. HIPDM-SPECT in patients with medically intractable complex partial seizures. *Arch Neurol* 1988;45:397–402.
7. Biersack HJ, Linke D, Brassel F, et al. Technetium-99m HM-PAO brain SPECT in epileptic patients before and during unilateral hemispheric anesthesia (Wada test)—report of 3 cases. *J Nucl Med* 1988;28:1763–67.
8. Lamanna MR, Sussman NM, Harner RN. Initial experience with SPECT imaging of the brain using 1–123 p-iodoamphetamine in focal epilepsy. *Clin Nucl Med* 1989;14:428–30.
9. Neiderinckx RD. Evolution of regional cerebral blood flow with 99m Tc-d, 1HM-/PAO and SPECT. *Neurosurg Rev* 1987;10:181–84.
10. Stefan H, Bauer J, Feistel H, Schuleman H, Neubauer U, Wenzel B, Wolf E, Neundorf B, Hunk WJ. Regional cerebral blood flow during focal seizures of temporal and frontocentral onset. *Ann Neurol* 1990;27:162–66.
11. Holmes MD, Kelly K, Theodore WH. Complex partial seizures. Correlations of clinical and metabolic features. *Arch Neurol* 1988;45:1191–93.

· · · · · ·
SITUATION-RELATED (SEIZURES)

Situation-related seizures are synonomous with provoked seizures and acute symptomatic seizures. The term is more common in Europe than in the United States. Three etiological subgroups are defined:

- *Febrile convulsions* (see this heading)
- *Seizures arising from an underlying systemic disorder*
  - Metabolic: Hypoglycemia, hypocalcemia, hyponatremia, hypercalcemia, hypoxia, dehydration, etc.
  - Endogenous toxin: Renal insufficiency, hepatic insufficiency.
  - Exogenous toxin: Alcohol-related or alcohol-withdrawal seizures, tricyclic antidepressants, neuroleptics, antihistamines, cocaine, other CNS stimulants, cytotoxic drugs, or contrast media (1–4).
- *Seizures due to direct cerebral insult*
  - Seizures may occur contemporaneously with ischemic or hemorrhagic stroke; frequently within the first week.
  - Head trauma and its aftermath may induce seizures.
  - Hypertensive encephalopathy, including eclampsia, can provoke seizures.

Treatment of a situation-related seizure is directed toward the underlying cause. Brief periods of AED therapy may be warranted, but long-term treatment should be reserved for cases in which the provoking factors cannot be eliminated.

References

1. Alldredge BK, Lowenstein DH, Simon RP. Seizures associated with recreational drug abuse. *Neurology* 1989;39:1037–39.
2. Choy-Kwong M, Lipton RB. Seizures in hospitalized cocaine users. *Neurology* 1989;39:425–27.
3. Levey AI, Weiss H, Yu R, Wang H, Krumholz A. Seizures following myelography with iopamidol. *Ann Neurol* 1988;23:397–99.
4. Messing RO, Closson RG, Simon RP. Drug-induced seizures: a 10–year experience. *Neurology* 1984;34:1582–86.

· · · · · ·
SKIN ERUPTIONS AND TOXIC DERMATOSES

These exanthems may present as local or diffuse morbilliform or urticarial eruptions during the second week of treatment, but will resolve when AEDs are discontinued or even despite continuation. They occur with all

AEDs, in approximately 3–10% of cases, more frequently with rapid increases in AED dose (1). They may be the first sign of:

- Hypersensitivity syndrome (see Anticonvulsant/antiepileptic drugs (AEDs)).
- Generalized rashes.
- Bullous dermatoses:
  - Lyell's syndrome or subacute necrotising epidermolysis which affects skin and mucus membranes, producing large confluent bullae with a "scalded" appearance. Death occurs in one-fourth to one-third of cases.
  - Stevens-Johnson syndrome or exudative erythema multiforme, with cutaneous and mucus membrane maculo-vesicular eruptions or bullous eruptions.

Because of the danger of bullous dermatoses, all skin eruptions must be carefully followed when a new drug is started. The offending drug should be stopped and should not be restarted (2).

Other skin eruptions and manifestations include:

- Nodular erythema;
- Acne: seen with prolonged treatment with phenobarbital, primidone, and the oxazolenediones.
- Pigmented patches (chloasma): due to prolonged treatment with phenytoin;
- Hirsutism: with phenytoin.

References

1. Chadwick D, Shaw MDM, Foy P, Rawlins MD, Turnbull DM. Serum anticonvulsant concentrations and the risk of drug induced skin eruptions. *J Neurol Neurosurg Psychiatry* 1984;47:642–44.
2. Schmidt D, Kluge W. Fatal toxic epidermal necrolysis following reexposure to phenytoin: a case report. *Epilepsia* 1983;24:440–43.

SLEEP

Seizures are more frequent during sleep in some patients (1,2), a fact often confirmed by EEG monitoring (3,4). In 1962 a classification of seizures according to hour of onset was proposed (5).

SLEEP STATE

By EEG criteria, 4 stages of sleep have been identified (6):

- *Slow wave sleep (NREM)*
  - Stage 1: Corresponds to sleep onset with the appearance on EEG of vertex sharp waves (5% of total sleep time).
  - Stage 2: Decrease in muscular activity with increase in cutaneous resistance; EEG recording shows discontinuous slow activity with the appearance of K complexes and sleep spindles (50–55% of total sleep time).
  - Stage 3: Diffuse delta activity at 0.5–2 Hz involving less than 20% of a 30 second epoch (10% of total sleep time).
  - Stage 4: Delta activity at 0.5–2 Hz occupying more than 50% of the 30 second epoch (10–15% of total sleep time).
- *Rapid eye movement sleep (REM) (paradoxical sleep):* Low-voltage desynchronized pattern associated with rapid conjugate horizontal eye movements; decrease in muscle tone, irregular cardiac and respiratory rhythm (occupies 25% of total sleep time). REM sleep lasting 90–100 minutes appears in 4–5 cycles during the night.

SLEEP AND EPILEPSY

- *Epilepsies of sleep* are epilepsies in which seizures appear preferentially during sleep. These are found mainly in idiopathic partial and generalized epilepsies:
  - Generalized tonic-clonic epilepsies: about 30% (6) with seizures seen during sleep.
  - Idiopathic partial epilepsies of childhood (see Benign epilepsies).
  - An epileptic syndrome of childhood with continuous spike and slow wave discharges during sleep, called "electrical status epilepticus of sleep" (ESES syndrome) (see Aphasia; Landau-Kleffner syndrome).
- *Activation of epileptic phenomena during sleep* (4,7,8)
  - Sleep architecture depends on the EEG and clinical characteristics of the epileptic syndrome and the frequency of seizures. Although sleep architecture may be normal interictally, paradoxical sleep may be disorganized or interrupted by arousals.
  - Polysomnography has identified several links between sleep and seizures (8):
    i. In idiopathic generalized epilepsies, seizure incidence increases during slow wave sleep and decreases during REM sleep.

During sleep, EEG discharges tend to decrease in duration and polyspikes appear.

ii. In specific symptomatic generalized epilepsies, there is an activation during the first two phases of slow wave sleep, and a decrease in activity during the third and fourth phases. Typically, there is no REM sleep.

iii. In nonspecific symptomatic generalized epilepsies, such as West syndrome, the EEG shows a hypsarrhythmic pattern that disappears during REM sleep. In Lennox-Gastaut syndrome, there is an increase in spike and slow wave activity during the first two phases of sleep and a decrease during the third and fourth phase of slow wave sleep. Tonic seizures usually appear during slow wave sleep.

iv. In partial epilepsies, especially idiopathic forms, slow wave sleep predisposes to generalization. In epilepsies associated with lesions, multifocal localization may appear. In certain childhood epileptic syndromes, continuous spike and slow wave activity may be recorded during sleep. The diagnostic value of a sleep tracing has been calculated to be increased by about a third. Early sleep is most useful for diagnosis: 46% of abnormalities appear in the first half hour of recording, 57.3% after 2 hours, 73% during the first 3 hours (8).

DIFFERENTIAL DIAGNOSIS OF NONEPILEPTIC PAROXYSMAL EVENTS DURING SLEEP

- *Sleep walking* is semi-purposeful ambulation for which the patient is amnestic, associated with automatisms and occuring during NREM sleep, often on coming out of stage 4 NREM (delta) sleep.
- *Night terrors* (see this heading), common in young children, also occuring during NREM sleep.
- *Sleep paralysis* associated with the hypnagogic hallucinations of narcolepsy.
- *Paroxysmal dystonic phenomena* seen in choreoathetotic seizures and dystonias in which the EEG recording is normal. These symptoms may respond to treatment with carbamazepine (9).
- *Periodic limb movements of sleep* (nocturnal myoclonus) (10,11) may respond to triazolam, L-Dopa, or dextropropoxyphene.
- *Psychogenic seizures* arising in the early nighttime period, during wakefulness, drowsiness, or soon after arousal from sleep.

ANTIEPILEPTIC MEDICATION AND SLEEP STRUCTURE

In general, AEDs increase stage 1 and 2 sleep and decrease REM sleep. Benzodiazepines shorten sleep onset and prolong early sleep cycles. Some benzodiazepines, e.g., nitrazepam, may decrease or eliminate REM sleep.

RECORDING

- *Recording of nocturnal sleep allows*
  - Analysis of sleep architecture.
  - Activation of different seizure or types during the various sleep phases.
- *Sleep recording during the day* can be extremely useful in children since stages 1 and 2 are often captured. Sleep deprivation may be more effective in eliciting ictal phenomena.
- *Drug-induced sleep recordings:* Medications without effect on the EEG (beyond their effect on producing sleep such as hydroxyzine or chloral hydrate) may be useful in the rapid induction of stages 1–3 of sleep.
- *Sleep after sleep deprivation* may be revealing (12). Recording for 20–40 minutes may be used in conjunction with other activation procedures, such as hyperventilation or photic stimulation. Increased diagnostic yield from recording after sleep deprivation may reach 26% (13).

References

1. Langdon-Down M, Brain WR. Time of day in relation to convulsions in epilepsy. *Lancet* 1929;2:1029–32.
2. Patry FL. The relation of time of day, sleep and other factors to the incidence of epileptic seizures. *Am J Psychiatry* 1931;87:789–813.
3. Gibbs FA, Biggs EL. *Atlas of electroencephalography.* Vol 1. Cambridge, MA: Addison-Wesley, 1950.
4. Janz D. The Grand Mal epilepsies and the sleep-waking cycle. *Epilepsia* 1962; 3:60–109.
5. Glossary of standardized terminology for sleep and biological rhythm research. *Sleep* 1980;287–88.
6. Billiard M. Epilepsies and the sleep-wake cycle. In: Sterman MB, Shouse MN, Passouant P (eds.). *Sleep and epilepsy.* New York: Academic Press 1983:269–86.
7. Degen R, Niedermeyer E. Epilepsy, sleep and sleep deprivation. Amsterdam: Elsevier, 1984.
8. Declerck AC. Interaction between sleep and epilepsy. *Eur Neurol* 1986;25 (Suppl 2):117–27.

9. Lugaresi E, Cirignotta F, Montagna P. Nocturnal paroxysmal dystonia. *J Neurol Neurosurg Psychiatry* 1986;49:375–80.
10. Coleman RM, Pollack C, Weitzman EM. Periodic movements in sleep (nocturnal myoclonus). Relation to sleep disorders. *Ann Neurol* 1980;8:416–21.
11. Kaplan PW, Allen RP, Buchholz D, Walters JK. A double-blind, placebo-controlled study of the treatment of periodic limb movements in sleep using carbidopa/Levodopa and propoxyphene. *Sleep* 1993;16(8):717–23.
12. Mattson RH, Pratt KL, Calverly JR. Electroencephalograms of epileptics following sleep deprivation. *Arch Neurol* 1965;13:310–15.
13. Logothetis J, Milonas I, Bostantzopoulos S. Sleep deprivation as a method of EEG activation. *Eur Neurol* 1986;25 (Suppl 2):134–40.

● ● ● ● ● ●
SLEEPWALKING

Sleepwalking is not an epileptic phenomenon but is a parasomnia arising during the transition from non-REM sleep to REM sleep. Epileptic seizures characterized by nocturnal sleepwalking are seen in adults and adolescents. Distinction may be made on clinical and EEG characteristics (see also Sleep).

Reference

Pedley TA, Guilleminault C. Episodic nocturnal wanderings responsive to anticonvulsant drug therapy. *Ann Neurol* 1977;2:30–35.

● ● ● ● ● ●
SOMATOMOTOR (SEIZURES)/ FOCAL MOTOR (SEIZURES)

Somatomotor seizures are characterized by clonic, tonic, or more rarely atonic (see Inhibitory (S)) motor activity involving all or part of one side of the body without affecting consciousness. A seizure focus may be located in the primary motor cortex.

Seizures may also be seen with symptomatic or cryptogenic partial epilepsies, as well as in benign epilepsy of childhood with centro-temporal spikes (see also Rolandic (S,E)).

• • • • • •
SOMATOSENSORY (SEIZURES)

Seizures characterized by somesthetic manifestations: formication, sensation of pins and needles, buzzing, electric, cold or heat, burning or pain (1,2). They are usually associated with motor phenomena. They may remain fixed or have a jacksonian march. They may be:

- unilateral with variable spread: in a contralateral sensory strip;
- bilateral involving the trunk, lower limbs, and face with a focus in the secondary somatosensory area;
- associated with proprioceptive problems in the case of parietal foci;
- they may cause headaches or migraines.

References

1. Mauguière F, Courjon J. Somatosensory epilepsy: review of 127 cases. *Brain* 1978; 101:307–32.
2. Blume WT, Jones DC, Young GB, et al. Seizures involving secondary sensory and related areas. *Brain* 1992;115:1509–20.

• • • • • •
SPELLS

A spell is a nonspecific term used by patients and physicians alike to describe a paroxysmal disturbance in well-being. This may include the sudden onset of sensory, motor, autonomic, psychic, or emotional changes due to a variety of causes. In addition to seizures, syncope, panic attacks, or hypoglycemia, for example, may produce sudden malaise prompting a visit to a physician.

Much effort may be necessary to determine whether these episodes are ictal in nature in order to lead to appropriate management. A hastily and incorrectly applied diagnosis of seizure may have significant social, professional, and medical implications, and great care may be needed in the diagnosis and evaluation of "spells."

Reference

Kaplan PW. Spells: syncope, seizures and other episodic disorders. In: Stobo JD, Hellmann DB, Ladenson PW, Petty BG, Traill TA (eds.). *The principles and practice of medicine*, 23rd edition. *Disorders of the nervous system. Spells: syncope, seizurs and other episodic disorders*. Stamford, CT: Appleton & Lange, 1996, Chapter 13.

• • • • • •
SPHINGOLIPIDOSES

Sphingolipidoses are disorders of lipid metabolism in which seizures are but one part of a complex clinical tableau. This group of disorders includes the glucosyl-ceramidoses (gangliosidoses and glucosyl cerebrosidoses), galactosyl ceramidoses (Fabry's disease, metachromatic leukodystrophy), phosphoryl ceramidoses, cytosidoses.

Diagnosis may be suspected on clinical grounds, but is secured by demonstration of a specific enzyme deficit.

• • • • • •
SPORTS

Involvement in team sports may have a beneficial effect on patients with epilepsy, improving social integration (1,2). Sports do not worsen epilepsy. Relations between sports and seizures may be addressed as follows:

THE EFFECT OF SPORTS ON SEIZURES

- Hyperventilation can precipitate some forms of seizures, particularly absence seizures in predisposed individuals. However, the homeostatic effect caused by metabolic acidosis and hypoxia from physical exertion is markedly different from the effect produced from hyperventilation in the resting patient, such that hyperventilation in response to exercise usually does not provoke seizures.
- Sustained hypoxia or hypoglycemia during sustained, vigorous physical exercise may rarely precipitate seizures.
- Repeated head injury in certain violent sports, such as rugby, boxing, or martial arts, may lead to epilepsy.
- A rare individual may demonstrate exercise-precipitated seizures (2).

THE RISK OF ACCIDENT DURING SPORTS

There is apparently little increase in frequency of sporting accidents in children with epilepsy compared to normal children. When accidents do occur in children with epilepsy, they are often unrelated to seizures. Special care must be taken with sports for which a seizure could be catastrophic, including aquatic sports (3) and climbing or flying sports.

PRACTICAL SUGGESTIONS

In poorly controlled epilepsies, potentially dangerous sports should be avoided. These include water sports, bathing, fishing, sail boarding, sailing, and underwater sports; sports involving access to heights, e.g., rock climbing, horseback riding, mountain bicycling, flying; mechanical sports; automobile or motorcycle riding. The majority of patients with epilepsy can practice sports normally (4); approximately 20% require assistance or surveillance. For individuals with reasonably controlled epilepsy, participation in most sports is to be encouraged.

References

1. van Linschoten R, Backx FJ, Mulder OG, Meinardi H. Epilepsy and sports. *Sports Med* 1990;10:9–19.
2. Denio LS, Drake ME, Makalnis A. The effect of exercise on seizure frequency. *J Med* 1989;20:171–76.
3. Pearn J, Bart R, Yamaoka R. Drowning risk to epileptic children: a study from Hawai. *Br Med J* 1978;ii:1284–85.
4. Livingston S, Berman W. Participation of epileptic patients in sports. *JAMA* 1973;224:236–38.

• • • • • •
STATUS EPILEPTICUS

DEFINITION

"A condition characterized by an epileptic seizure that is sufficiently prolonged or repeated at sufficiently brief intervals so as to produce an unvarying and enduring epileptic condition" (1). More recently, it has been generally accepted that status epilepticus is present when single seizures last for more than 30 minutes with or without impairment of consciousness; or repeated seizures last over 30 minutes with impairment of consciousness between seizures (2).

CLASSIFICATION (3)

Generalized status epilepticus

GENERALIZED CONVULSIONS

- Tonic-clonic convulsions;
  - Generalized tonic-clonic seizures from the outset are seen with the generalized idiopathic epilepsies and acute cerebral insults due to metabolic, toxic, or infectious agents;

- May occur after partial seizures (secondarily generalized) and are seen in symptomatic partial epilepsies or in patients with a recent focal cerebral lesion (traumatic or vascular);
- Tonic seizures: May be seen in children with generalized symptomatic epilepsies (4).
- Clonic seizures: May occur in young children with severe febrile convulsions in the absence of emergency treatment, or with an acute severe cerebral insult.
- Myoclonic seizures:
  - Do not impair consciousness and resolve spontaneously. They are seen in juvenile myoclonic epilepsy;
  - Occur in symptomatic generalized epilepsies and in end-stage progressive myoclonic epilepsies. They also occur in acute encephalopathies due to toxic, anoxic, metabolic, or infective causes.

GENERALIZED NONCONVULSIVE SEIZURES

- Absence status epilepticus:
  - Is seen with idiopathic generalized epilepsies; rarely with absence epilepsies of childhood or adolescence. It usually appears in patients over the age of 50–60 years (5). The clinical picture varies from brief, intermittent absences to a more continuous alteration in behavior and cognition with mild psychomotor retardation or even catatonia. An acute confusional state is often present, frequently with subtle eye blinking and clonic movements of the face. The EEG may show bilateral, synchronous, continuous or intermittent spike or polyspike and slow wave activity, rarely at 3/second.
  - Symptomatic generalized epilepsies, particularly the Lennox-Gastaut syndrome, may present with prolonged obtundation lasting from several hours to days that may be difficult to distinguish from interictal behavior states.
- Atonic status epilepticus in young children is extremely rare.

FOCAL STATUS EPILEPTICUS

- Simple partial:
  - Somatomotor:
    - Consists of repeated partial motor seizures occurring several times per hour. It occurs with partial epilepsies or an acute insult to the motor cortex;

> - ◆ Ongoing rhythmic jerking movements involving one limb or half the body associated with focal spike and slow wave activity on the EEG, are seen with lesions of the contralateral cortex (e.g., vascular, neoplastic, or traumatic).
> - ◆ Consisting of aphasia or other language problems that may persist postictally (6).
- Partial complex: Partial status epilepticus presenting with confusion may originate from the frontal or temporal lobes (7). Incidence may be underestimated (8) with unfortunate results (9). Lasting EEG paroxysmal lateralized epileptiform discharges have been reported in the elderly (10).

Unilateral status epiletricus is rare and is seen in the newborn and young children.

ETIOLOGY

- Fifty percent of patients with status epilepticus have chronic epilepsy. Usually symptomatic, they are typically generalized (epileptogenic encephalopathies) or partial epilepsies involving the frontal lobe (11). They also occur with trauma (12) and herald an underlying tumor (13). Status epilepticus often occurs following abrupt cessation of AED treatment or with subtherapeutic AED levels, but may also be seen in patients with low seizure thresholds despite "therapeutic" AED levels.
- Fifty percent of cases occur in patients with acute cerebral insult without a history of epilepsy; e.g., trauma, infections, cerebrovascular events, metabolic disturbances (hypoglycemia, hypocalcemia, dehydration, water intoxication, hepatic and renal insufficiencies), and toxicity (e.g., isoniazid, intrathecal penicillin, radiological contrast media (14), alcohol).

TREATMENT

This includes use of the benzodiazepines, phenytoin, barbiturates, and general anesthesia, usually in the intensive care setting. Patients with refractory generalized status epilepticus may be effectively treated with pentobarbital coma, often with vasopressor support (15). Intercurrent problems such as infection, cerebral edema, and ventilatory support must be addressed.

SEQUELAE

The morbidity and mortality depend on the underlying cause as well as the duration of status epilepticus.

- Mortality: 6–8% in children (16,17), 10% in adults (18) (probably because of inclusion of elderly patients with a poor prognosis).
- Morbidity: Often a worsening of a previous neurological deficit or appearance of new permanent deficit. Partial complex status epilepticus or generalized status epilepticus rarely results in cerebral edema, hypoxic ischemic insult, and significant neuronal death (20,21).

References

1. Gastaut H. *Dictionary of epilepsy. Part 1: Definitions.* Geneva: World Health Organization, 1973.
2. Engel J Jr. Status epilepticus. In: *Seizures and epilepsy.* Philadelphia: F.A. Davis, 1989:256–57.
3. Gastaut H. Classification of status epilepticus. In: Clifford Rose F (ed.). *Research progress in epilepsy.* Kent, UK: Pitman, 1983:39–45.
4. Sommerville ER, Bruni J. Tonic status epilepticus presenting as confusional state. *Ann Neurol* 1983;13:549–51.
5. Dunne JW, Summers QA, Stewart-Wynne EG. Non-convulsive status epilepticus: a prospective study in an adult general hospital. *Quart J Med* 1987;62:117–26.
6. Knight RT, Cooper J. Status epilepticus manifesting as reversible Wernicke's aphasia. *Epilepsia* 1986;27:301–304.
7. Williamson PD, Spencer DD, Spencer SS, Novelly RA, Mattson RH. Complex partial status epilepticus: a depth-electrode study. *Ann Neurol* 1985;18:647–54.
8. Tomson T, Svanborg E, Wedlund JF. Non-convulsive status epilepticus: high incidence of complex partial status. *Epilepsia* 1986;27:276–85.
9. Roberts MA, Humphrey PRD. Prolonged complex partial status epilepticus: a case report. *J Neurol Neurosurg Psychiatry* 1988;52:586–88.
10. Terzano MG, Parrino L, Mazzucchi A, Moretti G. Confusional states with periodic lateralized epileptiform discharges (PLEDs): a peculiar epileptic syndrome in the elderly. *Epilepsia* 1986;27:446–57.
11. Janz D. Status epilepticus and frontal lobe lesions. *J Neurol Sci* 1984;1:446–57.
12. Janz D. Conditions and causes of status epilepticus. *Epilepsia* 1961;2:170–77.
13. Oxbury JM, Whitty CWM. Causes and consequences of status epilepticus in adults. A study of 86 cases. *Brain* 1971;94:733–44.
14. Obeid T, Yaquab B, Panayiotopoulos C, Al-Jasser S, Shabraan A, Hawas N. Absence status epilepticus with computed tomographic brain changes following metrizamide myelography. *Ann Neurol* 1988;24:582–84.
15. Yaffe K, Lowenstein DH. Prognostic factors of pentobarbital therapy for refractory generalized status epilepticus. *Neurology* 1993;43:895–900.
16. Phillips SA, Shanahan RJ. Etiology and mortality of status epilepticus in children. A recent update. *Arch Neurol* 1989;46:74–76.
17. Dunn DW. Status epilepticus in children: etiology, clinical features, and outcome. *J Child Neurol* 1988;3:167–73.
18. Delgado-Escueta AV, Wasterlain C, Treiman DM, Porter RJ. Management of status epilepticus. *N Engl J Med* 1982;306:1337–40.
19. Towne AR, Pellock JM, Ko D, DeLorenzo RJ. Determinants of mortality in status epilepticus. *Epilepsia* 1994;35:27–34.

20. Stone JL, Hughes JR, Barr A, Tan W, Russel E, Crowell RM. Neuroradiological and electroencephalographic features in a case of temporal lobe status epilepticus. *Neurosurgery* 1986;18:212–16.
21. Meldrum BS. Metabolic factors during prolonged seizures and their relation to nerve cell death. *Adv Neurol* 1983;34:261–75.

● ● ● ● ● ●
STEREOENCEPHALOGRAPHY (SEEG)

Stereoencephalography (SEEG) is a technique of electroencephalography employing recording wires implanted directly into the brain. This methodology was developed by Talairach, Bancaud, and the group at Sainte-Anne (1,2) and developed further in the Americas (3,4). SEEG has been used in the preoperative evaluation of epilepsies (5,6). Practice at most seizure centers now involves the use of SEEG in surgical candidates for whom the noninvasive evaluation fails to fully localize a surgical target.

References

1. Bancaud J, Talairach J, Geier S, Scarabin JM. *EEG et SEEG dans les Tumeurs Cérébrales et l'Epilepsie.* Paris: Edifor, 1973.
2. Talairach J, Bancaud J, Szikla G, Bonis A, Geier S, Vedrenne C. Approche nouvelle de la neurochirurgie de l'épilepsie. Methodologie stéréotaxique et résultats thérapeutiques. *Neurochirurgie* 1974;20(Suppl 1):1–240.
3. Crandall PH, Walter RD, Rand RW. Clinical applications of studies on stereotactically implanted electrodes in temporal lobe epilepsy. *J Neurosurg* 1963;20:827–40.
4. So N, Gloor P, Quesney LF, Jones-Gotman M, Olivier A, Andermann F. Depth electrode investigations in patients with bitemporal epileptiform abnormalities. *Ann Neurol* 1989;25:423–31.
5. Engel J Jr, Rausch R, Lieb JP, Kuhl DE and Crandall PH. Correlation of criteria used for localizing epileptic foci in patients considered for surgical therapy of epilepsy. *Ann Neurol* 1981;9:215–24.
6. Spencer SS, Spencer DD, Williamson PD, Mattson RH. The localizing value of depth electroencephalography in 32 patients with refractory epilepsy. *Ann Neurol* 1982;12:248–53.

● ● ● ● ● ●
STRESS

Although difficult to quantify, stress during activities of daily living appears to increase seizure frequency in idiopathic epilepsies (1–3). The link between stress and epilepsy is, however, only statistical. Consistent precipitation of seizures by stress should raise a suspicion for psychogenic seizures (see also Induced (S)).

References

1. Gastaut H, Tassinari CA. Triggering mechanisms in epilepsy. *Epilepsia* 1966; 7:85–125.
2. Temkin NR, Davis GR. Stress as a risk factor for seizures with epilepsy. *Epilepsia* 1984;25:450–56.
3. Webster A, Mawer GE. Seizures frequency and major life events in epilepsy. *Epilepsia* 1989;30:162–67.

• • • • • •
STURGE-WEBER (SYNDROME)

Sturge-Weber syndrome (1) is a congenital disorder of cutaneous pigmentation (phacomatosis) characterized by leptomeningeal and cutaneous angiomas associated with calcium deposition in perivascular tissue and blood vessels.

Epilepsy occurs in 90% of cases, is seen early in the course, and may be the presenting feature. Seizures may be focal or generalized. Sometimes seizures are prolonged. Despite occipital cortex involvement, visual seizures are rare.

In Sturge-Weber syndrome, the EEG shows more or less widespread unilateral cortical suppression of rhythms with focal spike and wave discharges during seizures.

Seizures of the Sturge-Weber syndrome may respond to AED therapy. In certain severe forms, seizures may contribute to the intellectual deterioration and may be an indication for hemispherectomy (2). Pial angiomatosis and occipital calcification without cutaneous angiomas may represent *formes frustres* of Sturge-Weber syndrome, perhaps resembling epilepsy with occipital calcifications (3).

References

1. JH Menkes. Tumors of the nervous system. In: *Textbook of child neurology,* 3rd edition. Philadelphia: Lea and Febiger, 1985:575–76.
2. Hoffman HJ, Hendrick EB, Dennis SM, Armstrong D. Hemispherectomy for Sturge Weber syndrome. *Child's Brain* 1979;5:233–48.
3. Chevrie JJ, Specola N, Aicardi J. Secondary bilateral synchrony in unilateral pial angiomatosis: successful surgical treatment. *J Neurol Neurosurg Psychiatry* 1988;51:663–70.

• • • • • •
SUICIDE

The rate of suicide and attempted suicide in patients with epilepsy is 4–5 times greater than in the general population (1). Suicide accounts for 0.8–1.6% of deaths in patients with epilepsy (2). Risk factors include youth, isolation and introversion, psychopathic tendencies, and poor social adjustment. Further risk is added by depression and acute or chronic psychosis (3). Seizure frequency and the psychosocial environment do not appear to be major risk determinants (4).

Suicide attempts during seizures are highly unusual, but it may be difficult to distinguish certain delirious behaviors from a suicide attempt.

References

1. Barraclough B. Suicide and epilepsy. In: Reynolds EH, Trimble MR (eds.). *Epilepsy and psychiatry.* London: Churchill Livingstone, 1981.
2. Hawton K, Fagg J, Marsack P. Association between epilepsy and attempted suicide. *J Neurol Psychiatry* 1980;43:168–70.
3. Matthews WS, Barabas G. Suicide and epilepsy. A review of the literature. *Psychosomatics* 1981;22:515–24.
4. Mendez MF, Lanska DJ, Manon-Espaillat R, Burnstine TH. Causative factors for suicide attempts by overdose in epileptics. *Arch Neurol* 1989;46:1065–68.

• • • • • •
SURGERY IN EPILEPSY

According to the NIH consensus report (1), surgical therapy for epileptic conditions is underutilized; nonetheless "epilepsy surgery centres are appearing like mushrooms after a long period of cool weather and much rain" (2). In the United States, there are potentially 54,000 surgical candidates, whereas only relatively few are operated on yearly (3). Surgical intervention may be indicated if uncontrolled seizures persist for 2–5 years, despite trials of all the first-line AEDs, as well as polypharmacy of these agents (with therapeutic levels). The rationale is that AED therapy may be decreasingly effective with prolongation of poorly controlled seizures associated with a decline in the patient's medical and social condition. Surgery is mainly indicated in adults, but is increasingly used to treat adolescents and children (4–6). There are 2 goals to therapy:

- *Curative:* To eradicate seizures by resection of the seizure focus when the latter is well defined and limited (see Corticectomy);
- *Palliative:* To improve seizure control and quality of life and to diminish certain seizure types, e.g., drop attacks. The purpose may not be to eliminate all seizures (see Callosotomy; Hemispherectomy).

References

1. National Institutes of Health Consensus Development Conference Statement. Surgery for epilepsy. *Epilepsia* 1990;31:806–12.
2. Dasheiff RM. Epilepsy surgery: is it an effective treatment? *Ann Neurol* 1989;25:506–509.
3. Ward AA Jr. Perspective for surgical therapy of epilepsy. In: Ward AA Jr, Penry JK, Purpura D (eds.). *Epilepsy.* New York: Raven Press, 1983.
4. Ojemann GA. Surgical therapy for medically intractable epilepsy. *J Neurosurg* 1987;66:489–99.
5. Engel J Jr (ed.). *Surgical treatment of the epilepsies.* New York: Raven Press, 1987.
6. Green RC, Adler JR, Erba G. Epilepsy surgery in children. *J Child Neurol* 1988;3:155–66.

• • • • • •
SYMPTOMATIC (EPILEPSY)

Symptomatic epilepsies are acquired. They may be due to pre- or perinatal insult, such as infection, anoxia, or severe metabolic disturbance, which leads to generalized seizures. Examples include West syndrome, early myoclonic encephalopathy, or Lennox-Gastaut syndrome. Structural lesions sustained through trauma or acquired by cerebrovascular compromise, intracranial hemorrhage, or tumor, for example, may lead to recurrent focal seizures and a focal epilepsy. Focal epilepsies may secondarily generalize (see also Classification of seizures and epilepsies).

• • • • • •
SYNCOPE

Syncope is loss of consciousness resulting from global cerebral ischemia (1). Syncopal reactions depend on the severity and duration of ischemia:

*   *Para-syncopal autonomic phenomena* include pallor, profuse sweating, bradycardia, hypotension, hypersalivation, epigastric discomfort, nausea, and vomiting. These may precede the syncopal episode.
*   *Simple syncope* consists of loss of consciousness with a fall, hypotonia, pallor, and upward eye deviation. Consciousness is rapidly regained.
*   *Convulsive syncope* is a form of syncope leading to generalized hypertonia with tonic spasms and opisthotonos followed by myoclonic jerks predominantly involving the proximal upper extremities (2,3). Convulsive syncope can be distinguished from generalized tonic-clonic seizures with a careful history of the episode.

EEG recording (1), with provocative tests, such as tilt table testing, Valsalva maneuver, carotid sinus massage, or ocular compression, may reveal:

- A cardiac pause with or without clinical manifestations but without changes on EEG.
- Runs of bilateral synchronous diffuse monomorphic delta activity with simple syncope.
- With convulsive syncope (3), a stereotyped sequence of events is seen including bilateral synchronous runs of slow waves with intervening periods of suppression occurring simultaneously with a tonic spasm. Concurrent with clonic movements, the EEG shows hypersynchronous slow waves accelerating rapidly and changing to a normal tracing.

Distinguishing an epileptic seizure from syncope may be difficult. The patient is often alone during the loss of consciousness, witnesses may misinterpret events (especially with convulsive syncope), and patients may describe malaise before generalized seizures. Occasional patients with complex partial or atonic epilepsy may fall without convulsive movements. Additionally, syncope may trigger an epileptic seizure in predisposed individuals (4). Epileptic seizures may rarely induce cardiac dysrhythmias that result in syncope (5–7)(see also Arrhythmia; Autonomic (S); Drop attacks).

References

1. Gastaut H, Fischer-William S. Electroencephalographic study of syncope. Its differentiation from epilepsy. *Lancet* 1957;23:1018–25.
2. Kempster PA, Balla JI. A clinical study of convulsive syncope. *Clin Exp Neurol* 1986;22:53–55.
3. Lin J T-Y, Ziegler DK, Lai CW, Bayer W. Convulsive syncope in blood donors. *Ann Neurol* 1982;11:525–28.
4. Battaglia A, Guerrini R, Gastaut H. Epileptic seizures induced by syncopal attacks. *J Epilepsy* 1989;2:137–45.
5. Fincham RW, Shivapour ET, Leis A, Martins JB. Ictal bradycardia with syncope: a case report. *Epilepsia* 1989;30:706.
6. Tamara A, Di Luzio A, Rutecki PA. Complex partial seizures associated with asystole. *Epilepsia* 1989;30:705.
7. Radtke RA. Cardiac asystole: an epileptic arrhythmia? *Epilepsia* 1989;30:705.
8. Howell SJL, Blumhardt LD. Cardiac asystole associated with epileptic seizures: a case report with simultaneous EEG and ECG. *J Neurol Neurosurg Psychiatry* 1989;52:795–98.

●●●●●●
SYNDROMES (EPILEPTIC)

An epileptic syndrome is characterized by a constellation of signs and symptoms (1). The syndromes enumerated in the international classification of epilepsies were defined using pragmatic and conceptual approaches, emphasizing the distinction between generalized and partial epilepsies, idiopathic and symptomatic epilepsies, seizure type, age of onset, and precipitating factors.

The international classification, therefore, consists of apparently heterogeneous entities, juxtaposing rare syndromes with common ones, well-defined syndromes with less clearly defined ones. The syndromic classification is open to question (2), but has its practical applications. For a given patient, it allows the selection of appropriate treatment and determination and prognosis (3). More precise classification of syndromes will be possible as more is learned about the pathogenesis of the various forms of epilepsy.

References

1. Commission on Classification and Terminology of International League Against Epilepsy. Proposal for revised classification of the epilepsies and epileptic syndromes. *Epilepsia* 1989;30:389–99.
2. Aicardi J. Epileptic syndromes in childhood. *Epilepsia* 1988;29(Suppl 3): S1–S5.
3. Dreifuss FE. Classification of epilepsies: influence on management. *Rev Neurol* (Paris) 1987;143:375–80.

●●●●●●
SYSTEMIC LUPUS ERYTHEMATOSUS

Systemic lupus erythematosus (SLE) is a rare side effect of AEDs (1–4): phenytoin, diones, barbiturates, ethosuximide, primidone, carbamazepine, pheneturide, and valproate. AED-induced SLE resembles idiopathic lupus erythematosus but rarely is associated with CNS involvement. Although idiopathic and drug-induced lupus may coexist, disappearance of lupus after stopping AEDs confirms a drug-induced etiology.

References

1. Dorfmann H, Kahn MF, de Seze S. Lupus iatrogène iduit par les anticonvulsivants. *Sem Hôp Paris* 1972;48:2991–3000.
2. Lee SL, Chase PH. Drug induced systemic lupus erythematosus: a critical review. *Sem Arthritis Rheum* 1975;5:83–103.
3. Hannedouche TH, Godin M, Fillastre JP. Lupus induits médicamenteux. *Sem Hôp Paris* 1989;65:2195–2203.
4. Asconapé JJ, Manning KR, Lancman ME. Systemic lupus erythematosus associated with use of valproate. *Epilepsia* 1994;35:162–63.

TAURINE

The role of taurine (an inhibitory amino acid) in epileptogenesis is uncertain (1). Taurine has an antiepileptic effect in certain animal models and taurine concentrations in certain epileptic foci in man are reduced (2). Serum concentration of taurine in patients with epilepsy is variable (3). Some patients appear to have slow excretion (4). Taurine administration has provided favorable results in certain human epilepsies (5–6), but its long-term results are disappointing (1).

References

1. Durelli L, Mutani R. The current status of taurine in epilepsies. *Clin Neuropharmacol* 1983;6:37–48.
2. Van Gelder NM, Sherwin AL, Rasmussen T. Aminoacid content of epileptogenic human brain. Focal versus surrounding regions. *Brain Res* 1972; 40:385–93.
3. Goodman HO, Shihabi Z, Oles KS. Antiepileptic drugs and plasma and platelet taurine in epilepsy. *Epilepsia* 1989;30:201–207.
4. Goodman HO, Counoly BM, McLean W, Resnick M. Taurine transport in epilepsy. *Clin Chem* 1980;26:414–19.
5. Bergamini L, Mutani R, Delsedima M, Durelli L. First clinical experience on the antiepileptic action of taurine. *Eur Neurol* 1973;11:261–69
6. Fukuyama Y, Ochiai Y. Therapeutic trial by taurine for intractable childhood epilepsies. *Brain Develop* 1982;4:63–69.

TAY-SACHS (DISEASE)

Tay-Sachs disease has also been referred to as infantile amaurotic familial idiocy and type GM2 infantile gangliosidosis. It is a sphingolipidosis (see also Sphingolipidoses), due to a deficit of N-acetyl-beta-hexosaminidase A activity (1).

Transmission of Tay-Sachs disease is by an autosomal recessive gene, with an increased incidence in Ashkenazy Jews. Onset is usually at age

4–7 months, with apathy, progressive blindness, and psychomotor retardation. From birth, there may be sound-induced clonic movements with a prolonged refractory phase, but without EEG correlate. Seizures supervene at about two years, are frequent, and are of variable types. Myoclonic seizures are common.

The EEG in patients with Tay-Sachs disease shows high-voltage, disorganized background activity with poor reactivity to external stimuli and multifocal epileptiform discharges. Funduscopic examination often reveals a perimacular cherry-red spot. Visual evoked potential amplitude decreases during the course of the illness. Diagnosis can be made on clinical grounds, family history, and the demonstration of hexosaminidase A deficiency in cultures of fibroblasts (2).

References

1. Pampiglione G, Privett G, Harden A. Tay-Sachs disease: neurophysiological studies in 20 children. *Dev Med Child Neurol* 1974;16:201–208.
2. Specola N, Vanier MT, Goutières F, Mikol J, Aicardi J. The juvenile and chronic forms of GM2 gangliosidosis: clinical and enzymatic heterogeneity. *Neurology* 1990;40:145–50.

• • • • • •
TELEMETRY

EEG telemetry is a neurophysiological technique allowing laboratory EEG recording at a distance from the patient (1). Patients are free to move about their room during the recording. This system is designed to transmit an EEG signal and is frequently coupled with video recording. On-line computer analysis may provide automatic seizure or EEG spike detection (2). Many different techniques are utilized at various centers (3), but the central goal in all is to capture and analyze behavior and EEG during a seizure or seizure-like event. Information gained may be useful in distinguishing seizures from pseudoseizures (4), classification of seizure type (5), or localization of a seizure focus prior to possible surgery (6,7).

References

1. Penry JK, Porter RJ, Dreifuss RE. Simultaneous recording of absence seizures with video tape and electroencephalography. A study of 374 seizures in 48 patients. *Brain* 1975;98(3):427–40
2. Gotman J. Automatic recognition of epileptic seizure in the EEG. *Electroenceph clin Neurophysiol* 1982;54:530–40.
3. Gumnit RJ (ed.). Advances in Neurology, Vol. 46: *Intensive Neurodiagnostic Monitoring.* New York: Raven Press, 1986.

4. Desai BT, Porter RJ, Penry JK. Psychogenic seizures. A study of 42 attacks in six patients, with intensive monitoring. *Arch Neurol* 1982;39(4):202–209

5. Delgado-Escueta AV, Bascal FE, Treiman DM. Complex partial seizures on closed-circuit television and EEG: a study of 691 attacks in 79 patients. *Ann Neurol* 1982;11:292–300.

6. Kaplan PW, Lesser RP. Long-term monitoring. In: Daly DD, Pedley TA (eds.). *Current practice of clinical electroencephalography,* 2nd edition. New York: Raven Press, 1990:513–34.

7. Lesser RP, Fisher RS, Kaplan P. The evaluation of patients with intractable complex partial seizures. *Electroenceph clin Neurophysiol* 1989;73:381–88.

• • • • • •
TEMPORAL LOBE (SEIZURES; EPILEPSIES)

Temporal lobe epilepsies are characterized by simple or complex partial seizures, or secondary generalization, in various combinations. The EEG frequently reveals unilateral or bilateral temporal spikes. Onset is usually during childhood or in early adulthood and is rare after 35 years of age. Seizures are seen in flurries, often unpredictably. The following clinical features are common with temporal lobe seizure foci (1–6):

• Simple partial seizures characterized by autonomic symptoms or psychic symptoms and certain sensory phenomena: olfactory, auditory, and vertiginous. An ascending epigastric sensation is common.

• Complex partial seizures frequently involve arrest of ongoing activities (2) (see also Complex partial seizures) followed by lip-smacking, swallowing, and other automatisms. Behavioral automatisms are not the first, or the most prominent, ictal feature. Seizures typically last more than one minute. Postictal confusion with amnesia is usual.

Temporal lobe seizures and complex partial seizures are not synonymous. Complex partial seizures may arise from extra-temporal locations. More than half of temporal lobe seizures are partial simple, and do not impair consciousness; ictal discharges are limited to the temporal regions. When alteration in the level of consciousness supervenes, the seizure lasts longer and involves not only automatisms, but also focal motor manifestations (40% of cases) and, frequently, secondary generalization. Seizure discharges spread to both temporal lobes and/or extra-temporal structures (3–6). The interictal EEG may be normal, show a marked or mild asymmetry of background activity, spikes, or sharp waves. Synchronous or asynchronous unilateral or bilateral spike and slow waves may be recorded in the temporal regions or more diffusely.

The EEG may show different patterns during the seizures, including unilateral or bilateral interruption of background activities, low amplitude fast activities, rhythmic temporal or multifocal spike or spike and slow wave discharges. EEG abnormalities and the clinical seizure may occasionally occur independently.

Temporal lobe seizures are classified as limbic or neocortical. Limbic seizures involve the hippocampus, amygdala, parahippocampal gyrus, and related structures; hippocampal seizures account for at least 80% of temporal lobe seizures (7). Limbic seizures are characterized by an ascending epigastric discomfort, nausea, marked autonomic features (borborygmus, pallor, sweating, facial flushing, apnea, pupillary dilation), fear or panic, and olfactory or gustatory hallucinations (see also Autonomic (S)). Seizures may be complex at the onset. Most frequently, the etiology is one of hippocampal (mesial temporal) sclerosis; less frequently, gliomas, angiomas, cavernomas, or traumatic or infectious lesions.

Neocortical temporal lobe seizures result from foci in lateral temporal cortex. Seizures are usually simple partial in nature with auditory illusions or hallucinations, a dream-like state, disturbance of visual perception or language. Seizures evolve to complex partial or secondarily generalized seizures when the discharge spreads to and beyond mesial temporal structures. The interictal EEG shows unilateral or bilateral spikes in the temporal region.

Temporal lobe seizures are particularly amenable to surgical therapy, provided that they originate unilaterally (8).

References

1. Commission on Classification and Terminology of the International League Against Epilepsy. Proposal for revised clinical and electroencephalographic classification of epileptic seizures. *Epilepsia* 1981;22:489–501.
2. Maldonado HM, Delgado-Escueta AV, Walsh GO, Swartz BE, Rand RW. Complex partial seizures of hippocampal and amygdalar origin. *Epilepsia* 1988;29:420–33.
3. Bossi L, Munari C, Stoffels C, Bonis A, Bacia T, Talairach J, Bancaud J. Somatomotor manifestations in temporal lobe seizures. In: Akimoto H, Kazamatsuri H, Seino M, Ward Jr AA (eds.). *Advances in Epileptology, XIIIth Epilepsy International Symposium.* New York: Raven Press, 1982:29–32.
4. Duchowny M, Jayakar P, Resnick T, Levin B, Alvarez L. Posterior temporal epilepsy: electroclinical features. *Ann Neurol* 1994;35:427–31.
5. King DW, Ajmone Marsan C. Clinical features and ictal patterns in epileptic patients with EEG temporal lobe foci. *Ann Neurol* 1977;2:138–47.
6. Munari C, Bancaud J, Bonis A, Stoffels C, Szilka G, Talairach J. Impairment of consciousness in temporal lobe seizures: A stereo-electro-encephalographic study. In: Canger R, Angeleri F, Penry JK (eds.). *Advances in Epilepsy. XIth Epilepsy International Symposium.* New York: Raven Press, 1980: 111–14.
7. Harbord MG, Manson JI. Temporal lobe epilepsy in childhood: reappraisal of etiology and outcome. *Pediatr Neurol* 1987;3:263–68.
8. Glaser GH. Treatment of intractable temporal lobe—limbic epilepsy (complex partial seizures) by temporal lobectomy. *Ann Neurol* 1980;8:455–59.

• • • • • •
THETA ACTIVITY (SEE ALSO EEG)

This EEG frequency range of 4–8 Hz is called the theta band. Frontal, fronto-central, and midline central 5–6 Hz activity is normal in young adults, especially at the onset of drowsiness. High-voltage rhythmic theta activity can also be seen during transition periods between wakefulness and drowsiness in children. Waking predominance of posterior theta activity is abnormal in adults, indicating a diffuse dysfunction.

• • • • • •
TOLERANCE

The concept of drug tolerance involves the diminished pharmacological effectiveness of a drug when used at a constant dose. The clinical manifestations of AED tolerance are:

- Decreased effectiveness of a drug with the reappearance or increased frequency of seizures. This may take place over a prolonged period of time, from several days to months. A transient reappearance of seizures at a particular dose may not necessarily represent tolerance.
- There may be a decrease in the undesirable side effects experienced early in the course of treatment.

There are several types of tolerance:

- There may be tolerance to pharmacokinetic, metabolic, or peripheral factors. Carbamazepine, for example, also induces its own metabolism by increasing hepatic microsomal enzyme activity, leading to a shortened half-life and lower blood levels. This type of tolerance is limited to the first month of treatment.
- Central or pharmacodynamic tolerance is reflected by a more or less rapid decrease in effectiveness and is frequently seen with acetazolamide and the benzodiazepines. It occurs in 50–75% of cases during the first 6 months of treatment. Rarely, it may be seen with other AEDs. Tolerance to undesirable side effects seen early in the course of treatment is much more common, but may follow a variable time course. The metabolic mechanisms involved in functional tolerance are hypothetical and complex and may only be partly applicable to man.

Reference

Frey HH, Froscher W, Koella WP, Meinardi H (eds.). *Tolerance to beneficial and adverse effects of anti-epileptic drugs.* New York: Raven Press, 1986:1–180.

● ● ● ● ● ●
TONIC (SEIZURES) (1)

Tonic seizures are characterized by a sustained muscular contraction. These seizures are seen predominantly in children in the context of symptomatic generalized epilepsies, but may also be seen in adults during status epilepticus. Clinical evolution can be sudden or gradual over several seconds. Tonic seizures involve the trunk, the limbs, or both. If a tonic seizure ends with a few clonic jerks, it may be difficult to distinguish from a tonic-clonic seizure. Intermediate forms may present with asymmetric distribution, hemitonic seizures, or seizures with subtle motor signs. Falls, often with injuries, are frequent (2). As a rough clinical rule, tonic and tonic-clonic seizures produce scars on the back of the head, and atonic seizures on the front of the head because of the respective patterns of falling. Tonic seizures may be associated with alteration in the level of consciousness and autonomic disturbances, but unconsciousness may not be obvious with tonic seizures lasting only a few seconds.

The EEG correlates of tonic seizures are either suppression or rhythmic discharge at about 10 Hz, or a low-voltage discharge at approximately 20 Hz.

References

1. Gastaut H, Roger J, Ouachi S, Timsit M, Broughton R. An electroclinical study of generalized epileptic seizures of tonic expression. *Epilepsia* 1962;3:56–58.
2. Egli M, Mothersill I, O'Kane M, O'Kane F. The axial spasm. The predominant type of drop seizures in patients with secondary generalized epilepsy. *Epilepsia* 1985;26:401–15.

● ● ● ● ● ●
TONIC-CLONIC (SEIZURES)
(GRAND MAL SEIZURES)

Seizures are characterized by an evolution through three phases:

TONIC PHASE

This lasts 10–20 seconds. There is sudden loss of consciousness, stiffening, flexion and then extension of the torso with forward flexion of the head, elevation of the eyebrows, rolling back of the eyes within the orbits, mouth opening, elevation of the shoulders, and flexion of the forearms; followed by an opisthotonic posturing, closing of the mouth (with possible tongue or cheek biting), thoracic and abdominal muscle contraction, a sustained expiratory ictal cry, and limb extension. There may be marked autonomic features, including tachycardia, hypertension, mydriasis, flushing or cyanosis (due to apnea), sweating, sialorrhea, and bronchial hypersecretion.

CLONIC PHASE

This lasts approximately 30 seconds. The tonic phase gives way to rhythmic contractions of the limbs and facial muscles (with possible tongue and cheek biting) that progressively slow to approximately 1–2 per second before giving rise to the third phase.

POSTICTAL PHASE

A few seconds after the last jerk, there is a brief tonic phase with trismus (and possible tongue biting), urinary incontinence, and deep, labored breathing. With resolution of the cyanosis, the patient remains immobile and hypotonic (postictal unconsciousness). There is gradual lightening of coma followed by postictal confusion, lethargy, or sleepiness during which the patient may be confused, incoherent, and amnestic.

On EEG, the tonic phase is accompanied by an electrodecremental EEG pattern lasting 1–3 seconds followed by rapid rhythmic activity at approximately 20 Hertz slowing down to 10 Hertz. This rapid repetitive discharge progressively becomes interspersed with slow waves, and the polyspike and slow wave discharges of the clonic phase. The end of the seizure is characterized by suppression and slower frequencies in the theta and delta range that increase in frequency and decrease in amplitude. All ictal and postictal phases are symmetric, synchronous, and bilateral.

Rarely, generalized tonic-clonic seizures may be associated with:
- preservation of consciousness (very rarely);
- asymmetric motor manifestations with a versive component;
- a brief malaise or visual blurring at seizure onset.

Tongue biting and urinary incontinence do not occur with every seizure. Tonic-clonic seizures may be seen in idiopathic generalized epilepsies or symptomatic epilepsies. In partial epilepsies, secondary generalization may be so rapid that the partial onset is missed.

• • • • • •
TOXICITY

Toxicity may be due to intake of too high a dose of AEDs, an unusually slow metabolism of the drug, medication interaction, or intercurrent illness. Toxic effects may be acute, subacute, or chronic (see also Anticonvulsants/antiepileptic drugs (AEDs)).

• • • • • •
TRANSIENT GLOBAL AMNESIA (1)

This condition, usually seen in patients over the age of 50, is characterized by confusion and loss of memory for periods ranging from minutes to hours. A patient appears alert, has normal speech, and may carry out complex tasks such as driving, but remains amnestic for the period. Recovery is gradual and usually complete. Recurrence is not uncommon. Purported causes include migraine and cerebrovascular disease (2). No convincing epileptic cause has been proven.

References

1. Fisher CM, Adams RD. Transient global amnesia. *Acta Neurol Scand* 1964; 40(Suppl 9):1–83.
2. Kushner MJ, Hauser WA. Transient global amnesia: a case-controlled study. *Ann Neurol* 1985;18:684–91.

• • • • • •
TRANSIENT PAROXYSMAL DYSTONIA IN INFANCY (1)

This disorder consists of axial contraction and opisthotonos for several minutes without impairment of consciousness. The seizure frequency varies from once a day to once a month. The EEG is normal. Seizures appear between the first and fifth month of age, may remit spontaneously, or may become progressively worse between the sixth and twenty-second month. The differential diagnosis includes infantile spasms, tonic seizures, paroxysmal nocturnal dystonia, and "dystonia" due to gastroesophageal spasm (2).

References

1. Angelini L, Rumi U, Lamperti E, Nardocci N. Transient paroxysmal dystonia in infancy. *Neuropaediatrics* 1988;19:171–74.
2. Wyllie E, Wyllie R, Rothner AD, Morris HH. Another paroxysmal disorder in the differential diagnosis of seizures in infants: diffuse esophageal spasms. *Ann Neurol* 1988;24:328.

• • • • • •
TREATMENT

The goal of treatment for epilepsy is to decrease seizures and improve the quality of life for the patient. Treatment may take several forms, including AEDs, surgical intervention, rectification of provoking factors for seizures (e.g., alcohol abuse). There are also dietary therapies (see Ketogenic diet) and psychologically-based treatments (see Biofeedback) for epilepsy. AED therapy is the most important of these treatments.

Although not curative, AEDs suppress or decrease the frequency of seizures. Since some epilepsy syndromes remit with time, drug treatment is not necessarily life-long. Before starting treatment, the following points should be considered:

- The diagnosis of epilepsy should be established since AEDs will not necessarily benefit the imitators of epilepsy.
- Consideration should be given to the risk-benefit ratio associated with treating a single seizure in a patient with a normal EEG (see Isolated (S)).
- Treatment is usually initiated in patients with more than one spontaneous seizure. Some clinicians would also treat single seizures with interictal EEG epileptiform abnormalities.
- Initial therapy is best effected with monotherapy, for example, ethosuximide for absence seizures, valproate for generalized epilepsies, carbamazepine for partial epilepsies. Monotherapy provides the most favorable ratio of efficacy to side effects. A minority of patients with epilepsy will benefit from more than one drug.
- Start with low doses and work up gradually, achieving the full daily dose over a few weeks of treatment. This minimizes severe side effects upon initiation of treatment.
- Try to limit dosage frequency to two per day, and simplify the regimen to improve compliance (see Compliance).
- Selectively measure serum AED levels to assess compliance, toxicity, and efficacy.
- Advise the patient to contact the physician immediately should any serious adverse effect arise after initiating treatment.
- Approximately two-thirds of patients will have no further seizures and no side effects (1). In these cases, the same AED regimen should be continued. The physician should encourage compliance by regularly scheduled outpatient visits.
- If the patient continues to have seizures: verify that the patient is correctly following the prescription; confirm that the diagnosis of epilepsy is correct; gradually increase the chosen medication as long as the patient does not develop toxicity, even if the blood level is above the so-called therapeutic range.

- If seizures continue, add a second AED and gradually stop the first, trying in succession monotherapy with first-line AEDs. As alternatives, for example, ethosuximide may be used in absence seizures; phenobarbital, phenytoin, carbamazepine for other generalized seizures; valproate or phenytoin for partial seizures.
- If monotherapy fails, then after each medication has been pushed to the maximum tolerable dose, use two concurrent first-line AEDs or in the case of myoclonic epilepsies, a first-line AED with a benzodiazepine. Only 10–20% of patients failing monotherapy can adequately be controlled by polypharmacy.
- If seizure control is not reached in two years, consider seizure surgery.
- Stopping treatment (2–5): in some cases the most effective treatment is reduction or discontinuation of treatment. Many patients with severe and long-standing epilepsy have endured a gradual increase in AED dosage. Excessive polypharmacy may produce marked side effects and limit the ability to bring a single effective AED to the maximum dose. In this circumstance, one should consider reduction in AED dose over several months. The least effective medication or the most toxic may be chosen as candidate for initial reduction. Certain patients who have obtained seizure control over a long period of time do not wish to stop treatment. In these instances, potential benefits and risks of medication reduction should be discussed, but patients should not be forced off medications for the sake of principle. There is a small risk of psychopathology following AED withdrawal (5).

Discontinuation of therapy should be considered if patients have been seizure-free for several years (6,7). The medication taper period may extend from weeks to months (2) with a 30% relapse rate (3). That might be higher with rapid AED taper (4). Patients and families should be willing to accept this risk. Driving should be restricted during a discontinuation of AED and for a reasonable period thereafter.

References

1. Homan RW, Miller B, and the Veterans Administration Epilepsy Cooperative Study Group. Causes of treatment failure with antiepileptic drugs vary over time. *Neurology* 1987;37:1620–23.
2. Duncan JS, Shorvon SD. Rates of antiepileptic drug reduction in active epilepsy current practice. *Epilepsy Res* 1987;1:357–64.
3. Callaghan N, Garrett A, Goggin T. Withdrawal of anticonvulsant drugs in patients free of seizures for two years. A prospective study. *N Engl J Med* 1988;318:942–46.

4. Malow BA, Blaxton TA, Stertz B, Theodore WH. Carbamazepine withdrawal: effects of taper rate on seizure frequency. *Neurology* 1993;43:2280–84.

5. Ketter TA, Malow BA, Flamini R, White SR, Post RM, Theodore WH. Anticonvulsant withdrawal-emergent psychopathology. *Neurology* 1994;44:55–61.

6. Holmes GL. Stopping antiepileptic drugs in children: when and why? *Ann Neurol* 1994;35:509–10.

7. Shinnar S, Berg AT, Moshé SL, et al. Discontinuing antiepileptic drugs in children with epilepsy: a prospective study. *Ann Neurol* 1994;35:534–45.

● ● ● ● ● ●

TUBEROUS SCLEROSIS (BOURNEVILLE'S DISEASE; ADENOMA SEBACEUM)

Tuberous sclerosis (Bourneville's disease) is a hereditary, neurocutaneous phacomatosis with autosomal dominant transmission and variable penetrance, presenting frequently with seizures. Seizures may appear before the onset of cutaneous abnormalities (1). Clinical features include adenoma sebaceum involving the malar regions of the face, areas of dark pigmentation on the trunk and the extremities, peri-ungual fibromas, and café-au-lait spots. Mental retardation is frequent.

Tuberous sclerosis is usually associated with severe epilepsy, often presenting as infantile spasms (2), although partial motor, complex partial, and tonic-clonic seizures may also be seen (3). The clinical picture may evolve into Lennox-Gaustaut syndrome. Slowly developing forms of the disease may present with less severe seizures beginning in late childhood or adolescence. Early onset of seizures and the severity of epilepsy correlate with the greater degree of mental retardation (4).

The EEG in tuberous sclerosis is abnormal in 87% of cases (4) and shows a very disordered asymmetric background with multifocal and asynchronous epileptiform discharges. In patients without CNS manifestations, the EEG is normal (5). Imaging techniques such as CT head scan and MRI scans are helpful in early diagnosis as tubers may be identified; calcification and cortical atrophy are common (6,7,8). There is no clear topographic correlation between tubers and seizure foci (2,7,8). Cortical atrophy and ventricular dilation are more frequently seen with the severe epilepsies and with marked mental retardation (2).

References

1. Pampiglione G, Pugh E. Infantile spasms and subsequent appearance of tuberous sclerosis syndrome. *Lancet* 1975;2:1046.

2. Riikonen R, Simell O. Tuberous sclerosis and infantile spasms. *Dev Med Child Neurol* 1990;32:203–209.

3. Niedermeyer E, Naidu S. Degenerative disorders of the central nervous system. In: Niedermeyer E, Lopes da Silva F (eds.). *Electroencephalography. Basic principles, clinical applications and related fields,* 2nd edition. Baltimore: Urban & Schwarzenberg, 1987.

4. Lagos JC, Gomez MR. Tuberous sclerosis: reappraisal of a clinical entity. *Proc Mayo Clin* 1967;42:26–49.

5. Harvald B, Hauge M. The electroencephalogram in patients with tuberous sclerosis. *Electroenceph clin Neurophysiol* 1955;7:573–76.

6. Altman NR, Purser RK, Donovan Post MJ. Tuberous sclerosis: characteristics on CT and MR. *Imaging Radiology* 1988;167:527–32.

7. Cusmai R, Chiron C, Curatolo P, Dulac O, Tran-Dinh S. Topographic comparative study of magnetic resonance imaging and electroencephalography in 34 children with tuberous sclerosis. *Epilepsia* 1990;31:747–55.

8. Tamaki K, Okuno T, Ito M, Asato R, Konishi J, Mikawa H. Magnetic resonance imaging in relation to EEG epileptic foci in tuberous sclerosis. *Brain Dev* 1990;12:316–20.

● ● ● ● ● ●

TUMORS

Our present understanding of epilepsy secondary to tumors has been completely changed with the advent of CT and MRI head scanning. More and more frequently, tumors present with a single seizure leading to early investigation and diagnosis with CT head scan or MRI (1,2), often in patients with normal neurological exams (1). From 5 to 16% of patients with epilepsy are found to have tumors (3,4). The incidence of underlying neoplasm varies according to age: in children 0.2–0.3% (5), in adolescents 1% (6), in the young adult 12–16% (7), and in the older age group 10% (8). Among patients with known brain tumors, seizures may be seen in 40% (3).

- Clinical features: Tumor-associated seizures may be generalized tonic-clonic or partial. These include simple partial seizures, somatosensory seizures (7,8), sensory seizures (gustatory and olfactory), versive seizures, and seizures with speech arrest. The wide and changing variety of clinical features is highly suggestive of a growing tumor. Partial or generalized status epilepticus as a presenting feature is not unusual (9).
- Progression: Seizures may occur (1) within the context of a long-standing medically refractory epilepsy (1), or will be uncovered during surgical resection of an epileptic focus (10). Status epilepticus rarely occurs (11).
- Seizure frequency is variable, depending on seizure location. Frequent seizures result from supratentorial tumors, especially in the

Rolandic, temporal, or parietal cortical regions. Tumor histology influences seizure frequency: with a seizure incidence of 80–90% for oligodendrogliomas, 60–75% for astrocytomas, 55% for meningiomas, 55% for metastases, and 35–40% for malignant gliomas.

References

1. Morris HH, Estes ML, Gilmore R, Van Ness PC, Barnett GH, Turnbull J. Chronic intractable epilepsy as the only symptom of primary brain tumor. *Epilepsia* 1993;34:1038–43.
2. Ramirez-Lassepas M, Cippolle RJ, Morillo LR, Gumnit RJ. Value of computed tomographic scan in evaluation of adult patients after their first seizures. *Ann Neurol* 1984;15:536–43.
3. Mouritzen Dam A, Fuglsang-Frederiksen A, Svarre-Olsen O, Dam M. Late-onset epilepsy: etiology types of seizures and value of clinical investigations, EEG and computerized tomography scan. *Epilepsia* 1985;26:227–31.
4. Aicardi J. Epilepsies as a presenting manifestation of brain tumors. In: *Epilepsy in children.* New York: Raven Press, 1986.
5. Loiseau P, Dartigues JF. Formes éléctrocliniques des épilepsies de l'adolescence. *Rev EEG Neurophysiol Clin* 1981;11:493–501.
6. Luhdorf K, Jensen LK, Plesner AM. Epilepsy in the elderly: etiology of seizures in elderly. *Epilepsia* 1986;27:458–63.
7. Mauguière F, Courjon J. Somatosensory epilepsy: review of 127 cases. *Brain* 1978;101:307–32.
8. Blume WT, Jones DC, Young GB, et al. Seizures involving secondary sensory and related areas. *Brain* 1992;115:1509–20.
9. Oxbury JM, Whitty CWM. Causes and consequences of status epilepticus in adults: a study of 86 cases. *Brain* 1971;94:733–44.
10. Spencer DD, Spencer SS, Mattson RH, Williamson PD. Intracerebral masses in patients with intractable partial epilepsy. *Neurology* 1984;34:432–36.
11. Steg RE, Frank AR, Lefkowitz DM. Complex partial status epilepticus in a patient with dural metastases. *Neurology* 1993;43:2389–92.

UNCINATE (SEIZURES)

An uncinate seizure is a partial seizure that begins with an olfactory hallucination followed by a dreamlike state. These seizures have been correlated to a focus in the anteromesial part of the temporal lobe or in the orbitofrontal region. Orbitofrontal cortex and mesial temporal cortex are linked by the uncinate bundle, giving the seizure type its name.

UNCLASSIFIABLE (SEIZURES, EPILEPSY)

All populations of people with epilepsy include a certain number of patients who cannot be classified because of the absence of sufficient information.

UNILATERAL (SEIZURES) (OR HEMIBODY SEIZURES)

Listed in the Classification of Seizures of 1970, the term "unilateral seizures" was not retained in the Classification of 1981. This seizure type referred to partial somatomotor seizures (see Somatosensory (S)/Focal motor (S)) or generalized seizures with an age-dependent electroclinical presentation—hemitonic or hemiclonic seizures (see Clonic (S)).

Reference

Gastaut H, Roger J, Faidherbe J, Ouachi S, Franck G. Non-jacksonian hemiconvulsive seizure. One-sided generalized epilepsy. *Epilepsia* 1962;3:56–68.

• • • • • • •
UNVERRICHT-LUNDBORG (DISEASE)

Unverricht-Lundborg disease was the first progressive myoclonic epilepsy to be described (1891) (1–3). The description included entities later defined as Baltic myoclonus and Lafora disease. Unverricht-Lundborg disease predominantly affects patients from Estonia, Finland, and southeast Sweden. Transmission is by an autosomal recessive mode, with age of onset between 6 and 14 years. The seizure disorder is characterized by spontaneous or provoked myoclonic jerks, generalized tonic-clonic seizures, myoclonic "cascade" seizures, and signs of cerebellar dysfunction (4). A late progressive dementia is invariable. Other phenotypic variants have been described elsewhere in the world.

References

1. Unverricht H. *Die Myoclonie.* Leipzig: Franz Deuticke, 1891:1–128.
2. Unverricht H. Über familiare myoclonie. *Dtsch Z Nervenheilk* 1895;7:32–67.
3. Lundborg H. *Die progressive Myoklonus. Epilepsie (Unverricht's Myoclonie).* Upsala: Almquist and Wiskell, 1903:1–207.
4. Kyllerman M, Sommerfelt K, Hedström, Wennergren G, Holmgren D. Clinical and neurophysiological development of Unverricht-Lundborg disease in four Swedish siblings. *Epilepsia* 1991;32:900–909.

VACCINATION

AS A CAUSE OF EPILEPSY

Smallpox (now eradicated) vaccination may cause encephalitis and epilepsy. Other vaccinations have been incriminated, but the risk is low (1). There is great difficulty in interpreting the role of vaccinations in the appearance of certain epilepsies, since age-dependent epilepsy syndromes (febrile convulsions, West syndrome) may coincide with a period of obligatory childhood vaccinations. Additionally, febrile reactions from vaccinations may provoke benign febrile seizures. Post-infectious encephalitis and encephalopathy may cause seizures and epilepsy, and therefore vaccinations against these diseases may provide protection against these causes of epilepsy (2–4).

VACCINATIONS IN PATIENTS WITH EPILEPSY

There are no contraindications for vaccinations against diphtheria, poliomyelitis, tetanus, or tuberculosis. Theoretically, vaccination against mumps is contraindicated.

References

1. Baraff JL, Shields WD, Beckwith L, Strome G, Marcy M, Cherry JD, Manclark CR. Infants and children with convulsions and hypotonic-hyporesponsive episodes following diphtheria-tetanus-pertussis immunization: follow-up evaluation. *Pediatrics* 1988;81:789–94.
2. Ogunniyi A, Osuntokun BO, Bademosi D, Aduja AOG, Schoenberg BS. Risk factors for epilepsy: a case-control study in Nigerians. *Epilepsia* 1987;28:280–85.
3. Griffin MR, Ray WA, Mortimer EA, Fenichel GM, Schaffner W. Risk of seizures and encephalopathy after immunization with the diphtheria-tetanus-pertussis vaccine. *JAMA* 1990;263:1641–45.
4. Zimmerman B, Gold R, Lavi S. Adverse effects of immunization. Is prevention possible? *Postgrad Med* 1987;82:225–29.

• • • • • • •
VALPROATE, SODIUM (DIVALPROEX SODIUM, DEPAKOTE®); VALPROIC ACID (VPA, DEPAKENE®)

Valproic acid is a carboxylic acid designated as 2-propylpentanoic acid. Depakene® is valproic acid; Depakote® is divalproex sodium and is a stable coordination compound made of sodium valproate and valproic acid in a 1:1 molar relationship. Overall, VPA is as effective as phenytoin, carbamazepine, or phenobarbital (1-4). It is a drug of choice in absence epilepsy, myoclonic epilepsy, and all idiopathic generalized epilepsies (5). It is clearly effective in West and Lennox-Gastaut syndromes (1) and in the partial epilepsies.

PHARMACOKINETICS (8)

Valproate is metabolized in patients by linear kinetics. Bioavailability is 86–100% of the oral dose. Peak plasma levels depend on the formulation. Plasma levels are maximal 1 hour after ingestion of the solution, 3–8 hours after ingestion of enteric-coated tablets, and occasionally more than 12 hours after meals. Protein binding is 90% for most serum concentrations, but less with serum concentrations above 120 mg/l and in the newborn (9). Half-life when used as monotherapy is 8–16 hours, but much prolonged in the newborn: 20–50 hours, and in the premature: 75 hours. A steady state is reached in 2 days. The volume of distribution (Vd) is 0.1–0.4 l/kg. Presence of valproate may delay the hydroxylation and the clearance of other drugs, particularly phenobarbital and the carbamazepine epoxide. There is a significant increase in free fraction of valproate in hypoalbuminemia, and if taken with acetylsalicylic acid or heparin. There is a marked decrease with other enzyme-inducing medications such as phenobarbital, carbamazepine, or phenytoin.

Suggested blood levels of valproic acid are 50–100 mg/l, or 300–600 micromol/l, although higher levels have been tolerated with improved seizure control.

SIDE EFFECTS (10)

The most common side effect of valproic acid is gastrointestinal discomfort, especially if therapy is initiated too rapidly. Weight gain, tremor, and mild sedation are common. Rare effects include skin rashes, hearing loss, symptomatic hyperammonemia, thrombocytopenia, and significant platelet dysfunction. Acute hepatitis is an extremely rare but dangerous side effect, often occurring without warning (11). It appears during the first 6 months of treatment, almost exclusively in children under the age of 3, especially with polytherapy. It is believed to be due to abnormal metabolism with the production of a markedly toxic metabolite. Since being recognized, the incidence of hepatitis has fallen. Reversible coma of uncertain mechanism is another rare side effect (12). Valproate is also known to produce a 1–2% incidence of spinal dysraphism in offspring of mothers taking the drug during the first trimester of pregnancy (13).

References

1. Bourgeois BFD. Valproate clinical use. In: Levy RH, Mattson R, Meldrum B, Penry JK, Dreifuss FE (eds.). *Antiepileptic drugs,* 3rd edition. New York: Raven Press, 1989:633–42.
2. Callaghan N, Kenny RA, O'Neill B, Crowley M, Groggin T. A prospective study between carbamazepine, phenytoin and sodium valproate as monotherapy in previously untreated and recently diagnosed patients with epilepsy. *J Neurol Neurosurg Psychiatry* 1985;48:639–44.
3. Chadwick D. Comparison of monotherapy with valproate and other antiepileptic drugs in the treatment of seizure disorders. *Am J Med* 1988;84 (Suppl 1A):3–6.
4. Turnbull DM, Howel D, Rawlins MD, Chadwick DW. Which drug for the adult epileptic patients: phenytoin or valproate? *Br Med J* 1985;290:815–19.
5. Wilder BJ, Ramsay RE, Murphy JV, Karas BJ, Marquardt K, Hammond ES. Comparison of valproic acid and phenytoin in newly diagnosed tonic-clonic seizures. *Neurology* 1983;33:1474–76.
6. Dean JC, Penry JK. Long term follow-up: valproate monotherapy in 30 patients with partial seizures. *Epilepsia* 1988;29:695.
7. Penry JK, Dean JC. Valproate monotherapy in partial seizures. *Am J Med* 1988;84 (Suppl 1A):14–16.
8. Zaccara G, Messori A, Maroni F. Clinical pharmacokinetics of valproic acid. *Clin Pharmacokin* 1988;15:367–89.
9. Gal P, Oles KS, Gilman JT, Weaver R. Valproic acid efficacy, toxicity and pharmacokinetics in neonates with intractable seizures. *Neurology* 1988;38:467–71.
10. Dreifuss FE, Langer DH. Side effects of valproate. *Am J Med* 1988;84 (Suppl 1A):34–40.
11. Dreifuss FE, Langer DH. Hepatic considerations in the use of antiepileptic drugs. *Epilepsia* 1987;28(Suppl 2):S23–S29.
12. Marescaux C, Warter JM, Micheletti G, Rumbach L, Coquillat G, Kurtz D. Stuporous episodes during treatment with sodium valproate: report of seven cases. *Epilepsia* 1982;23:297–305.
13. Lindhout D, Schmidt D. In-utero exposure to valproate and neural tube defects. *Lancet* 1986;2:1392–93.

• • • • • •

VALPROMIDE
(AMIDE OF VALPROIC ACID) (DEPAMIDE®)

Valpromide is rapidly transformed to valproic acid (see also Valproate). Valpromide has been used as an AED in Europe because of a prolonged action.

With the development of Depakene Chrono®, a long-acting form used in Europe, and the dangerous association of valpromide with carbamazepine resulting in excessive production of epoxide, valpromide is now used less often.

• • • • • •
VERSIVE (SEIZURES) (SEE ALSO GYRATORY (S,E))

Versive seizures are characterized by eye deviation involving the eyes alone (oculogyrate seizures), the head, or head and eyes. Occasionally there is truncal rotation (gyratory seizures) either ipsilateral or contralateral to the ictal discharge. Seizures are usually partial motor in type, with frequent secondary generalization. The following correlations have been identified (1–5):

- Rapid tonic deviation of the eyes alone or with head rotation—without loss of consciousness—correlates with a focus in the intermediate frontal cortex or contralateral mesial frontal cortex.
- Simultaneous eye and head deviation with loss of consciousness corresponds to an anterior, ipsilateral frontal focus.
- Tonic elevation and abduction of an upper extremity followed by deviation of the head and the eyes to the same side correlates to a contralateral (or less often ipsilateral) supplementary motor area focus.
- Tonic head and eye deviation with rapid eye blinking is associated with a focus in the contralateral parastriate occipital region.
- Sudden truncal gyration may indicate a focus in contralateral primary motor area.
- Curling up of the body suggests a parietal focus.
- CT scans may show no structural lesion.

References

1. McLachlan RS. The significance of head and eye turning in seizures. *Neurology* 1987;37:1617–19.
2. Lüders H, Lesser RP, Dinner DS, Morris HH, Wyllie E, Godoy J. Localization of cortical function: new information from extraoperative monitoring of patients with epilepsy. *Epilepsia* 1988;29:(Suppl 2):S56–S65.
3. Robillard A, Saint-Hilaire JM, Mercier M, Bouvier G. The lateralizing and localizing value of adversion in epileptic seizures. *Neurology* 1983;33:1241–42.
4. Wyllie E, Lüders H, Morris HM, Lesser RP, Dinner DS. The lateralizing significance of versive head and eye movements during epileptic seizures. *Neurology* 1986;36:606–12.
5. Meshram CM, Prubhakar S, Sawhney IMS, Dhand UK, Chopra JS. Rotatory seizures. *Epilepsia* 1992;33:522–26.

• • • • • •
VERTIGINOUS (SEIZURES)

Seizures may induce nonspecific dizziness or true vertigo, with a sense of rotation in space. Vertiginous seizures usually are associated with a posterior temporal focus or a focus in the antero-inferior parietal cortex.

Reference

Tartara A, Manni R, Mira E, Mevio E. Polygraphic study of vestibular stimulation in epileptic patients. *Rev EEG Neurophysiol Clin* 1984;14:227–34.

• • • • • •
VESTIBULOGENIC (SEIZURES)

Vestibulogenic seizures are partial seizures provoked by caloric vestibular stimulation.

Reference

Tartara A, Manni R, Mira E, Mevio E. Polygraphic study of vestibular stimulation in epileptic patients. *Rev EEG Neurophysiol Clin* 1984;14:227–34.

• • • • • •
VIGABRATIN (SABRIL®)

Vigabratin (gamma-vinyl GABA) was developed as an AED specifically designed to enhance GABA-mediated inhibition. Brain GABA levels are enhanced by the irreversible inhibition of GABA transaminase, thus preventing GABA breakdown (hence, the delay in the onset of AED activity after initiating vigabratin therapy). Animal models have shown an effect for partial and secondary generalized seizures, with no effect, or a possible worsening, in absence seizure models. Initial trials were halted because of the appearance of intramyelinic edema in studies of mice, rats, and dogs, a finding that was not noted in further studies on monkeys. There is, however, a possible teratogenic effect as demonstrated in the rabbit model.

More than 60% absorbed with an oral dose; T max: 1–2 hours; Vd = 0.6–0.8 L/kg; no protein binding. Although the T 1/2 = 5–7 hours, a pharmacological effect can be noted for more than 24 hours. 60–70% is excreted renally, unchanged. No therapeutic range has been established.

Side effects include fatigue, drowsiness, and dizziness in 10–20%. Behavioral abnormalities, including psychosis, are rare, but are more commonly seen in patients with a history of mental retardation and psychiatric problems. Because of this, more gradual institution of lower doses has been recommended.

Drug interactions include a decrease in phenytoin levels of 20–30%.

Drug trials have shown it to be effective in refractory, partial, and secondary generalized seizures, producing 75% reduction in seizure frequency in 40–60% of patients.

References

1. Gram L, Klosterskov P, Dam M. γ-vinyl GABA: a double-blind placebo-controlled trial in partial epilepsy. *Ann Neurol* 1985;17:262–66.
2. Rimmer EM, Richens A. Double-blind study of γ-vinyl GABA in patients with refractory epilepsy. *Lancet* 1984;1:189–90.
3. Loiseau P, Hardenberg JP, Pestre M, et al. Double-blind, placebo-controlled study of vigabratin (gamma-vinyl GABA) in drug-resistant epilepsy. *Epilepsia* 1986;27:115–20.

● ● ● ● ● ●
VIOLENCE

Aggressiveness can be defined as behavior with intent to damage. Violence represents aggressiveness with damage directed toward people or goods. Aggressiveness and violence have been considered to be part of the purported epileptic personality (1). Studies of this issue have been subject to selection bias (2), and no clear evidence exists that people with epilepsy are more violent than the baseline population. Isolated instances of violence in epilepsy have been noted during complex partial seizures. Such instances are rare, occurring in 14 of 5,400 patients in one study (3), and 10 of 699 seizures recorded in 79 patients in another study (4). In this latter study, 7 of the 10 episodes were due to patient struggling, rather than directed violence (5).

Violence in people with epilepsy has also been examined as a function of postictal delirium, psychosis, or behavior disturbance. Delinquency in patients with epilepsy is typically seen in men living in a poor socioeconomic environment with brain damage causing both seizures and diminished IQ. The prevalence of patients with epilepsy in prison is higher than that in the general population, although the proportion of serious crimes is no higher in this group (6).

Epilepsy itself appears not to be responsible for violent behavior (7). No clear link has been established between murder and epilepsy (8,9).

References

1. Pincus JH. Can violence be a manifestation of epilepsy? *Neurology* 1980;30: 304–307.
2. Kligman D, Goldberg DA. Temporal lobe epilepsy and aggression: problems in clinical research. *J Nerv Ment Dis* 1975;160:324–41.
3. Delgado-Escueta AV, Mattson RH, King L, et al. The nature of aggression during epileptic seizures. *N Engl J Med* 1981;305:711–16.
4. Stevens JR, Hermann BP. Temporal lobe epilepsy, psychopathology and violence: the state of evidence. *Neurology* 1981;31:1127–32.
5. Delgado-Escueta AV, Bascal FE, Treiman DM. Complex partial seizures on closed-circuit television and EEG: a study of 691 attacks in 79 patients. *Ann Neurol* 1982;11:292–300.
6. Whitman S, Coleman TE, Parmon C, Desai BT, Cohen R, King LN. Epilepsy in prison: elevated prevalence and no relationship to violence. *Neurology* 1984; 41:651–56.
7. Hermann BP, Schwartz MS, Whitmann S, Karnes WE. Aggression and epilepsy: seizure type comparisons and high-risk variables. *Epilepsia* 1980;22:691–98.
8. Treiman DM. Epilepsy and violence: medical and legal issues. *Epilepsia* 1986;27 (Suppl 2):S77–S104.
9. Walker EA. Murder or epilepsy? *J Nerv Ment Dis* 1961;133:430–37.

• • • • • • •

VISUAL (SEIZURES)

Seizures with visual manifestations may present with elementary hallucinations, structured hallucinations, or illusions. Blurring or decreased visual acuity has little specific localizing value.

- Elementary hallucinations consist of phosphenes, or more rarely scotomata or hemianopsia, involving the contralateral visual field with a focus in Brodmann's area 16 or 17.
- Structured hallucinations comprise objects, animals, people, and more or less complex scenes due to ictal involvement of visual association areas.
- Illusions (metamorphopsias) represent an alteration in the size or shape of objects. They may appear enlarged (macropsias), diminished (micropsias), or changed in position: vertical or horizontal lines are seen as being oblique, or with undulation of contour, change in color, dulling or heightening of color, the illusion of movement (generally acceleration), an impression of proximity or distance, change in relief, monocular diplopia or polyopia, or perseveration in time of the visual image. Illusions are usually due to parietal or parieto-occipital foci.

● ● ● ● ● ●
VOMITING

Vomiting may occur during a seizure (ictus emeticus), particularly in children with idiopathic partial epilepsies (1,2). If associated with visual disturbance or headache, migraine may be suspected, and in fact represents a more common etiology of this symptom complex. Vomiting may be the only sign heralding a seizure (3). Vomiting may follow a seizure, but may also be seen after vasovagal syncope (see also Abdominal (E)).

References

1. Jacome DE, Fitzgerald R. Ictus emeticus. *Neurology* 1982:32;209–12.
2. Panayiotopoulos CP. Vomiting as an ictal manifestation of epileptic seizures and syndromes. *J Neurol Neurosurg Psychiatry* 1988:51:1448–51.
3. Mitchell WG, Greenwood RS, Messenheimer JA. Abdominal epilepsy. Cyclic vomiting as the major symptom of simple partial seizures. *Arch Neurol* 1983; 40:251–52.

● ● ● ● ● ●
VON RECKLINGHAUSEN'S (DISEASE) (NEUROFIBROMATOSIS) (1–3)

This hereditary condition is characterized by skin pigmentation and firm benign neural tumors involving peripheral nerves, spinal and cranial nerve roots. With an incidence of 30 to 40 per 100,000, it is transmitted as an autosomal dominant trait or may occur sporadically. Mental retardation, usually mild, is seen in about 10% of patients. Seizures occur in a minority of patients.

References

1. von Recklinghausen F. *Ueber die multiplen Fibrome der Haut un ihre Beziehung zu den mutiplen Neuromen.* Berlin: A Hirschwald, 1882.
2. Crowe FW, Schull WJ, Neel JV. *A clinical, pathological and genetic study of multiple neurofibromatosis.* Springfield: Charles C. Thomas, 1956.
3. Riccardi VM. Von Recklinghausen's neurofibromatosis. *N Engl J Med* 1981;29:1–9.

WADA (TEST): SODIUM AMYTAL TEST (1,2)

The Wada hemispheric dominance test, named after Juhn Wada (2), is used to localize language and memory functions to a particular hemisphere in patients undergoing surgery for seizures. The test is performed by rapid injection of sodium amobarbital into an internal carotid artery, after angiographic catheterization of the artery. Selected angiography may be used to involve a more restricted area of hemisphere (3), but increased risk is entailed. The amobarbital is taken up into brain directly from the first pass of circulation, and essentially "anesthetizes" a portion of one hemisphere. With typical doses (100–200 mg), unilateral deficits last for 5–15 minutes. There is resultant contralateral hemiparesis with aphasia (dominant hemisphere) or no language disturbance (nondominant hemisphere). EEG shows ipsilaterally maximal delta activity. As judged by concurrent SPECT scans, hippocampal and posterior cerebral artery perfusion occurs in a minority of Wada studies (4), rendering interpretaion of memory deficits somewhat difficult (5,6). Nevertheless, Wada studies are useful empirically prior to seizure surgery for predicting the dominant speech hemisphere and for indicating unexpected contralateral memory dysfunction.

References

1. Blume WT, Brabow JD, Darley FL, Aronson AE. Intracarotid amobarbital test of language and memory before temporal lobectomy for seizure control. *Neurology* 1973;23:812–19.
2. Wada JA. A new method for determination of the side of cerebral speech dominance. A preliminary report on the intracarotid injection of sodium amytal in man. *Medicine and Biology* 1989;14:221–22.
3. Jack CR Jr, Nichols DA, Sharbrough FW, Marsh WR, Petersen RC. Selective posterior cerebral artery amytal test for evaluating memory function before surgery for temporal lobe seizure. *Radiology* 1988;168:787–93.
4. Jeffery PJ, Monsein LH, Szabo Z, et al. Mapping the distribution of amobarbital sodium in the intracarotid Wada test by use of TC-99M HMPAO with SPECT. *Radiology* 1991;178:847–50.

5. Powell GE, Polkey CE, Canaval AGM. Lateralization of memory functions in epileptic patients by use of the sodium amytal (WADA) technique. *J Neurol Neurosurg Psychiatry* 1987;50:665–72.
6. Loring DW, Lee GP, Meador KJ. The intracarotid amobarbital sodium procedure. False-positive errors during recognition memory assessment. *Arch Neurol* 1989;46:285–87.

• • • • • •
WEST (SYNDROME) (INFANTILE SPASMS WITH HYPSARRHYTHMIA)

West syndrome is an age-dependent epilepsy of infancy and early childhood with a typical triad of infantile spasms, severe mental retardation, and hypsarrhythmia (1). The incidence is 0.24 to 0.42 per thousand births (2). Males predominate in a ratio of 1.5 to 1; family history is positive in 6% of cases (3). Onset usually is between the age of 3 and 7 months, and rarely after the first year. They rarely persist beyond three years of age.

Clinical characteristics (4,5):

1. *Seizures (infantile spasms)* present with clinical expression with flexion or extension persisting throughout the spasm.

- flexor spasms are most frequent, with massive flexion of the head, trunk, upper and lower extremities;
- extensor spasms may involve extension of the neck, trunk, and extremities;
- mixed spasms alternately involve flexor and extensor muscles;
- atypical, limited, or *forme fruste* of spasms may show asymmetry or may be unilateral.

In each of the above seizure forms, the child may show impairment of consciousness, changes in respiration, crying at the end of the spasm or, more rarely, smiling, or eye deviation. Observation of repeated spasms is helpful in making the diagnosis.

Infantile spasms are usually seen upon waking or falling asleep. Initially sporadic, their frequency tends to increase over the course of the illness. Occasionally, they may resolve spontaneously (6). In addition to the tonic seizures, infantile spasms may show tonic-clonic, atypical absence, and partial motor seizures (7,8).

2. *Psychomotor retardation* may precede the spasms. Early in the course of West syndrome, there is loss of spontaneous smiling, apathy, diminished reactivity to external stimuli, then delay or loss of milestones and stereotyped activities.

3. *EEG characteristics:* According to Gibbs, hypsarrhythmia is the usual interictal pattern: there is an uninterrupted sequence of high amplitude

(300 microvolt) spike and slow waves of varying amplitude and localization seen asynchronously and diffusely over the scalp (1). During sleep, there are bursts of more or less synchronous irregular polyspike and waves on a highly disorganized background (4). Continuous recording (8) has revealed asymmetry, lateralization, suppression bursts, bilateral spike and slow wave discharges, and attenuation of activity (3). A temporal focus is also common (4). EEG recording during a seizure shows a high amplitude slow wave in the frontal regions followed by general suppression or rapid bilateral discharges, more rarely with slow spike and slow wave discharges (3).

DIFFERENTIAL DIAGNOSIS

- benign myoclonus in early infancy (9) shows similar characteristics; however, psychomotor development and the waking and sleep EEG are normal. Seizures disappear before the age of two without sequelae;
- early onset myoclonic encephalopathy (see Neonatal (S));
- early infantile epileptogenic encephalopathy with burst suppression (Ohtahara's syndrome) (see Neonatal (S));
- benign myoclonic epilepsy of infancy (see Benign (E));
- severe myoclonic epilepsy of infancy.

ETIOLOGY

Infantile spasms may be cryptogenic or symptomatic (10,11):

- *Symptomatic spasms* comprise most cases. Any cerebral insult occurring in the prenatal, perinatal, or postnatal period may lead to infantile spasms: these include anoxic-ischemic encephalopathy (see also Anoxia/hypoxia; Hypoxia), malformations (Aicardi's syndrome), the phacomatoses, abnormalities of cerebral migration, macrogyria or microgyria, Down syndrome, porencephaly, holoprosencephaly, or infections. More rarely, tumors, hemorrhagic syndromes, head trauma, inborn errors of metabolism, severe hypoglycemia, and toxins are implicated.
- *Cryptogenic spasms* (3). In this group, no identifiable cause can be determined (11–13).

TREATMENT

Corticosteroid therapy, particularly ACTH, is effective (7). There is some disagreement as to the formulation (natural ACTH versus synthetic corticosteroids), administration modality, associated medication, or duration of treatment (14). Treatment may be administered for 1 to 6 months.

Adjunctive AED therapy using benzodiazepines or sodium valproate has been advocated (15,16). In 30% of cases, there is relapse when treatment is stopped. EEG monitoring may be helpful in management.

Prognosis is serious:

- death occurs in 20% of cases (6);
- serious sequelae result in 30–50% of cases: mental retardation 70–85% of cases, Lennox-Gastaut syndrome or complex partial seizures (16);
- approximately 10% of children have a normal development. The best outcome is usually seen with cryptogenic forms of the syndrome (5–7,11).

Poor prognostic indicators include identifiable fixed or progressive lesions, the onset of spasms before the age of three months, other types of seizures (particularly in symptomatic cases) and atypical hypsarrhythmia. There is disagreement about the role of treatment, type, AED dose, or duration.

References

1. Dulac O, Chugani HT, Dalla Bernardina B. *Infantile spasms and West syndrome.* London: W.B. Saunders Co., 1994.
2. Riikonen R, Donner M. Incidence and aetiology of infantile spasms from 1960 to 1976: a population study in Finland. *Dev Med Child Neurol* 1979;21:333–43.
3. Kellaway P, Hrachovy RA, Frost JD, Zion T. Precise characterization and quantification of infantile spasms. *Ann Neurol* 1979;6:214–18.
4. Hrachovy RA, Frost JD, Kellaway P. Sleep characteristics in infantile spasms. *Neurology* 1981;31:688–94.
5. Fusco L, Vigevano F. Ictal clinical electroencephalographic findings of spasms in West syndrome. *Epilepsia* 1993;34:671–78.
6. Jeavons PM, Bower BD, Dimitrakoudi M. Long term prognosis of 150 cases of "West Syndrome." *Epilepsia* 1973;14:153–64
7. Lombroso CT. A prospective study of infantile spasms: clinical and therapeutic correlations. *Epilepsia* 1983;24:135–58.
8. Riikonen R. Infantile spasms: modern practical aspects. *Acta Paediat Scand* 1984;73:1–12.
9. Lombroso CT, Fejerman N. Benign myoclonus in early infancy. *Ann Neurol* 1977;1:138–43.
10. Matsumoto A, Watanabe K, Negoro T, Iwase K, Hara K, Miyasaki S. Infantile spasms: etiological factors clinical aspects and long term prognosis in 200 cases. *Eur J Pediatr* 1981;135:239–44.
11. Gastaut H, Gastaut JL. Regis H, Bernard R, Pinsard N, Saint Jean M, Roger J, Dravet C. Computerized tomography in the study of West's syndrome. *Dev Med Child Neurol* 1978;20:21–27.
12. Singer ND, Haller JS, Sullivan CR, Wolpert S, Mills D, Rabe EF. The value of neuroradiology in infantile spasms. *J Pediat* 1982;100:47–50.

13. Aicardi J. Current management of infantile spasms. *Int Pediatr* 1989;4:188–92.
14. Fois A, Lalandrini F, Balestri P, Giorgi D. Infantile spasms. Long term results of ACTH treatment. *Eur J Pediat* 1984;142:52–55.
15. Vassela F, Pavlincova E, Schneider JH, Rudin HJ, Karbowski K. Treatment of infantile spasms and Lennox-Gastaut syndrome with clonazepam. *Epilepsia* 1973;14:165–75.
16. Pavone L, Incorpora G, La Rosa M, Li Volti S, Mollica F. Treatment of infantile spasms with sodium dipropylacetic acid. *Dev Med Child Neurol* 1976; 58:828–32.
17. Kurokawa T, Goya N, Fukuyama Y, Suzuki M, Seki K, Ohtahar S. West syndrome and Lennox Gastaut syndrome: a survey of natural history. *Pediatrics* 1980;65:81–88.

• • • • • •
WILSON'S (DISEASE)

Wilson's disease is a disorder of copper metabolism with hepatic and neurologic sequelae. The incidence of epilepsy has been calculated to be about 6% in patients with Wilson's disease. Rarely heralding the onset of the disease, seizures appear more often to be triggered by the use of chelation treatment (penicillamine), which produces an abnormal mobilization of copper within the brain. In untreated patients, seizures appear toward the end of the process, some months before death. Seizures do not affect the prognosis.

Reference

Dening TR, Berrios GE, Walshe JM. Wilson's disease and epilepsy. *Brain* 1989; 111:1139–55.

• • • • • •
WITHDRAWAL (SEIZURES)

Withdrawal seizures arise either in the context of acute or chronic alcoholic intoxication (see Alcohol, effects of) or during withdrawal of certain AEDs (1,2). Barbiturate and benzodiazepine withdrawal are especially liable to provoke seizures, or even status epilepticus. It may be difficult to distinguish withdrawal seizures from a relapse of the epilepsy. Withdrawal seizures are usually generalized. Rarely, withdrawal seizures emerge in the newborn children of mothers on AEDs.

References

1. Spencer SS, Spencer DD, Williamson PD, Mattson RH. Ictal effects of anti-convulsant medication withdrawal in epileptic patients. *Epilepsia* 1981; 22:297–307.
2. Marciani MG, Gotman J, Andermann F, Olivier A. Patterns of seizure activation after withdrawal of antiepileptic medication. *Neurology* 1985;35:1537–43.

ZONE OF EPILEPTOGENESIS

The area of brain tissue from which epileptic seizures arise is the epileptogenic zone. Specific structural lesions such as scars or tumors are referred to as epileptogenic lesions. These focal lesions produce a primary epileptogenic zone, which in turn may produce distant epileptogenic zones (secondary epileptogenesis). (See also Focus, epileptogenic).

Reference

Engel J Jr. Terminology and classifications. In: *Seizures and epilepsy.* Philadelphia, F.A. Davis, 1989.

●●●●●●

ZONISAMIDE (EXCEGRAN®)

This sulfamide derivative has been shown to be effective in refractory partial epilepsies (1–3). Behavioral problems (4) and a dose-dependent impairment of cognition have been noted (5). Kidney stones have been reported as a side effect. For this reason, trials have been abandoned in the United States, but continue in Japan.

References

1. Wilensky AS, Friel PN, Ojemann LM, Dodrill CB, McCormick KB, Levy RH. Zonisamide in epilepsy: a pilot study. *Epilepsia* 1985;26:212–20.
2. Sackellares JC, Donofrio PD, Wagner JG, Abou-Khalil B, Berent S, Aasued-Hoyt C. Pilot study of zonisamide in patients with refractory partial seizures. *Epilepsia* 1985;26:206–11.
3. Peters DH, Sorkin EM. Zonisamide. A review of its pharmacodynamic and pharmacokinetic properties, and therapeutic potential in epilepsy. *Drugs* 1993;45:760–87.

4. Kimura S. Zonisamide-induced behavior disorder in two children. *Epilepsia* 1994;35:403–405.

5. Berent S, Sackellares JC, Giordani B, Wagner JG, Donofrio PD, Abou-Khalil B. Zonisamide (C-912) and cognition: results from preliminary study. *Epilepsia* 1987;28:61–67.